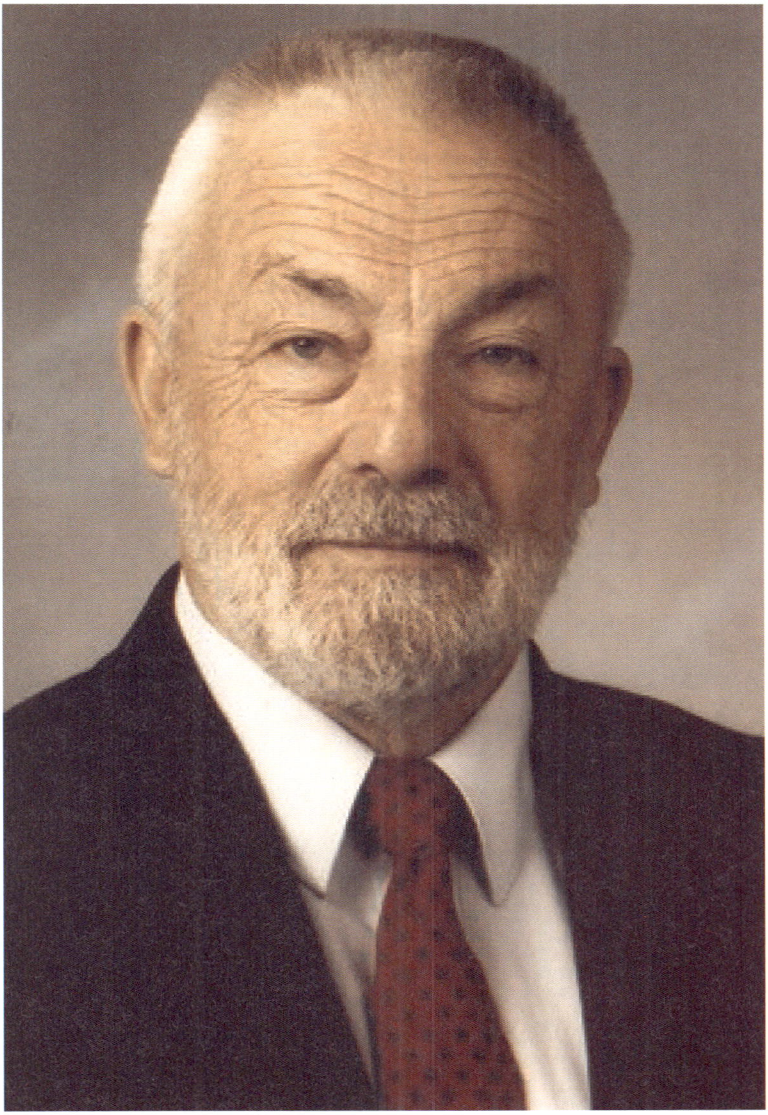

(1927 – 2016)

John M. King

N.Y.S. College of Veterinary Medicine

Cornell University

What a surprise! He did about 120,000 cases of necropsy during his lifetime!

John King's shout : common Phrases

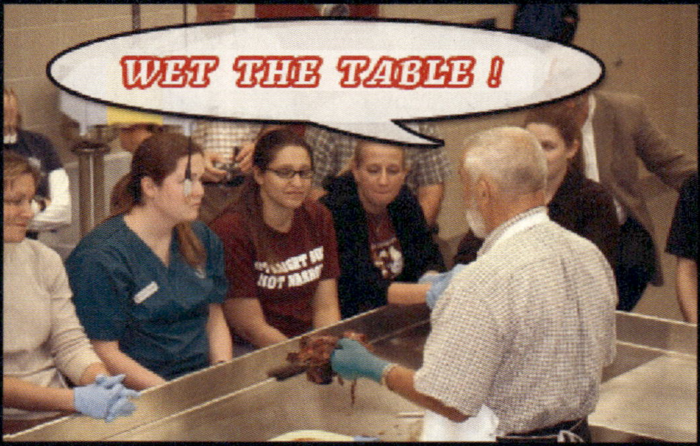

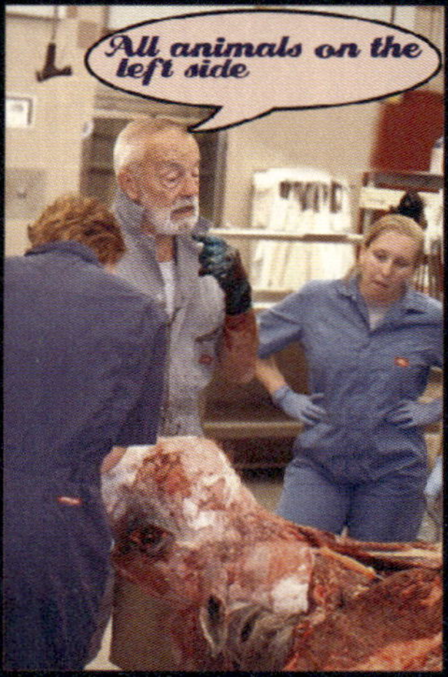

"Wet the table!"

"Ain't firm, ain't pneumonia"

"All animals on the left side"

"Mickey mouse stuff"

"No interest"

"God said so and everybody agrees"

"Do not read the history (until afterwards)"

"Drop dead as a doughnut!"

"Could it be a meteorite?"

"Maybe you should have been a truck driver"

"You need to know how to sharpen your knife"

"Baloney!"

John King's Witty Conclusion

존 킹의 재치있는 결론

"Sherlock holmes' lame excuse"

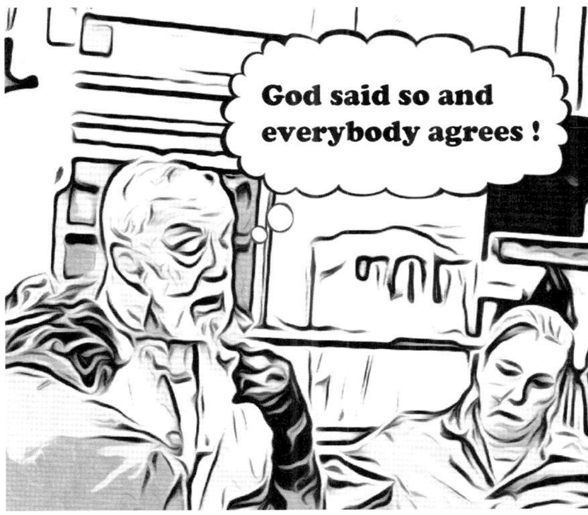

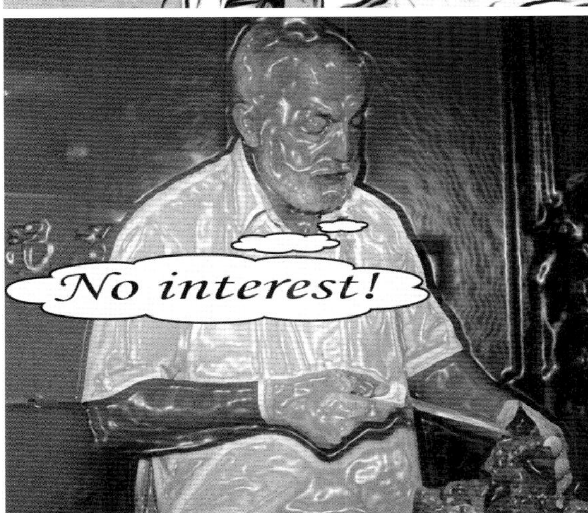

His clever jokes lifted our spirit and afforded great pleasure

The Title of

Wet The Table!
John M. King

First published February 2021
Written by Nam-Yong Park, Professor Emeritus,
Chonnam National University

Publisher : Sungtaek Jung

Price: 20,000 Won (20 USD)

ISBN 978-89-6849-808-4 (93990)

Published by Chonnam National University Press,
77 Yongbong-ro, Bukgu, Gwangju,
Republic of Korea, 61186
Tel: 82-62-530-0571/3, Fax: 82-62-530-0579
E-mail: cnup0571@hanmail.net

Printed and bound in the Republic of Korea

This collection Book of
John M. King's Stories
is dedicated to
John M. King,
Marie R. King
and
all acquaintance

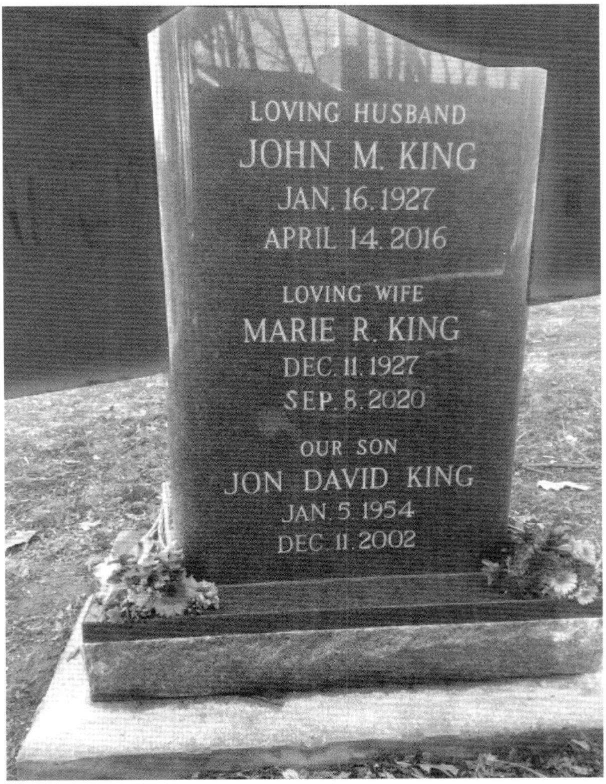
LOVING HUSBAND
JOHN M. KING
JAN. 16. 1927
APRIL 14. 2016
LOVING WIFE
MARIE R. KING
DEC. 11. 1927
SEP. 8. 2020
OUR SON
JON DAVID KING
JAN. 5. 1954
DEC. 11. 2002

184 Pleasant Grove Rd, Ithaca, NY 14580

Acknowledgments

Thanks to Chonnam National University authorities and
publishing press Gwangju, Rep. of Korea,
Bruce H. Williams, Donald J. Meuten and Ana Alcaraz
for their generosity.
Special thanks to Joseph Masangkay, Mun-il Kang,
Therese Collantes, Ho-myung Na for
their valuable helps and Paul Stromberg, Corrie Brown,
Keith Harris, Claus Buergelt,
Judy St. Leger, Peg Miller, John Edwards
for their benevolent spirits

Author's Note

I am not a disciple of Professor John King, a Cornell graduate. However, I respected and liked Professor John King a lot.

Mr. and Mrs. King did not feel so lonely in their old age. He always boasted many of his talented disciples as great assets. Among them, Helen Han Hsu and Ana Alcaraz played a role of adoptive daughter well.

I would like to express my sincere thanks to those who have provided me emails and photos: Corrie Brown, Anne Ryan, Richard Jakowski, William Cadwallader and et al.

Our Chonnam National University has an open recruitment system for book publication once a year. I was fortunate enough to pass the screening and publish this book.

Two hundreds published books will be purchased in person and donated to various libraries around the world, including Davis-Thompson Foundation.

Contents

Preface

Even without being a college professor, we often ask ourselves the following questions; What would be the right way to live, what are the most important issues in life, and how could we conclude our lives in a meaningful way?

In the course of our lives, we make relationships with many others. Out of them, I have no doubt that Prof. John King (1927-2016) was most distinctive and a role model for everyone around him. He was not only a veterinary pathologist like me and an outstanding teacher, but a practitioner of universal love with his professional knowledge.

When I first proposed the idea of publishing this book, as expected, he was quite reluctant. However, I persuaded him by saying that as a master of veterinary pathology, you should never leave your achievements unrevealed, and, most of all, you have to be a good example for the next generations with your life. He finally agreed after my sincere proposal to publish his work including bioinformation, pictures, and interviews even after his death.

Now, five years have passed since Prof. John King's demise at the age of 89, and, in September last year, his 70-year-long wife Marie R. King (1927~2020) also passed away at the age of 93. So I became more eager to keep the promise with him. However, it was not an easy task to publish this book together with a Korean translation of 'The Necropsy Book', which Prof. John King had permitted to do when he was alive.

For the publication of this book, I frequently exchanged correspondences with Prof. King when he was alive. He treated me as if his son in Korea a Korean like his son and he was happy to send me various documents he had collected. I thought hard about the title of this book and eventually decided it as 'WET THE TABLE!'.

This was the phrase he used to say before a necropy session in the necropy room at the Veterinary School of Cornell University.

Dr. Bruce Williams, Chairman of Davis-Thompson Foundation that promotes the education and development of veterinary pathology globally, estimated that Prof. King performed about 120,000 necropy cases over 50 years (1955~2005) and I cite a eulogy to Prof. King 'In Memoriam' that moved many people around the world as below.

"Legend" or "pillar" of pathology, but he was so much more. John was beyond larger than life. He was mythic, orphanage childhood, rubber boots, army paratrooper, 70-years marriage to his darling Marie. It was a magical story. His book "The Necropsy Book" -the best-selling volume ever written for veterinary pathologist- raised money not for his pocket, but for the education of veterinarians around world.

Prof. King liked to collect and record diverse items as an atypical hobby. The night before his death he drove a scooter, and his hearing was limited or impaired but he didn't need glasses. He was gifted with good eyes by God to become a talented veterinary pathologist. The "necropsy show & tell" Cornell website, which consists of about 45,000 photos including about 26,000 lesion images obtained from the numerous cadavers handled by him in the necropy room, is an open repository accessible to anyone around the world. It is a great treasure of veterinary medicine.

These days I feel we urgently need the knowledge and wisdom of Prof. King, who left such an immense achievement. About 5 million people have died by the end of this month due to the COVID-19 pandemic and the number is still rising. The United States is one of the countries most seriously affected because there are diverging interpretations of the pathological mechanism for various lesions caused by the viral infection and widespread vaccine reluctance due to some reports of post-vaccine myocarditis and thrombosis.

Finally, I would like to share an excerpt from 'The hill we climb' recited by Amanda Gorman, an African American girl, at the inauguration ceremony of President Joe Biden this year both in

English and Korean:

If we're to live up to our own time, then victory won't lie in the blade,
but in all the bridges we've made.
우리가 주어진 시간에 최선을 다해 산다면, 승리는 날카로운 칼날 위가 아닌,
우리가 만든 튼튼한 다리 위에 있을 것이니.

That is the promise to glade, the hill we climb, if only we dare.
이것이 바로 우리가 가고자 하는 곳, 바로 우리가 오르는 언덕이다.

It's because being American is more than a pride we inherit.
미국인이라는 것은 우리가 조상들에게 물려받은 자부심 이상의 것이다.

I know that like miss Gorman, both the late John King and his wife Marie, believed and longed for a more peaceful America, a dream that seemed impossible just a few years ago, but is now a reality. I hope that readers of this book will continue to uphold their dignity and pride, much like how John King carried his profession until the end.

Feb. 28. 2021

Nam-Yong Park, Professor Emeritus.
College of Veterinary Medicine
Chonnam National University
Gwangju, Republic of Korea

Precious Photos

• John king's first time to slaughter a cow at age 13

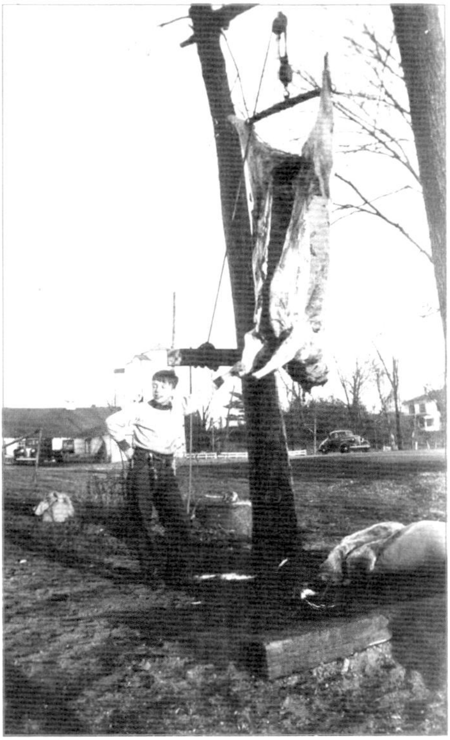

Picture 1. When I was seven years old my family split up by divorce and I was brought to Hillside School for boys five to fifteen years old, or actually from grades one through eight. We had eighty boys and ten adults. Each of us had to do a certain amount of work daily. As one of the older boys at thirteen in 1940, I was lucky to be allowed to do the slaughter of the farm animals and chickens. This was my first cow. I believe she was sterile and had to be killed. I had to kill her by knocking her out with a ten pound sledge hammer and cutting her throat. I had watched before, but I was alone for this one. The cow hanging by the hind legs with a whiffletree block and tackle was hauled up by a farm tractor as the horse team shied away from the odor of blood. I did not know what I was doing, but you can be sure I've learned since in doing necropsies at Cornell with all the farm species and many wild animals.

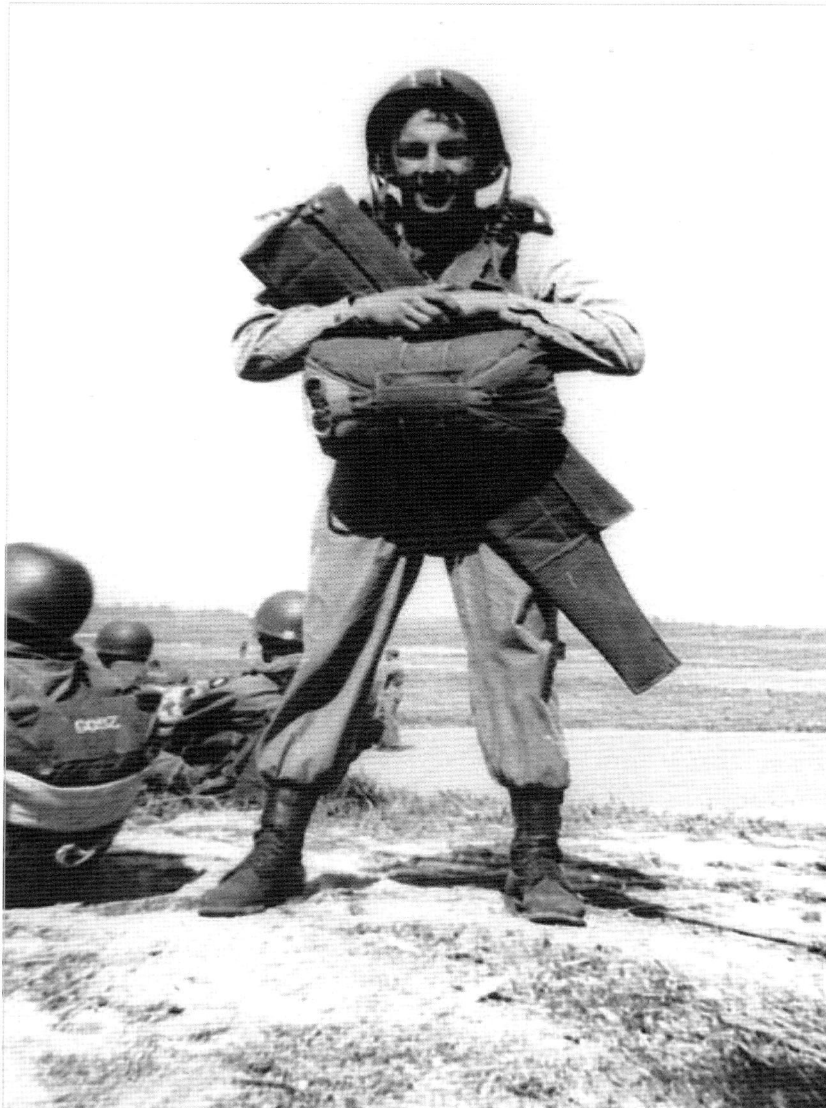

Picture 2. All set for a practice parachute jump over some beet field in Germany, 1946. The war was over for Japan, but they kept us busy in case.

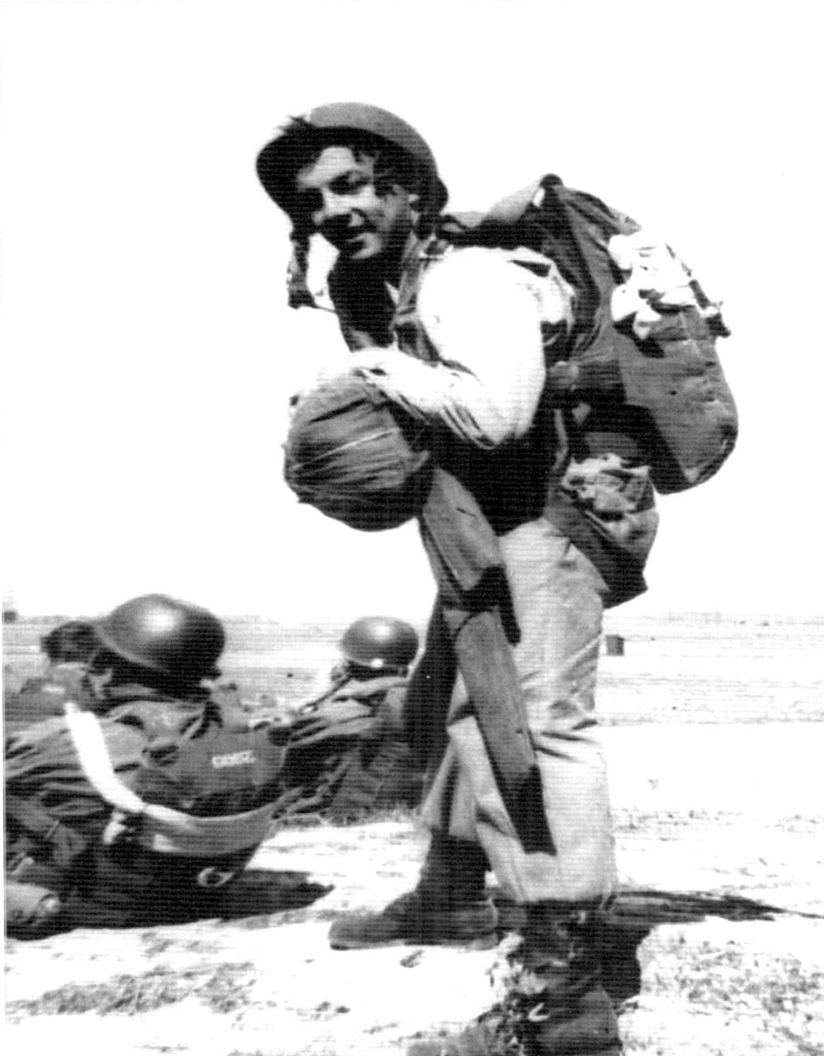

Picture 3. That is me ready to jump in Germany. I have a smile on my face, but the chute is too tight.

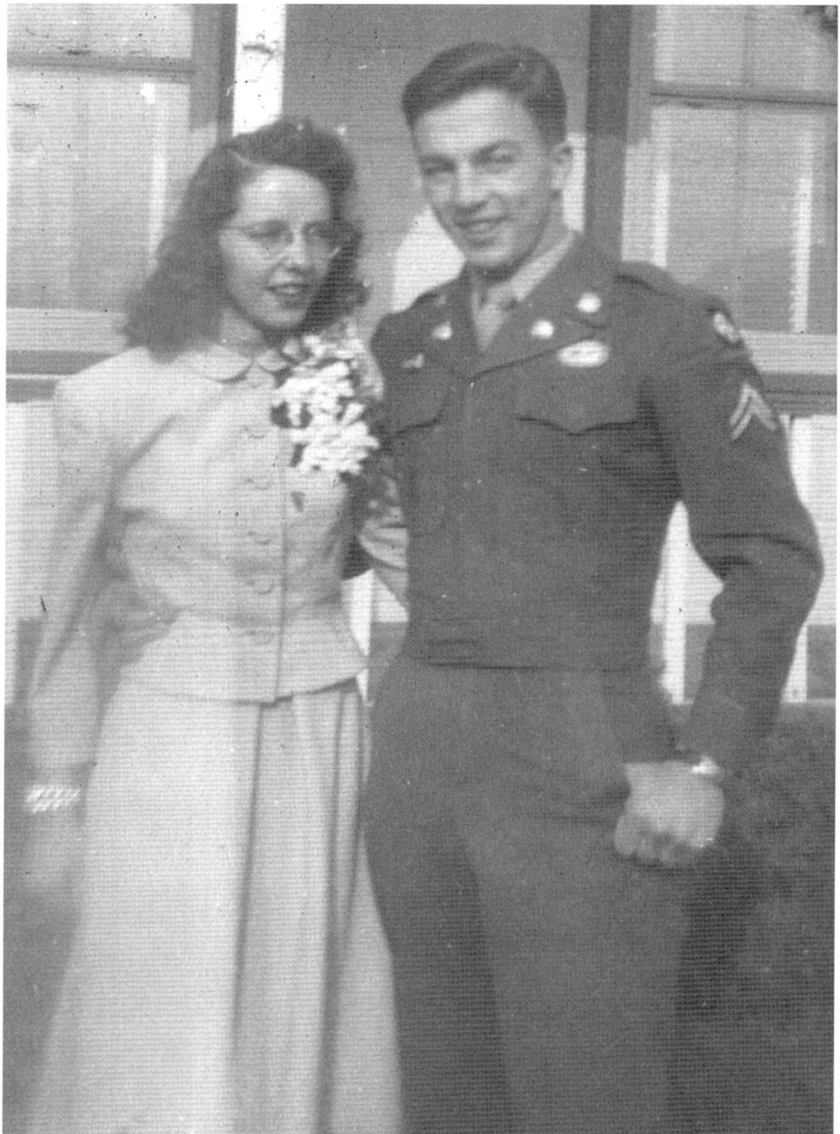

Picture 4. Marie and Cpl John M. King in front of Re's home December 14, 1947, our wedding day.

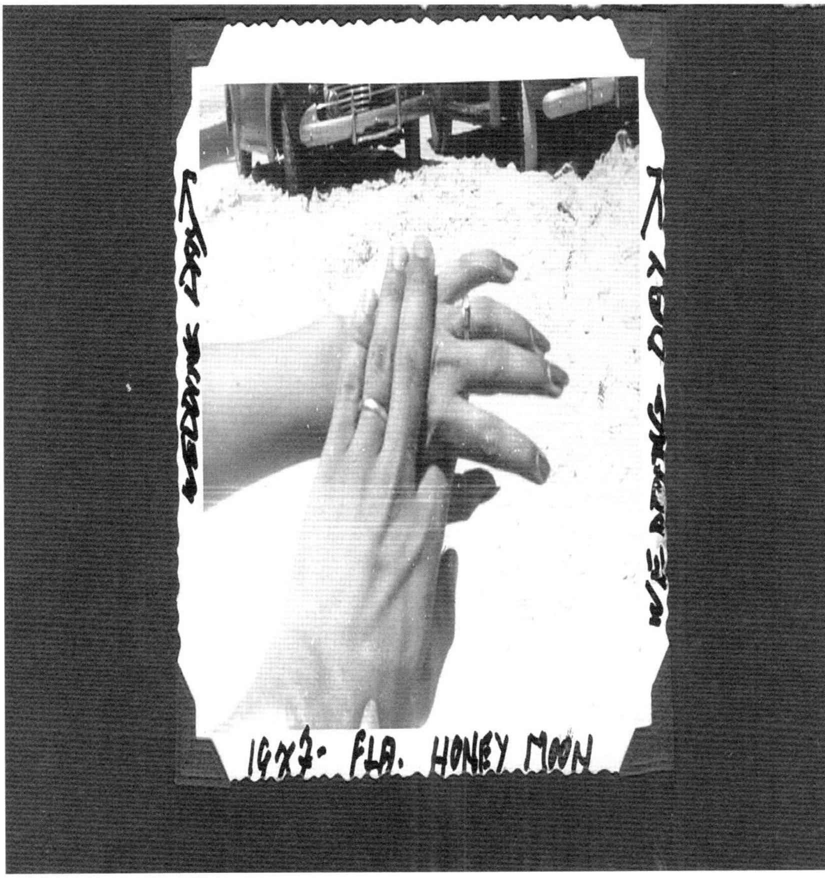

Picture 5. We had a Honeymoon in Daytona Beach, Florida in the summer of 1948 while I was still in the Army. Even went to a "fortune teller" who told us of a happy day to come. We would be together as of one day in December when I got my discharge. Now how did he know?

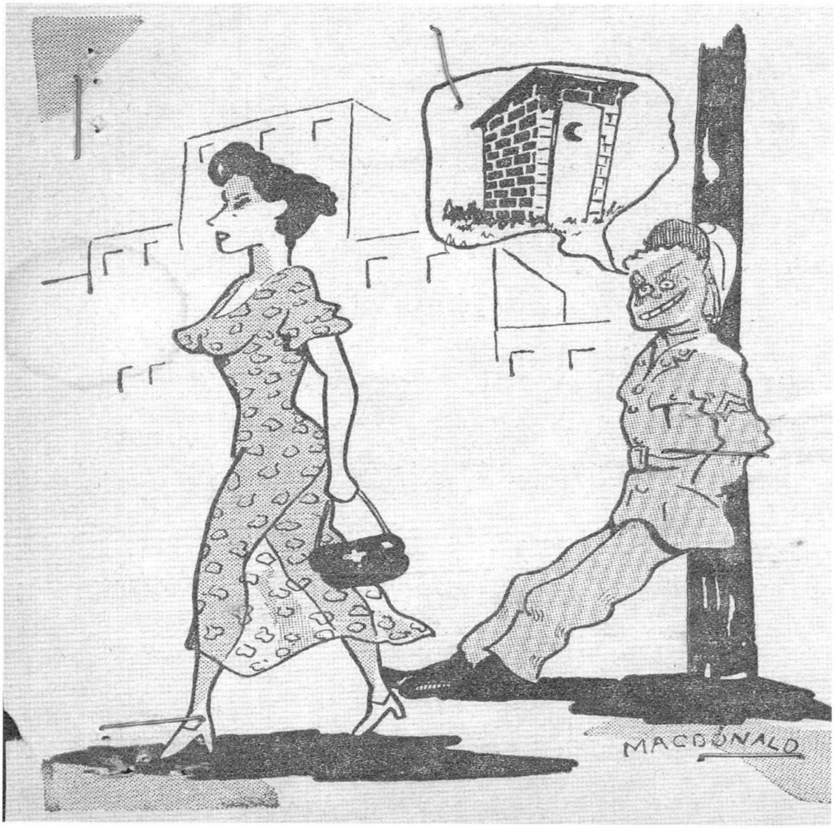

Picture 6. This cartoon gem came from the American Army's published newspaper Stars and Stripes when I was in Germany in 1945. It depicts a well endowed female as built like a brick outhouse. Really does not make sense, as my wife agrees, but I think it is great.

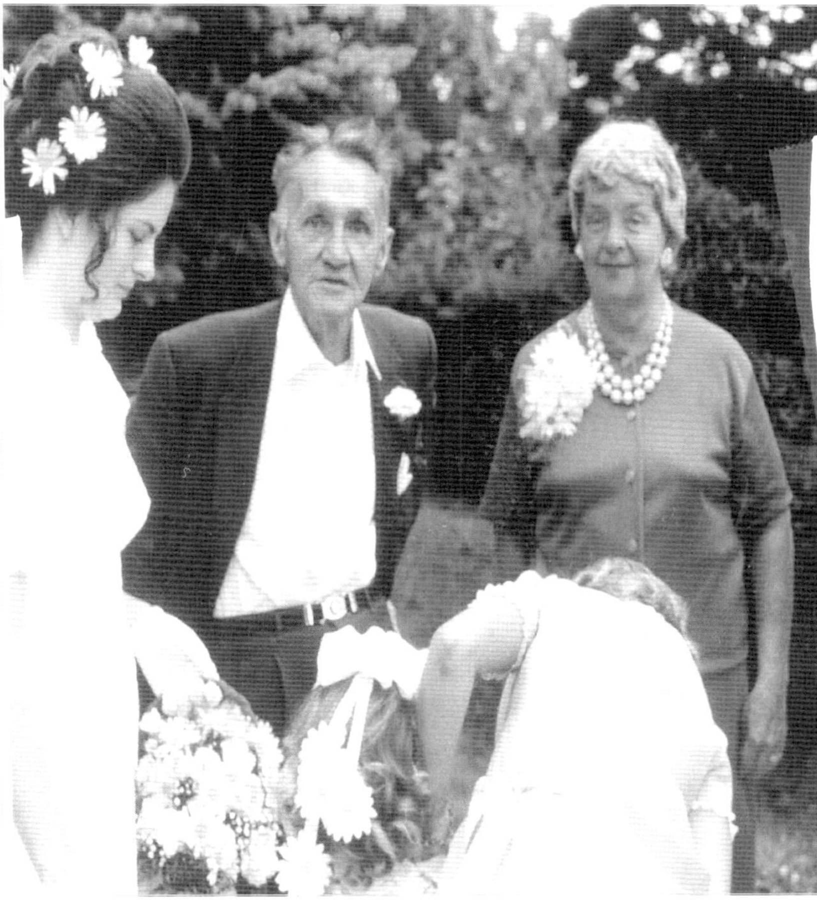

Picture 7. My Mom and Dad at Judy's wedding 1975.e

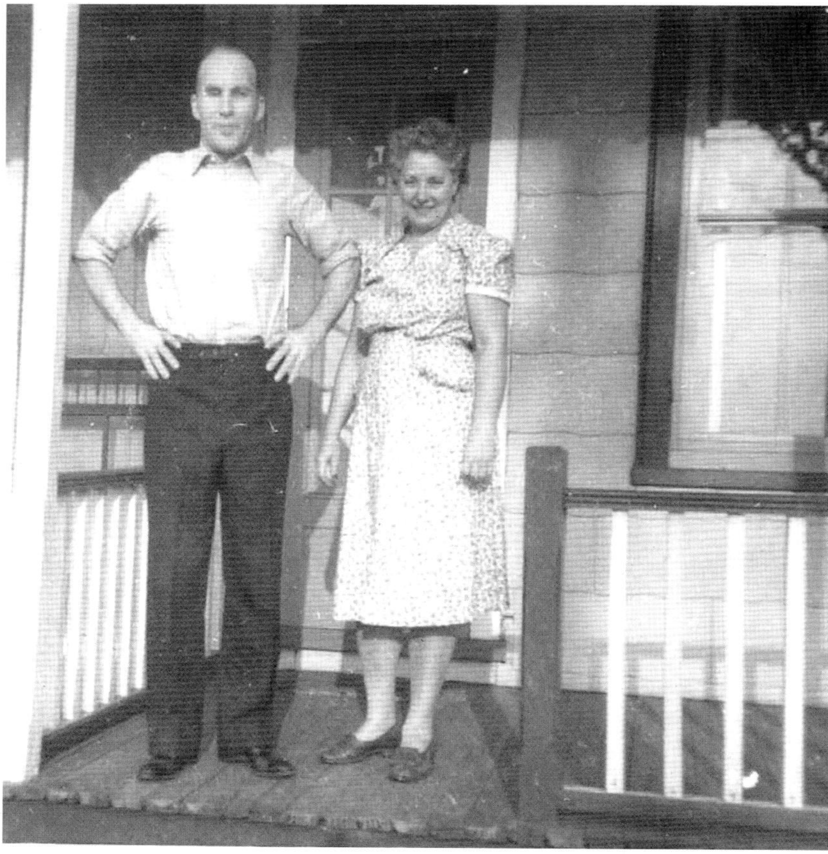

Picture 8. Marie's stepfather and Mother at 3115 Market Street, Wilmington, De, 1948

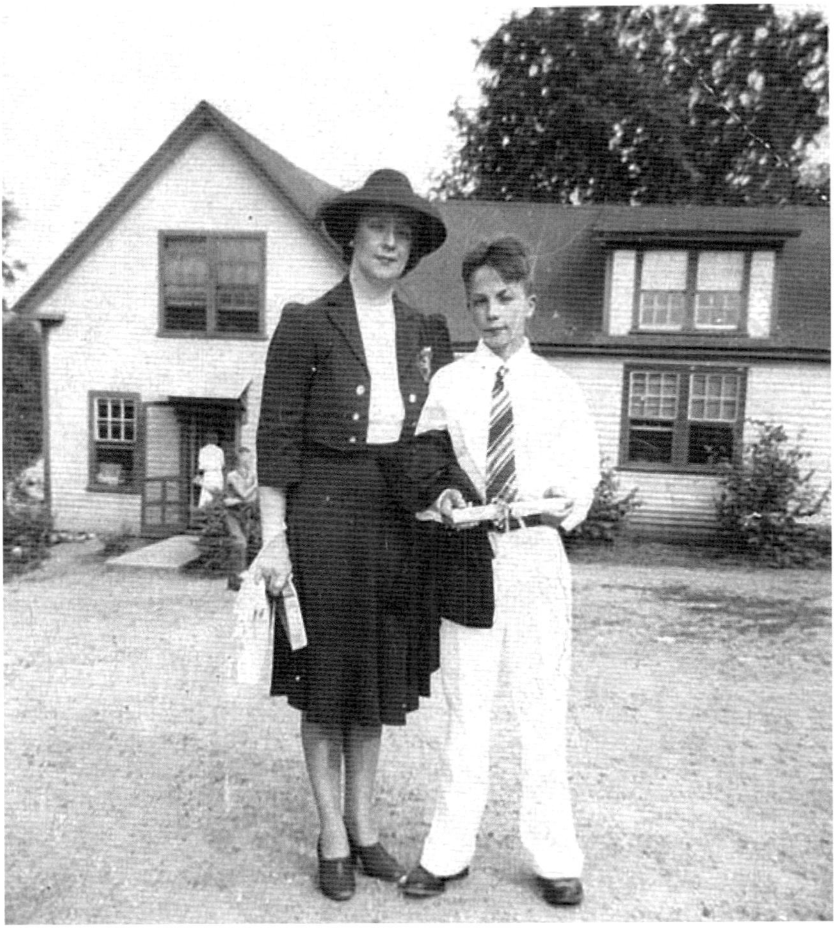

Picture 9. My Mother did come to Hillside from Boston for my eighth grade graduation in 1941. The Hillside first and second grade classroom is more behind my mother and the third, fourth and fifth grades are behind me.

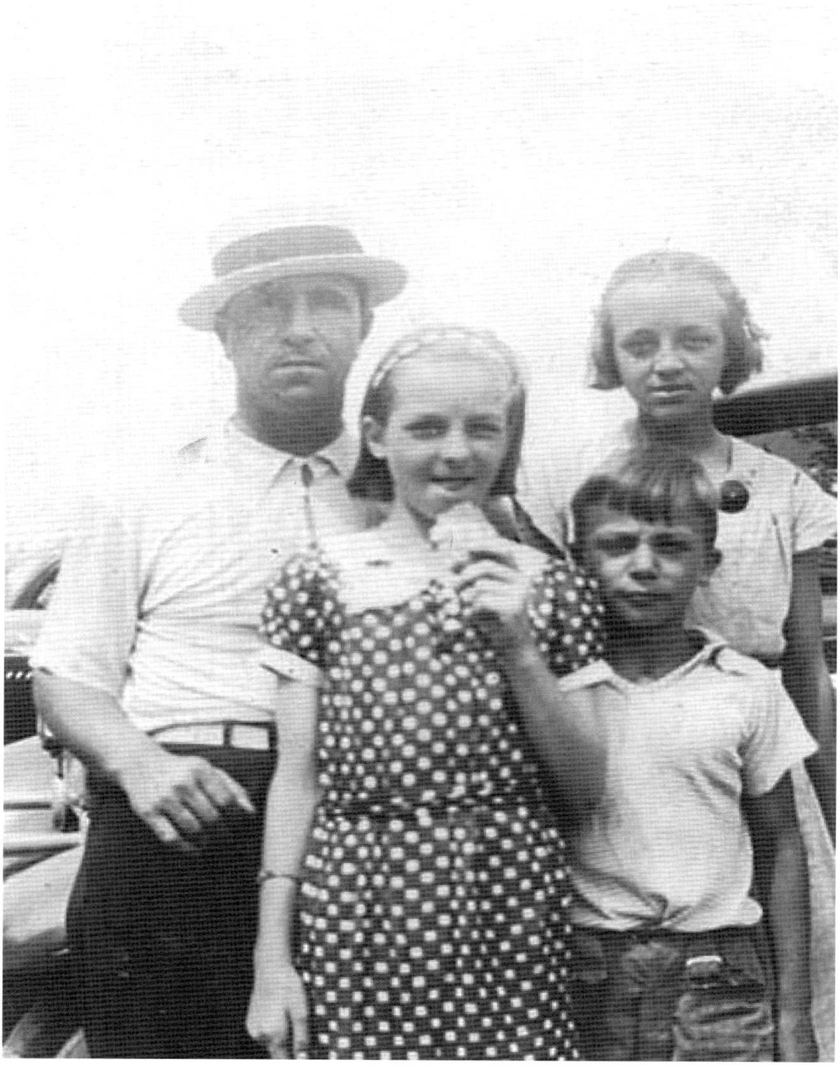

Picture 10. Two years after I got to Hillside School forty miles west of Boston, John Mason, a car owning friend of our Mother, brought my sisters, Ruth and June, to Hillside for a picture of all of us as Mother took the picture, in 1937.

First meeting with John King:
Interview with Marie King, April 8. 2017: by Nam-Young Park

Park *Mrs. Marie, it is the 1st anniversary of John's death. I remember being so shocked after reading your email about his death. It greatly saddens me that I was 1 week late to the news, as in South Korea, we seldom use Facebook and use Kakaotalk instead. Thus, it took me a while to check my Facebook account and read your message. I am very saddened to have broken my promise to attend his funeral.*

Let me have the story of your first meeting and final moment with John King, please

Marie Say about how to get there. Take well the story, we were like, Oh what I wanted to wanna say, We were with the ladies, from Young Women's Christian Association that was YWCA.

And then We were down with the young men who came back from the war or they were leaving from the war so we were there to just feed them coffee and donuts and talk or else the music was playing and they with wanna dance. The first word John ever said to me was 'Dance ma'am?' That's how we met. So that's good. And we were married for 68 years long time.

Park *Approximate 70years ago. Exactly 68 years*

Park *What was the most valuable treasure in your home? These medals?*

Marie That's right. So···, and these are all his medals. All of these things on it (Indirect) are medals that he got from all kinds of organizations that gave him recognition and someway

Park Good, Thank you

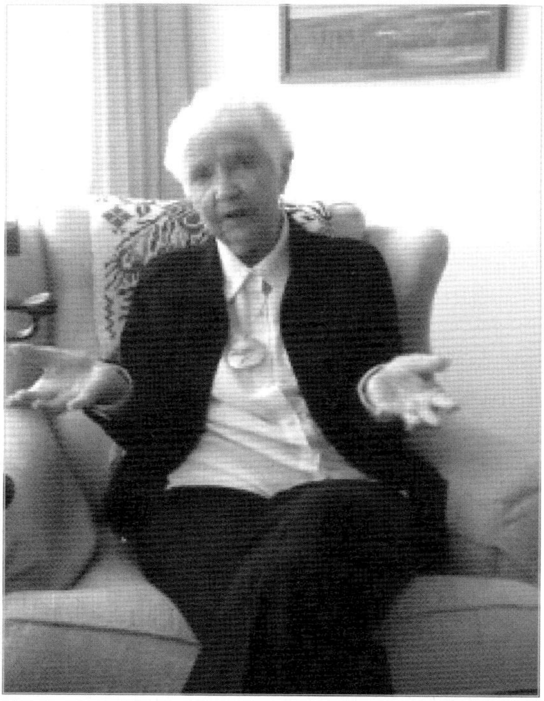

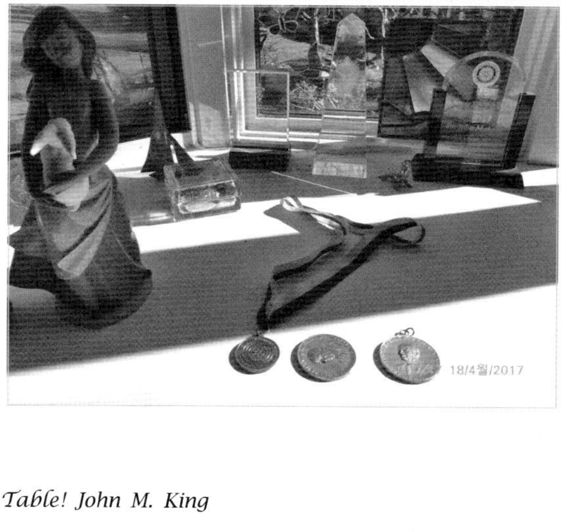

Time to Say Goodbye : John King's, Final Moment :

Interview with Marie King, Apr. 8. 2017 : by Nam-Yong Park

Park *I remember, on 8th November of 2014, a year and half before his decease, John and I went to visit the place where John King would be buried and the tomb of his mentor Professor Peter Olafson. Then, John showed me the tree which he planted to honor him and asked me, "Can you do the same for me when my time comes?" So I replied, "Of course. But, I said that it would make more sense to do it jointly with your old disciples."*

Park *Marie? May I have the story of the moment at death bed of John's?*

Marie That, um, a month, uh, before he died, he had a stent put in one of his coronary vessels because they thought maybe it would help him breathe better. Now, John, wasn't having trouble breathing, but he let him do it. And from that pool, the pole to be. Okay. So that was like a month before. Yes. And he put this, they put the stent in and, and then he came home from the hospital and he began to change.

He was doing very strange things. He would go out in the middle of the night and he would go, yes. And, and I really never knew where. But he would go out and then come back and, and I would try to say, there is no one, you know, out there, why are you going? And he would say, I'll find somebody. And when he would come back, he would go to bed next day in the evening, his same thing.

He took, he would take the scooter and he would drive around. So I had to. Put the police on his tail because I was afraid something would happen to him. But he came home one night after being gone for about four hours. Middle of the night. Yes. And he came in and he said he was very tired and he was going to bed.

He slept the whole next day. And the whole night that was like 24 hours straight. And when he woke up, he wasn't himself, he was not feeling good at all. So I sent him to the hospital and the hospital told me that I should stay at the hospital because they thought he was too sick to be left alone. So I stayed to that at the hospital.

Oh, maybe a day. And I asked them to bring him here to Kendall, put him in our health department and let me take care of him. And they did. And two weeks it took about two weeks later that he just went downhill a little bit every day. They. They gave him more faint. If he had great pain, I don't know why he pain, but he seemed to have it.

They made me in his chest. I'm not sure, but, um, it was worse every day and, and he just got to where he wasn't eating at all and he didn't know, and he wasn't speaking anymore. So I was, but I was there every day, almost all day long. Until the day he died and I was right there when he died and it was very peaceful.

He was not in any pain and there was no movement or anything that would make you feel like he's having pain. He just stopped breathing. So I say it was very peaceful.

Park *Peaceful. Yes, that's right. It's wonderful. So it was, it was the way to go. So at that time he's a pacemaker heart. There's no problem moving.*

Marie No, no problem. The thing is. When the last two weeks, you couldn't tell where he was having pain, but in the hospital, all of the nurses and doctors knew that he was here, maybe sometimes having a nightmare in the light, something that she would move on the beat the night or.

You know, in the daytime, he just, he just wouldn't would not be, you'd been feeling well. And then they gave him morphine to keep him quiet and to help him if he was having. And it was, it was, I want to say that it was peaceful and I'm grateful. Yeah. Yeah. Good.

Park *Certainly, death is a sad, but as loyal husband John will be preparing for you in the heaven, after 10 years more. Thank you.*

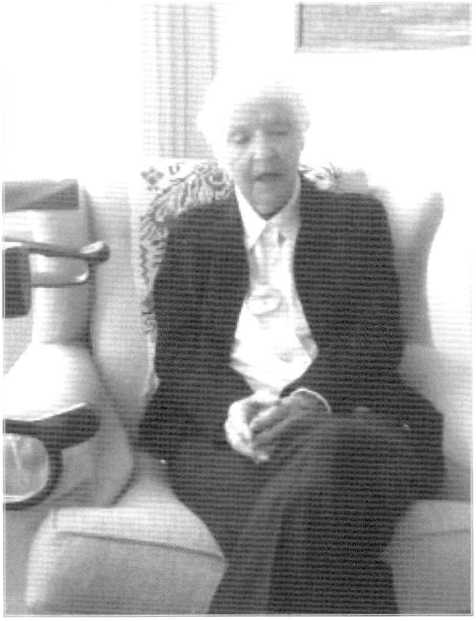

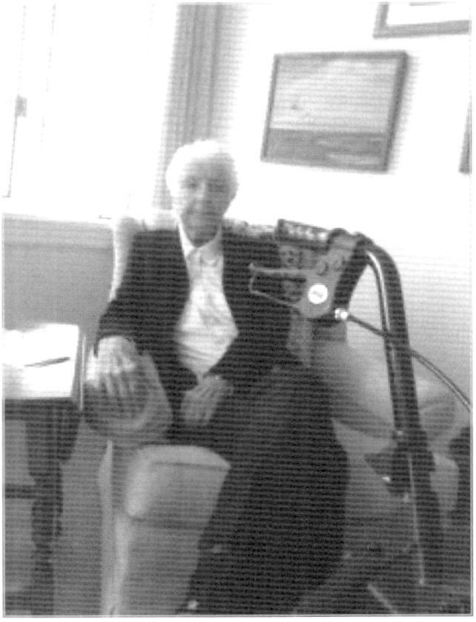

A Letter from John M. King :

His Biography and More

1 May 09

Dear Nam Yong,

It was very nice to receive your request for bio information, but I am still wondering why you are doing this for me. There are many others who I am sure deserve it much more. Because you have asked I am pretty much involved in doing it for you and not to be rude in ignoring of your wonderful request.

I will start with a few specific requests as you indicated. Enclosed in what I am sending you is a thick batch of notes and letters on my behalf when it came to the process of the Harold Casey Teaching Award. I enclose it but certainly wish to have it returned sometime as those were from dear friends. Other information I have also sent and a set of notes of True Stories of a Different Kind(TSDK) and a portion of the newer and really last edition of the Necropsy Book that I hope to have included into it. This will make it a rather thick book when it is finished and should include the 1) Necropsy Book (original), the 2) Helpful techniques the Necropsy Table, and 3) The True Stories of a Different Kind (also called Thirty Years at the Necropsy Table. I had give Bruce Williams a CD on the three combined edited (proof read) last year and he said it would be put last fall, but he mentioned hard economic times. I will actually try to get it published here if he doesn't get on the ball and do it under the C. L. Davis aegis.

The notebook affair with all the letters is a compilation from friends, even Deans, and graduate trainees and I have asked by letters written to them already (with your address also included) to several other friends, faculty, foreign acquaintances to write you directly to be used as you wish for the biography.

Now for your specific requests.

Father: John William H. King

Hamilton, Canada. Was born there in 1897 (?) and lived there until after WWI when he fought with the Canadian Army and on return met my mother and moved to Pittsburgh, Pa., USA. 4 sisters

Mother: Gladys McCain- born 1901 in Pittsburgh, Pa., Only child. Married about 1920.

Children: 3 daughters and then yours truly in January 16, 1927 as baby of family. One sister still living in Boston, Ma., USA.

Lived in and around Boston with family until 1935 when Mom and Dad split up. Three sisters lived with 3 different family members and I guess no one wanted a little rough 7 year old boy so I was put in a farm home for boys. Hillside School in Marlborough, Mass., in 1935.

First however, I went to a Mrs Crow's home with my sister, 2 years older for a time, about 8 children there, had rice three times a day, plus other things (?) I think. We all had only white flour snacks with neck and arm holes to wear every day. We were not allowed outside to play, but we considered it was great as we could see some children walk by our "home", but never see them again as Mrs. Crow said, they were all kidnapped. We were lucky to be with her. Apparently, we did not recognize they were the same children going to school, but with different clothes every day. Mrs Crow ate with a knife.

Dad never visited us but Mom did with candy in her pockets.

At the farm school, we all cried our first nights there, but we soon got over that to commiserate with new kids. Stayed there 10 years, weeding, picking beans, cutting wood as all furnaces were wood burners only. Had 3 dorms to heat in cold New England nights and when I got older there, I did all the fire keeping alone.

I learned a lot. 80 boys at the school all year unless you had a home you could go to for holidays. Never saw my father once in the 10 years and my mom only 2-3 times a year as the school was so far from Boston. All of 28 miles.

We kids did all the corn for the table and cow corn for the silage to feed the dairy cattle, about 60, which gave us all the milk we wanted and lots for selling to the dairy. I drove the milk truck to the milk dairy when I got old enough, 16, 17 and 18 until I joined the army, 1944-45.

I enjoyed every day on the way to high school in town, but in taking the milk early, especially in winter, my fingers were too cold to pass the test for my eight o'clock typing class.

Four years in the army was great as I got paid and now HAD MONEY. Got to Germany to join the parachute- school there in preparation to jump into Japan, but after the atom bomb went off, there was no need for us paratroopers. Guarded a few German prisoners and even the so-called Butcher of Lednice, Poland who had tried to commit suicide.

Married to Marie Ryan in 1947 while in the army.

Left into service in 1948 to climb electric power company in Wilmington, Delaware, my wife home. She worked as a laboratory technician at the Dupont Nemours hospital there, joined in the U.S.O (United Service Organization) to volunteer for dances with the soldiers attending the many different service schools being taught in the Aberdeen Proving Grounds. Saw some of the big German V2 rockets there. I met her at one of the dances and we were married 62 years ago in Delaware.

Went to the University of Delaware for a little over a year under the wonderful G.I. bill with tuition and fees paid and a stipend of $80.00. What a blessing.

Wrote to all the extant veterinary colleges for admittance, but only heard from Dean McElroy in Okla, advising me to keep up my grades and come to Okla.

Our best man at the wedding had a home in Tulsa, Okla. He died that year so we decided to go write them to finish the two years of prevet workout there and meet his folks also.

Five years in Okla A & M College allowed me to finish vet school in 1955. With my wife working and my enrolling late, at best a month every semester, and with the G.I. bill had a free veterinary education in effect.

Dr. Panciera was another Yankee who went to Okla from Rhode Island and he was at Cornell in 1955 and I decided to take a residency in Pathology with Dr. Peter Olafson and Charles G. Rickard at Cornell. Had 5 wonderful years at Cornell and then went to Washington State University for two years teaching and on to Carnegie- Mellon University in Pittsburgh as a veterinary pathologist for the Union- Carbide laboratory in Export, Pa.

A position in Teaching opened up at Cornell and in 1968, I moved back to Cornell to retire 30 years later in 1998 and as an Emeritus Professor since.

In all the time since DVM graduation I have spent about 6 whole years on sabbatical leaves and other shorter leaves at many foreign veterinary schools mainly in teaching veterinary students, faculty, graduate students and others from a large collection of Kodachrome pictures with discussions and doing necropsies when available.

My son, Jon David King was born in Okla while I was a veterinary student there in 1954. He has since graduated from Cornell in the School of Hotel Administration. Maybe my wife and I pushed him a bit here since graduation he took or made time to study building, home heat, air conditioning and ventilation and earn his much prized certificate in that endeavour to become one of the few certified men in that field in Ithaca.

His building efforts have been accomplished with just the two of us, with me as his assistant, in building two large, two apartment home including all plumbing and electrical work under strict Ithaca city codes. While doing these he realized I imagine that several of his older friends and his dad may need on the job medical help and thus complete training in Emergency Medical Service (EMS) classes for over a year to also certify as an EMT (Emergency Medical Technician).

Nam-Yong, I think all the above gives you an idea of my life which although a busy one have had much time to do other things, especially with my wife and son who unfortunately died unexpectedly at 48. He is surely missed.

I have had years with him at Sport Parachuting after my Army training and he and I did that for a while, but even more we had about 30 years together with my teaching rock face climbing almost every other weekend in good weather mostly in the Schwangunk Mountains 90 north of NY city.

To keep busy I have learned how from John Wilson about the Shaker religion he taught one evening and in a day with 15 students how to make the famous Shaker Oval Boxes. This effort takes up much of my free time in the winter season as a Snowbird in St. Augustine, Fl., USA.

I also enrolled in a class of about 50 students to take a 10 evening class on learning to play the fiddle. That is the use of violin in country music. It has been a great hobby also as it is all playing by ear and not reading a single note. My wife is amazed at my "lack of pride" in doing this but at least anyone who hears my music will recognize the tunes.

Although Prof. Peter Olafson hired me, Dr. Rickard, one of the best teachers I have known has been my singular teacher with Dr. Olafson around to keep me somewhat subdued. Working with Dr. Panciera in the Department as a co-worker was a tremendous experience. And I think kept me honest the most by his searching questions. They made me think of an answer in detail not just giving the cause or whatever but why that answer; what's the pathogenesis; what else would you expect to see in the animal. It was not in his nature to accept a simple answer.

It has not been a bed of roses I guess especially when called onto the carpet by the Dean. I used to teach such things as having a student stand up and I would pantomime choking them to illustrate trauma to the neck that might crush the thyroid glands with the victim living through this like a dog on a choke chain. Then I'd ask the student what would the "crushed" thyroids look like if they lived? That was to help distinguish simple atrophy from trauma with its fibrous components.

Of course this was related to the dean as having touched the student. Another example holding a student's wrist and hand in the proper position to sharpen our necropsy knives on sharpening stone.

An even more remarkable misunderstanding of a student complaint was the taking of a student's wrist in the necropsy room that had a scalpel in it and dropping (throwing) it (the scalpel) on the floor telling the student to use the probe knife to do the necropsy on a large animal. This was even after the student had had a week's experience supposedly doing them properly. I was not there the first 5 days of her rotation.

These were the most unpleasant efforts of the sort in my 50 years on the floor but in this day and age i imagine it might be expected from the different groups of students seen.

Maybe these last few comments can be excluded from what you receive as most of my experiences teaching have been fabulous. Maybe as I grew older I was less willing to put up with some things more than others.

It is to the credit of Cornell that during these fifty years we have had a veritable wealth of cases to work on. Of equal value has been Cornell's willingness to take pictures for teaching of anything and all we as trainees or trainers wanted to photograph, culture or histologically examine. I would guess that we did examine histologically at least 60-70 of all tissue we wanted to and certainly 95-100% of cases we needed to for diagnosis.

It is also fabulous that Cornell was financially able to have faculty enough to have "experts" available for most of the species and most of the systems to be examined as ophthalmology, dermatology, neurology, parasitology, anatomy, plant and chemical toxicology. Not only did we have them, but almost without exception, they were willing to discuss cases, lesions, results and other aspects with the pathologists doing the actual necropsies. Having interest residents in all fields certainly helped keep the interest up as well.

I believe the sharing by all concerned was one of the high points of Cornell College of Veterinary Medicine and Pathology. It is also necessary here to also give credit to the many other divisions at

Cornell who also gave all the help they were able as regards need to the pathologist such as the many animal specialists in chickens, cattle, swine, wildlife, poisonous plants, the virus research labs, ornithology, the meats lab, fish labs who actually went out of their ways to help.

I am proud to say I worked at such a school with such a strong faculty and student body.

Cornell's sabbatical leave program is above reproach and is in part a major plus in the excellence of the entire system.

I have never been denied such a leave when requested and took them whenever possible. This has allowed a fantastic opportunity for me as an individual to broaden my knowledge and help whenever I could. I was never told I had to do something or I could not do something during these trips.

The taking of a graduate degree at Cornell was another strong point in my training. I admit that even though I did not become fluent in street German or French it did help me understand a bit of their culture and answer a few questions asked although most foreign countries "wanted" to hear my medical English.

It allowed me some entrance to their world of pathology and animal science.

I think I've blown my horn enough so I will send this as is in hopes that is what you wanted.

A great picture or set of pictures in one is on its way when I receive it from my home in February. It has even a picture of me doing my first necropsy (slaughter cows I had to kill at that boys school in 1941)

Most respectfully,
John M. King
May 2009

John McCain King - Autobiography

Born in Boston at the Massachusetts General Hospital Jan 16, 1927.

Being raised in a farm type boys school, Hillside School, Marlborough, Massachusetts, from 1935-1945, probably was the start of my interest in Veterinary Pathology. My father, John Henry King, and my mother, Gladys McCain King, had separated and my three older sisters went to my grandparents and two aunts all being around Boston, Massachusetts.

It was a typical farm environment with lots of work for us kids and only eleven adults including two recently graduated lady teachers and Mrs. Sanford to teach all eight grades. We raised most of our own vegetables, pigs, chickens and dairy cows with two draft horses, Tom and Dolly, to do most of the tractor type work while us kids in first through eighth grades did the weeding, woodcutting, milking, lawn care, cleaning, waiting on tables, cleaning the dormitories ,etc. and all the farm work. With eighty boys from first to eighth grade it was a lot of work.

"Pop," Lemuel Sanford, was the superintendent and boss. Ana D. Davis was the secretary with Miss Betty, the nurse. We had one chef and I actually cooked for the chef when he was absent a couple of times. We also had two really old men, one black and one recluse who lived nearby and helped Pop whenever and wherever he needed them. We had a large, old, farm house for the older boys at the farm itself , two dorms for most of the younger boys and a cottage for a few boys and the nurse.

I stayed on after eighth grade as the oldest boy there and attended high school in Marlborough. It was a long walk and bus ride every school day.

As the oldest, I had more responsibility than the other boys. This allowed me to help care for any sick animals when Pop called a local veterinarian from Wellesley. I was his gopher at the time of his visits. Incidentally, he was a Middlesex College Veterinary College graduate and wrote a wonderfully entertaining and informative book titled "The Hoss Doctor." It got me started. His name was Dr. R.J. Dinsmore.

My mother paid for my room and board for a short while, but then a very wonderful Daughter of the American Revolution lady, Miss Grace Cummings paid my way for almost the entire ten years I was there.

I enlisted in the army in late 1944, but was deferred until my high school graduation in June 1945.

After Basic training in Camp Croft, South Carolina in June, I went to New Jersey and was shipped out to LeHavre, France to a replacement depot (Repple Depple) near Frankfort, Germany when I was immediately transferred to the 508th Parachute Infantry Regiment. I volunteered for airborne training in Heddernheim, Germany. They were training for the invasion of Japan. I was fortunate to get into the jump training program at the tag end of one class so I only had five days total of training including my first five jumps.

As an eighteen year old, I was having the time of my life. President Roosevelt died while I was learning to jump in Germany and then the atomic bomb ended the war, so there was no move to Japan.

On return to the United States in 1946, we were at Fort Bragg, Fayetteville, North Carolina with the 82nd Airborne division. During all the time in the army, I took all the specialized detached schooling I was allowed to take. I even met my wife to be, Marie Ryan from Wilmington, Delaware, when she came to the USO dances at the Aberdeen Proving Grounds, Maryland where I was enrolled in a track and wheel vehicle electrician course. We were married on December 14, 1947. Our son, Jon David King, was born January 5, 1954 but died unexpectedly December 12, 2002.

After four years in the Service, my professional career started thanks to the wonderful GI Bill that gave me forty eight months of college education for my forty eight months in the Army. Fantastic.

I started in at the University of Delaware and when an army buddy died in Oklahoma, Re and I transferred to Oklahoma Agricultural and Mechanical College, Stillwater, Oklahoma. I got into their Veterinary College the next year, 1952.

I graduated in 1955 from Oklahoma A&M College now called Oklahoma State University. A 1953 graduate from OSU and a good friend, Roger Panciera was at Cornell then studying with Dr. Peter Olafson, Dr. Charles Rickard and Dr. Ken McEntee, and Roger advised me to go there with him for Veterinary Pathology graduate work. Great advice as another buddy, also a Yankee, Dr. Robert Kenney, who graduated from OSU in 1954 and was at Cornell said to come, also. I worked three months (79 days) in Tulsa, Oklahoma in a small animal hospital before heading to Cornell in 1955 under the three professors named above.

The Cornell Graduate School into which I had stumbled required the passing of two foreign languages. That was often a real stumbling block for all of us as veterinarians, but in the long run I'd have to say it was worthwhile. Another very big difference at Cornell from many graduate schools elsewhere is that there are no required courses by the graduate school itself, but you must of course take and pass successfully whatever courses your graduate committee decrees . You must pass the two languages rule, submit a perfectly finished and typed thesis signed by your major professor and your minor professors. Now a graduate member appointed by the graduate school must also sign for the graduate work.

Last, but not least, the graduate student must have earned six residence units of graduate work with at least two completed on the Cornell campus. There were no specific graduate course credit requirements, but your major and minor professors were free to require you to take whichever course they thought you needed, what grades were expected and other requirements for the degree before they would sign your PhD final examination acceptance paper. I thought then, and still do, that it was a very hard set of requirements, but much better than just concentration on course work and grades. The work requirement in teaching, doing necropsies almost twenty four hours a day and studies for the pathology board examination were more to the point of becoming a veterinary pathologist.

The five years also encompassed the time for study and passing of the rather detailed, lengthy examination for the American College of Veterinary Pathologists which I accomplished in 1961 with my thesis, approved, PhD degree from Cornell University, Ithaca, New York in 1963.

Putting all the work and education together allowed me to take an Assistant Professor position teaching at Washington State University School of Veterinary Medicine, Pullman, Washington for 1961 and 1962.

Needing a change of pace and a chance to make more money and gain experience in a different genre of pathology I accepted a position as a toxicology pathologist at Carnegie- Mellon University in Pittsburgh, Pennsylvania in 1963. Many laboratory animals as rats, mice, rabbits and primates, over a fourteen year period, were involved with the chemical testing of Union Carbide chemicals and other companies following governmental dictum for safety in man, animals and the environment. Again clinical pathology was as important as the gross and histopathology for each animal.

After six years of toxicology I returned to Cornell as an Associate Professor teaching undergraduate veterinary students and residents, both from the states and foreign countries. I still continued the histological and gross pathology toxicological studies by mail and many on-site visits to Pittsburg for eight years.

In the early days of my training, the two residents shared the necropsy and clinical pathology duties at Cornell on a weekly basis with Dr. Rickard as the pathologist in case we needed help. Over the years it has changed with a heavier load of animals and more professional help.

I joined the American VeterinaryMedical Association in 1961 and the American College of Veterinary Pathologists in 1963.

Graduate Pathology Teaching Endeavors

Show and Tell was started in my career and actually consisted of my wheeling a wheelbarrow full of yesterday's great lesions to demonstrate them to the seniors in Drs. Fox, Robert's and Fincher's eight o'clock classes. These demonstrations increased and finally reached a heavy, voluntary attendance of about one hundred students, faculty and guests every Friday at four. Specimens were saved from any interesting and worthwhile cases including wildlife and all domestic animals. The specimens were saved in a walk-in cooler in Klotz solution to maintain most of the color and pliability.

As a well appreciated aside of this, the best specimens would be saved for a few weeks before the yearly scheduled **Cornell Road Show and Tell** trip to the Southeastern Pathology Annual Conference held each May in Tifton, Georgia.

The specimens would be presented at six different veterinary schools along the eastern shore one year and the six inland schools the next year. At each school along the way, the specimens were demonstrated at eight to twelve o'clock in the morning after an overnight stay. The pathology specimens were kept in the laboratory refrigerators overnight. At noon, after the demonstration, the van with residents, students and myself would drive to the next veterinary school. The hosts provided for the lunches, dinners and board at each school. Fabulous for all.

The schools visited along the way were invited to save specimens for us as a quiz of unknowns as for sure our hundreds of specimens were unknown to them. It was a very good learning experience for all.

The **Olafson Short Course**, a general, 40 hour intensive, diagnostic pathology course, was given at Cornell each year with the many knowledgeable, in- house faculty pathologists. They gave a fifty's, Fox's and Roberts

minute presentation of their expertise in one of the many facets of Veterinary Pathology to include: Gross and Histopathology, Neuropathology, Avian Disease, Ophthalmological Pathology, Dermatopathology, Reproduction Pathology, Electron Microscopy, Woodchuck Pathology, Myopathy, Renal Pathology, Parasitology, Clinical Pathology and others. Most of these teaching efforts were given yearly for almost thirty years, from 1968 to 1998.

Another important aspect of my professional efforts was the

availability and opportunities for regular sabbaticals and leaves-of-absence for **Professional improvement** in venues other than the United States. This totaled more than eight years of professional teaching and learning via necropsies in more than thirty different countries. Most were initiated by my contact with visiting veterinary graduate students and faculty who would invite me to their universities and facilities. My primary function was to demonstrate the necropsy technique and teach using a well organized presentation and discussion of lesions from my very large kodachrome collection.

Over the years, the humane euthanasia methods as needed turned out to be an important set of demonstrations in many locations as was knife sharpening. It is no fun to necropsy any animal with a dull knife.

Mornings were usually arranged for in-house necropsies and afternoons for the kodachrome presentations. My wife, a keen birder, accompanied me on most of these sabbaticals and other leaves.

The host country usually took care all of our expenses for room, board and transportation and even the airfare, as often we were not paid otherwise. This was no hardship as Cornell still paid my professorship half pay while on full year sabbatical leave. Several countries insisted on paying me which was certainly appreciated.

A list of the venues visited for research, teaching and professional improvement of all types are included below with approximate times.

It should also be stated that while most of my efforts were towards the aims above, a very important part of pathology is the actual visit by the pathologist to the farm or location where the animal or animals had died. It is not that the owner or clinician would not have given a good history

for the animal, but instead, the pathologist, after finishing the actual dissection, will be more secure in what to look for than others. He or she will be able to concentrate their efforts to fit the necropsy to the environment.

This approach also allowed the visiting pathologist to be more easily acquainted to the area in general and discuss the cases in detail.

All of the following countries visited were by official governmental or academic invitation to conduct diagnostic necropsies on animals submitted for such in the mornings and presentation and discussion of kodachrome pictures of lesions usually by systems and discussion of techniques needed for diagnosis.

There were also visits to various locations where diseases had occurred . Owners, students and various faculty usually attended.

Students, faculty and others usually served as interpreters for most of the presentations as needed.

Thankfully, most understood English pathological terms and would rather hear my slow, distinct English pronunciation as it is quite an important language in most countries worldwide in the fields of science, economics and medicine.

I have been lucky to be at Cornell during most of these years with its freedom of teaching and its broad base of animals as well as its competent teaching and, equally important, willing faculty. The eight years of foreign study, research, teaching of veterinary students, residents and guests of techniques and methods for humane slaughter and processing for necropsy and histopathologic studies of the many thousands of cases which has been conducted similar to those done at Cornell, with open discussion pretty much at all times which is not always allowed elsewhere. The invitations from the various countries and institutions have pretty much expressed their wish that my presentations be continued in like manner with almost no restrictions to my methods. This was very much appreciated in both directions.

Publication and Research

Newfoundland, June 1958, and June 1963

This primary research effort, while still a graduate student, was directed at finding the cause of the

yearly death rate of 75-80% of the caribou calves. It was

successfully determined in 1963 as being

caused by Canadian lynx predations. Its control consisted of the elimination of the lynx by trapping and removal from the calving grounds.

Many individual publications have been produced as a co-author with the majority associated with toxicology while working at Carnegie-Mellon University. Books include two **Atlases of General Pathology** published in Taiwan. **Volume I** was published in 1976 by the Joint Commission on Rural Reconstruction and the Pig Research Institute of Taiwan and written by J. M. King, F. S. Hsu, C. B. Hong and R. C. T. Lee . **Volume II** was published in 1983 by The Council for Agricultural Planning and Development Executive Yuan and the Pig Research Institute of Taiwan with pictures and detailed discussions for each by J.M. King and Robert C.T. Lee.

The first **Necropsy Book** was written in 1970, by J.M. King, L. Roth, D.C. Dodd and Marian Newsom, and was primarily on necropsy technique. Four more editions with additional text on aids to diagnosis on common domestic animal and wildlife lesions have been published over the years, with the same authors and the original drawings by Marian Newsom by the C.L. Davis Foundation in Gurnee, Illinois, also including the fifth edition in 2010.

A sixth edition of The Necropsy Book is expected to be published in 2012. In general, the

Necropsy Book concerns the actual techniques for performing a complete necropsy of almost any

animal with the Newsom diagrams for ease and completeness. Common lesions and their actual locations are shown diagrammatically and discussed briefly based on their gross appearance for ease of identification in the later printings.

Fifty Years at the Necropsy Table (True Stories of a Different Kind) was published in 2010 by the C.L. Davis **Foundation**. It is a text book of over one hundred stories, by J.M. King, of the finding of new, surprisingly common and unique lesions often including the discussion of the needed visit to the actual farm or facility where the animal died in order to make the most proper diagnosis.

Cornell Web Page

A very important addition to all the published information listed above is the time consuming, wide coverage of the actual lesions which have amounted to the taking of over **45,000 kodachrome** pictures of the lesions found. Approximately 27,000 have been digitized and put on a Cornell web page: http://w3.vet.cornell.edu/nst and are **free** to everyone worldwide with computer and internet access.

It has been a major effort starting with Dr. John Leukowitz, the computer programmer and expert who developed the program. It allows almost instant downloading, by anyone, of the individual pictures or groups of pictures as he programmed the web page to identify each picture by web page number, necropsy case number, species and age if known, tissue, gross or histologic diagnosis, simple gross appearance, morphological diagnosis, etiologic diagnosis, cause, final diagnosis or comment. All items may not have all the descriptors filled in, if they are not known, but the pictures will often speak for themselves. The space for comment is fairly large as it is often my personal reason for taking the picture.

Dr. Lois Roth was my chief assistant for taking many of the actual pictures while Dr. Jim Britt in the Arkansas Diagnostic Lab and Dr. Linda Parrish of Kendal, Wisconsin, Susan Williams and Cindy LaCroix at Cornell did the main typing and correcting of much of the texts and the digitizing of most of the pictures. Dr. John Edwards of Texas and Dr. Coos Coetzer, Praetoria, South Africa contributed great groups of the pictures.

The Web Page is in receipt of about 2,000-4,000 hits a day from all over the world.

Countries Visited

Taiwan I June 1975-March 1976

Hong Kong
Thailand
India

Kenya
South Africa
Israel
Finland

Morocco	September 1979
Taiwan II	March-May 1981
Australia	August 1983-July 1984
New Zealand	July 1984
Switzerland I	September 1989
Egypt	November 1989
Lichtenstein	February 1990
France	February 1990
Germany	March 1990
Italy	April 1990
Brazil I	March-June 1990
Greece	November 1992
Spain I	November 1992
Spain II	November-December 1995
Argentina I	August-December 1996
Brazil II	December-Christmas 1996
Chile	January-February 1997
Brazil III	March 1997
Trinidad & Tobago	April 1997
Mexico	January-February 1998
Brazil IV	July-August 2003
Argentina II	August-September 2003
Switzerland II	April-September 2004
Peru	September-October 2005
Peru	2008
Korea	April 2008
Taiwan III	April 2010

Antique Veterinary Instruments and Museum

Started in 1975, this author, to remind the public what little the veterinary profession had to work with initially compared to the present, has collected ten to fifteen thousand veterinary instruments and paraphernalia for cleaning, wire brushing, waxing and mounting into museum quality glass fronted wooden display cases with individual identification of name of the item, probable manufacture source and use, if not self explanatory. The name of the veterinarian or person who donated, used or informed me about the items is typed on acid free paper and laminated for protection and mounted on or near the items.

Twenty-odd cases are mounted on the wall along the corridor near the Cornell veterinary library. The original cases were designed by Dr. Roger Panciera, Oklahoma State Veterinary College, Stillwater, Oklahoma, and Dr. Bruce Calnek, Cornell University. These multiple display cases have been registered with the American Veterinary Medical History Society with the continued efforts of the Secretary-Treasurer Susanne Whitaker.

These boxes, and subsequent boxes, have been made by J.M. King and are constructed of wood boards salvaged from a barn on the Elmira Road out of Ithaca. These boards came from a now disintegrating barn which in 1946 housed some dairy cattle that died from Bovine Virus Diarrhea ten to fourteen days after the ambulatory clinician, Dr. Frances Fox, and his students accidently transmitted the first known cases IN THE WORLD OF THIS DISEASE.

The latter boxes with many instruments and paraphernalia, as can reasonably be displayed within, have been donated to many small town museums and historical societies that would take them. A few larger cases have been donated to several larger museums such as the New York State Farmers Museum in Cooperstown, New York, The American Museum of Veterinary Medicine outside of Philadelphia, PA and the new Veterinary Museum at the school in Stillwater, Oklahoma. Some of the many duplicate instruments have been donated to individuals who have indicated their desire to build showrooms for such.

The multiple Cornell display cases have been registered with the American Veterinary Medical History Society with the continued efforts of its Secretary-Treasurer, Susanne Whitaker.

Recognition

Several stunning awards have come my way including the Olafson Medal from Cornell in1998 and the Inaugural John M. King award from the C. L. Davis Foundation in 2006. Both were for Veterinary Pathology.

Two endowed awards in my name have been given to a resident in training at the Veterinary College in Stillwater, Oklahoma by Dr. L. Roth and Tom Johnson and the other was given by Dr. Kenneth Gumaer for a resident at Cornell University in Ithaca, New York. All are gratefully appreciated for their generosity and commitment to Veterinary Pathology worldwide.

This fabulous journey through life could only have been accomplished by the many friends, colleagues, students, faculty and acquaintances throughout the world who have made it possible and are too numerous to mention individually.

Recalling 10 Years at Hillside (1935-1945) :

John M. King

O.K. I'm tired of always making the choices she says. Hell don't worry how you know I love and eat everything you cook. Well not this time you tell me what's for supper so to stop the discussing I agree and her fish on Friday; Baked beans on Saturday; Chicken on Sunday and has every other Monday. Thus the first Friday was O.K. but she refused the other dogs request sayin she should have known I'd never to the standard Hillside fare as Hillside is what explained half of my idiosyncrasies in our (now 53 years) married life.

This type of comment all started in 1933 when my mom and dad split up and three older sisters went to live with family and I was placed at the Hillside School for Boys in that year. I think Mom was supposed to pay $ 20.00 per week but shortly later I heard I was a freebie. So I started a great 10 years of my life.

Hillside School started by the Drinkwater Sisters in a town further west in Massachusetts was moved to Robin Hill Rous in Marlborough, Mass. early in the century when a lake was put in. It's a 330 acre dairy farm area with a great several acre pond, rice farm area with the Assabet river running through it and the main buildings and school rooms at the top of the hills with lots of fields, pasture and woods pretty much scattered around the dairy farm and between the farm and the main buildings.

80 boys from 6-14 years were the major inhabitants year round and one or two stayed to attend high school locally. Only a few adults were there to care for and teach the first to eight grade of school in three classrooms so only three teachers were available with an imported teacher now and then to cover was necessary.

People will be coming and going through this story so at least a few of the stationary objects should be described as a starting point.

The whole school area of 330 acres starts a mile or so from Hardy's comers where in time I'd get a school bus owned and driven by a Marlboro undertaker Mr. Feighe. Of course sometimes I'd get out of high school class early and waited at the undertaker's garage for the bus back to Hardy's Corners. I would spend some time hunting for slightly bloody sheets left in the road accident rattan body carriers, a slight suggestion of my future interests.

As Hillside was only a grade school only a few of us stayed for high school and the daily hike to get the public school bus to town, 2-3 miles away. A rough cold walk some days in New England. When I reached 16, I drove the pickup truck to the Hillside dairy (No relation to our school) early in the morning and stayed for high school but never passed the 8 block typing class as my hand didn't thaw out until 10 A.M. on the road to the bus I found a great sheath knife that was fantastic and I hid it while I went to high school and on my return pick it up and threw it at a tree as we were all half native, weren't we? No way, and an early toss that didn't stick broke the blade off. Now watch a teenager cry.

Another half mile or so along the characteristic stone walled road the school starts with several breaks in the stone allowing some horse drawn sleighs and wagons into the woods where periodically Pop Sanford and we boys would harvest a few trees for our primary heat source for all the school buildings. Pop would tell us what trees to cut down or more correctly Pop would tell "Old Jack" who would have been assigned to oversee gangs of us boys who would do much of the tree felling and trimming and cutting up. The little kids would load the sleigh in the winter with the smaller pieces and the older boys in charge of the axes, saws and horse work did the more difficult and hard, heavy work. Many teams fell in love with one crosscut saw (no chain saws then) and faithfully learned to sharpen and care for them. Some had the same feeling for the sledge hammer and wedges in their care. The single fitted axes were likewise gems cared for individually.

We did have only one wet stone grinder that as little kids we vied heatedly to be the one or ones to turn the crank sharpener.

Most everyone tried however best to work up to using the axe, driving the horses or driving one horse in snaking one log out of the swamp areas whatever to dry ground to be piled for further transport.

The sleigh or wagon used depended on the season would only haul the 10 or 16 feet sections to the strong walls and the pack truck would make the longer trip by road to the tractor powered saw at the farm where the long pieces were sawn shorter. We had a stationary single cylinder for years for the saw but it was replaced by the power take off and belt of a tractor.

The problem here was that we only had a single tractor at anyone time and it had to be switched to many jobs. A sorry take is we had a Dougie and Wallace Turner with us and when I was a sophomore Dougie was a freshman at high school waiting for Wally to graduate from 8th grade. Dougie and I came home from high school at 1:30 as usual and Pop had told us to get the tractor hooked up to the saw. It was winter and the tractor would start so I harnessed Dolly one of the 2 or 3 draft horses we had at any one time and hauled the tractor up the little hill at the back of the farm to push it down for a start. We hauled it up by zigzagging to make it up the hill easy on the horses. Pop came about this time and gave us holy heaven for mistreating the horse, etc. He made me put up the horse away and for Dougie to leave the tractor as we had other chores we left it like that. As it was Friday night no problems but we needed the tractor for wood sawing Saturday. Dougie got up Satuday A.M. looked at his tractor, went back to bed and refused to come with us to breakfast. After breakfast, Miss Betty' who knew Pop's family in Connecticut and came to Hillside with Pop in 1927, I think was the school nurse and lived in Matthew's Cottage, our infirmary, came to the farmhouse as that was her duty also keeping it clean etc., by supervising the boys in overseeing the farm house. She found Dougie in complete amnesia and we never heard how he turned out. On inspection thet ractor's block had frozen and broken. Poor Dougie. The work the boys all did was based on a check list.

In Memoriam
for John King (1927-2016)

Bruce H. Willians, DVM
JPC, Chairman of Davis-Thompson Foundation

A giant's heart was stilled recently and its silence will reverberate forever within our profession. It was far larger the most, filled with a love of pathology, a love of learning, of students and of teaching, and a love of challenging both young and old minds alike.

It was a heart whose generosity filled our textbooks with his observations without the need for recognition, that filled our lectures with his images without the need for attribution, and whose "Necropsy Book" - the best-selling volume ever written for veterinary pathologists - raised money not for his pocket, but for the education of veterinarians around the world.

John M. King's peers called him a "legend" or a "pillar of pathology", but he was so much more. John was beyond larger than life, he was mythic. His childhood in an orphanage where his only shoes were a pair of rubber boots, his service in as a U.S. Army paratrooper in Nazi Germany and his life-long love-affair and 70-year marriage to his darling Marie - even without veterinary pathology, it was a magical story.

Everyone who knew John has stories of him to tell, and some are probably even true. Some of us were blessed to know John a bit more than just his public persona, and our stories can only paint a pale picture of the influence he had on our lives and careers. But knowing John, he would rather have me impart story or two, rather than perform a dry-as-dust recitation of accolades from his amazing career.

I said that without the pathology, his story would still be amazing - but oh, the pathology! John was the unrivalled master of observation and perhaps the finest pure pathologist our field has ever known. His library was the necropsy floor, and his books were the endless stream of autopsied animals divulging their secrets to his knife or the knives of his students under his watchful eye. For 50 years, he saw with those crisp blue eyes alone what most pathologists, backed by the steady

progress of technology, could or would not. Unlike most of us, who have assimilated the mass of our professional knowledge from books and the work of others, John learned it all on the necropsy floor. Although few of these discoveries were published at the time, they populate textbooks today, largely through the hundreds, maybe even thousands of his students around the world, who learned from him and later proved them to be true during their own careers.

John's curiosity was his defining feature. but perhaps even more important was his unflagging questioning of literally everything. He was not someone to accept an explanation simply because it was in print or was cited by a prominent pathologist. Seeing John's hand go up in the middle of one of your lectures meant that the podium was about to become your hot seat, much to John's and the audience's delight. More importantly, he imbued this truth-seeking into his thousands of students, encouraging them to challenge even what he was teaching them.

I believe that it is this simple trait which has resulted in so many of his graduate students becoming renowned teachers on their own, as well as professors of veterinary pathology, outstanding researchers, and leaders of our profession.

In his later years, he wouldn't interrupt your lecture but he would let you know at the end. On a lecture trip I made with him to Korea a number of years ago, I thought I was doing pretty well until a week later when I received a 24-page handwritten letter from John of all of the things I had "gotten wrong". I felt terrible about it, until another more senior teacher than I admitted he had gotten one of 26 pages. (It isn't as bad as it sounds – John's handwriting was "unique" at best and try as he might, he could only fit about 10-12 lines onto a sheet of lined paper.) I still have that letter and it is one of my fondest possessions.

The necropsy room was not only his library, but it was also his theater. He was a master showman, always playing to packed houses. Even at 5PM on a Friday afternoon, at his "Show and Tell" sessions, the risers were always packed and it was standing room only. This wasn't just a Cornell phenomenon – "Show and Tell" toured the country as well. Each spring he would pack a truck with grad students and barrels of tissue in Klotz solution, sloshing his way down the East Coast and the South hitting every vet school from Ithaca to finally Texas A&M where the tissues were frayed and broken from the thousands of exploring hands they had encountered in between.

Many pathologists who only knew John from afar were put off by the size of John's personality. For those of us who were able to know him, we knew John's bluster to be far more a part of his myth than grounded in any truth. One of my favorite stories about John concerned his mentor Dr. Peter Olafson, who had "owned" the Cornell necropsy floor before John. When John took over that responsibility, each Friday afternoon he would help the frail and nearly blind Dr. Olafson to a seat at the edge of the necropsy table in front of a hundred or more students and faculty. John, an amazing pathologist by now in his own right, would simply describe the lesions for Dr. Olafson, who would either comment on the case, or wave his hand for John to describe another lesion.

John never offered a dissenting opinion, and his kindness and obvious love and respect for Dr. Olafson was not lost on a packed house. Later in his career, John was the driving force in instituting the Olafson Medal, an award given to pathologists around the world who have made distinguished contributions to the field in the combined disciplines of diagnostics, teaching and research. After many years, and only after stepping down from the committee, he was unanimously given the award for which he had steadfastly refused to allow himself to be considered.

To see John with the students was to see the real man. Students loved John and he loved them back. No question was beneath him, and his time was always theirs. John had some rough edges to be true, but they were necessary as a defense for the softest, kindest heart imaginable. Passing years were not always kind to John's unfiltered nature; however, the tremendous diversity of those in our profession who love him shows that good people will always triumph over progressively narrowing sensibilities. Sadly, on this day, I would rather hear one of John's "Williams, just what good ARE you?" than a compliment from anyone else I know.

God, John loved to teach – anywhere and anyone. My glass tabletop still proudly bears scratch marks from when he would hold court with non-pathologist dinner guests and my kids, showing them bezoars, blister beetles, and other bits of magic from his "Black Box" - a battered old suitcase with a chain leash for a handle into which he had piled a career's worth of portable oddities and treasures that didn't require fixation. One of John's favorite pastimes was giving young (and old) booksmart pathologists the "pathology catechism"... over a 100 questions about veterinary pathology that aren't in any textbook. I took it several times, always failing miserably (and later pretending to after I had memorized a copy he left lying around) to his great delight. While a correct answer would bring a twinkle to his eye and a paternal smile, he loved wrong answers best, because he knew a spirited discussion was in the offing. John loved the argument, because in his later years, when he was no longer in the necropsy room, that was where he would learn something new (not that it would change his long-held views on pathology, but he delighted in learning new things almost as much as he did in teaching). At the 2012 ACVP meeting, where he was invited to talk as a "Pillar of Pathology", rather than recounting the high points of his unrivaled career as expected, John decided to give the assembled guests a part of the "catechism" instead. The ACVP

learned that day what we all had known for so long – you never know what John was going to say, but it was always entertaining.

John didn't know everything, and he was the first person to tell you this fact. There were few questions he probably had never considered, and he knew the ones that had him stumped. When you asked him one of these, he would just smile and simply raise his index finger to the sky and say "Ask him". And his later years, he would tell me "Ask him yourself, because I'm too close to doing it for real".

Now that my friend John is gone, I know that God is going to be busy for a while.

… Bruce H. Williams, DVM (JPC)

More Photos from John King : Life and Practice

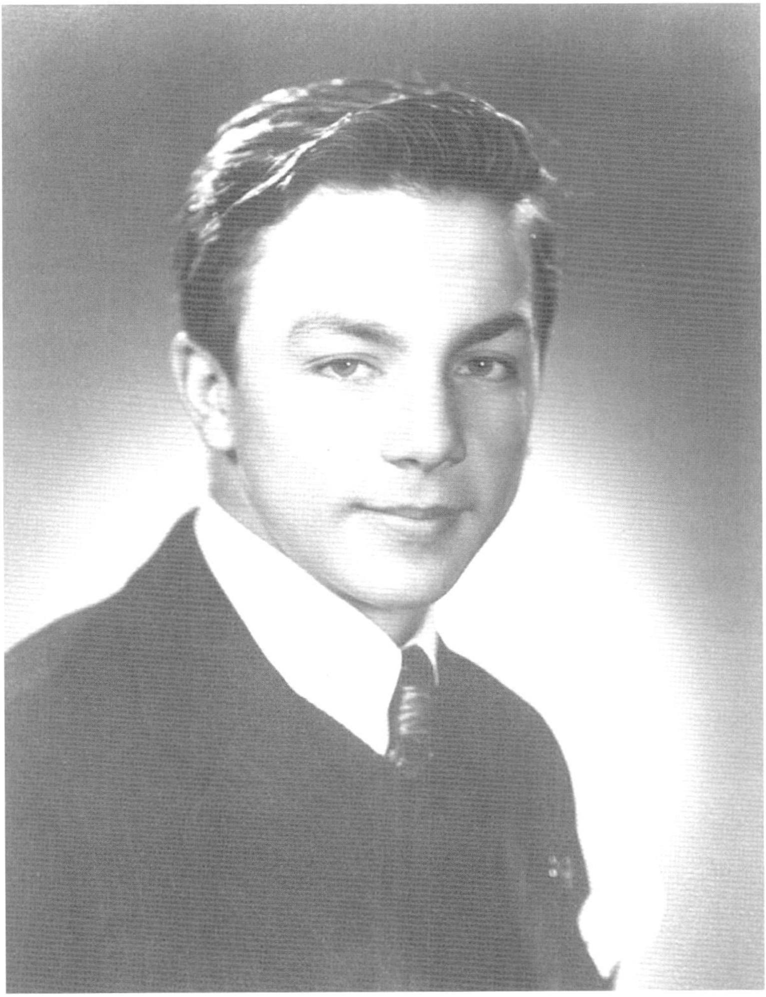

Picture 11. My high school graduation picture at Marlboro High School, Massachusetts, in 1945. I took a college course for those years never knowing where I would ever get the funds for college. However, immediately after Marlboro High School the US Army took care of that. My forty-eight months of army life entitled me to forty-eight months of the G.I. Education Bill for veterans. What a blessing for all who used it.

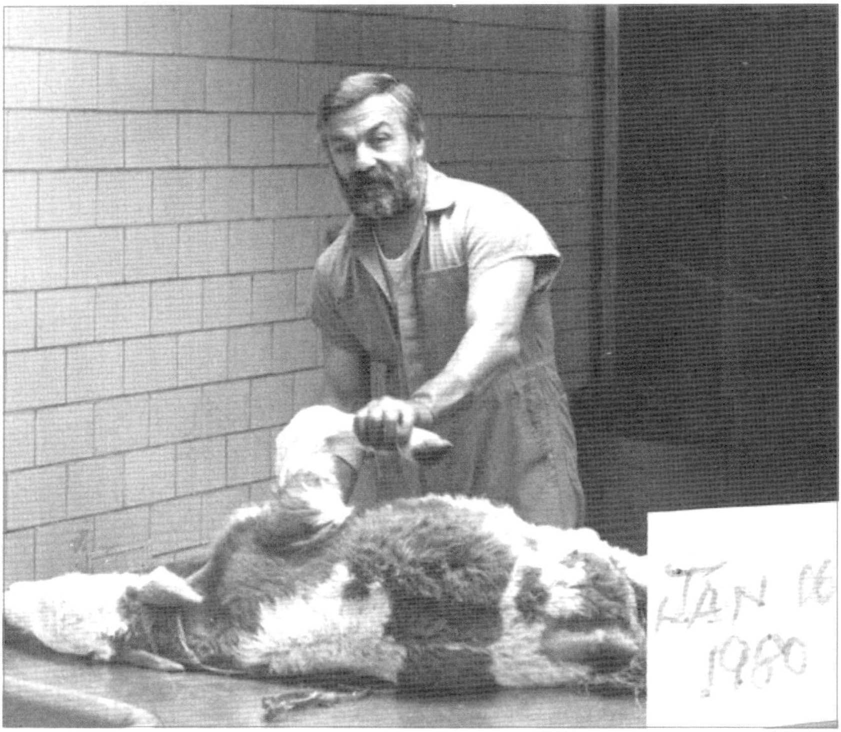

Picture 12. Here I am at fifty three on my birthday doing a necropsy on a calf. It's on a hydraulic table in our new necropsy room at the Cornell Veterinary College in 1980. Nice having good gloves and coveralls, but better yet to have a sharp knife and the hydraulic table to go up and down to make it a pleasure to do the necropsy.

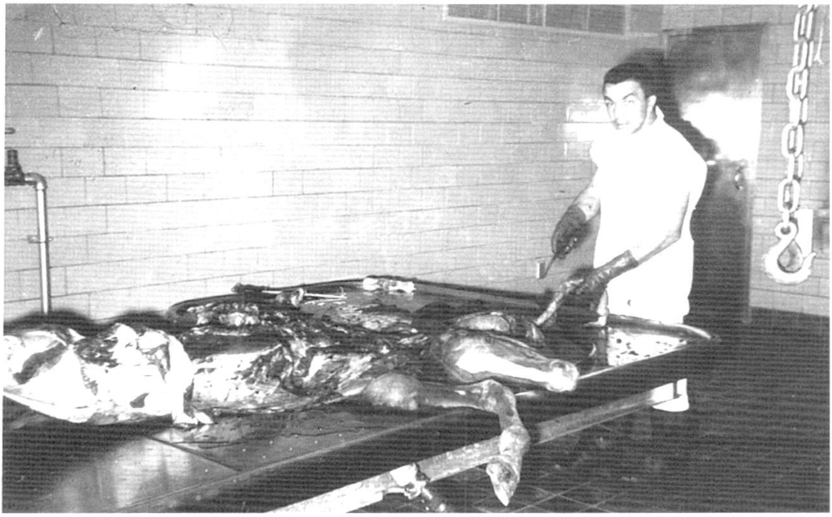

Picture 13. still dressed in coveralls, knee boots, rubber gloves and a sharp knife to do the necropsy at the hydraulic table. I even used a ceiling strong hoist for the heavy work at Cornell. Over the years I would imagine we averaged about 2,500 animal necropsies a year, all species and a complete necropsy (animal autopsy) including the brain in most cases. Probably we did as many large animals as small animals. Chickens and small research animals were done in other facilities. This foal was the last one I did in 1960 as a graduate student at Cornell.

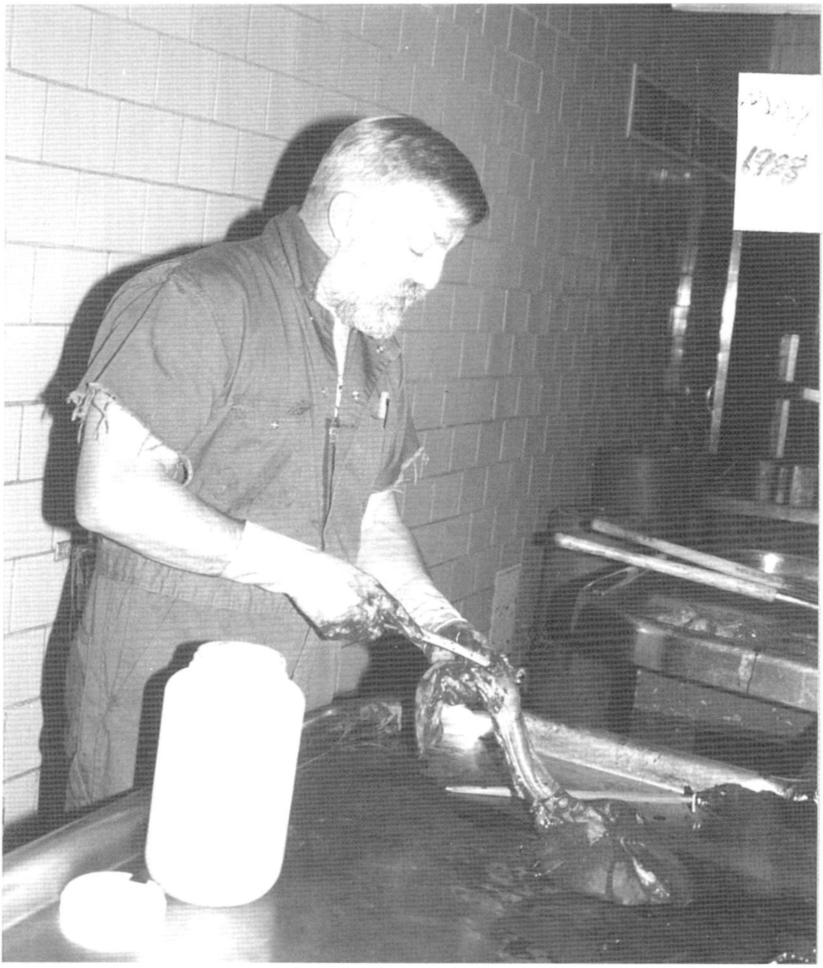

Picture 14. Here I am trimming out the tissue to place in the necessary gallon jug of formalin solution for preservation and histological preparation. Underneath the trachea being opened is the very necessary sharpening steel needed to dress the knife blade now and then to keep it sharp. It is absolutely not easy to cut even soft tissue with a dull knife.

I am demonstrating necropsy technique and proper tissue collection to a high school class. I would talk about what I was doing as I was doing it otherwise the students would be more concerned with the blood and odors involved and not the reasons for the animal being dead. I would explain what I hoped to find at all stages of the necropsy and why. It really worked for all ages of onlookers.

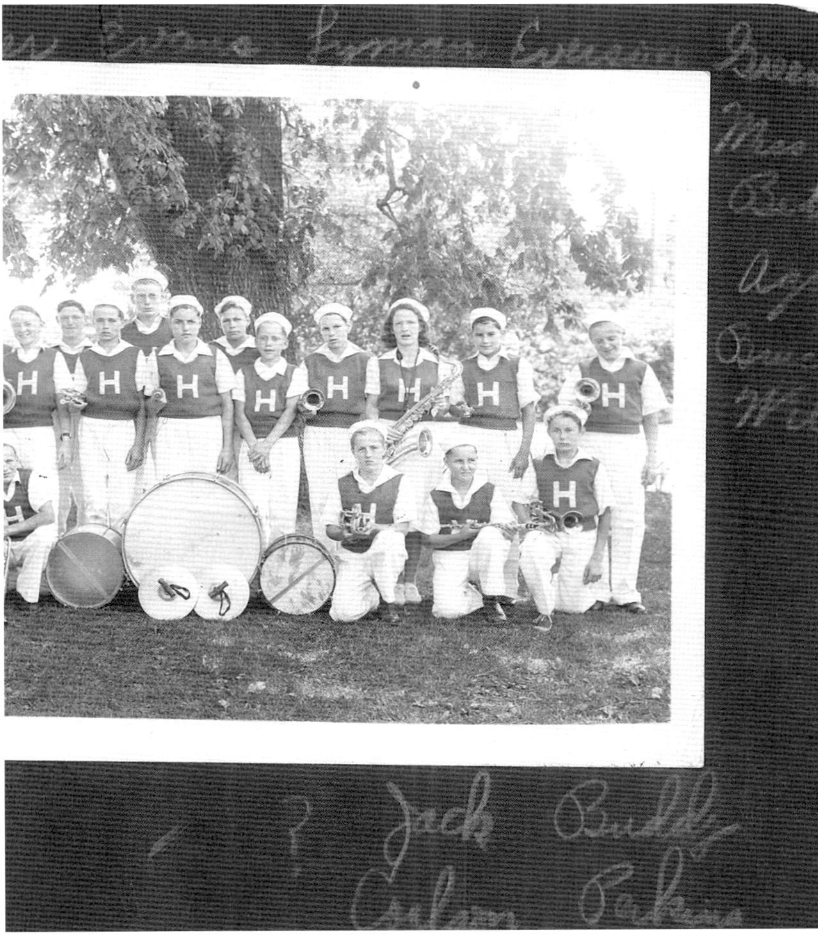

Picture 15. Of course we had a Hillside Band and our great initialed sweaters were made for us by Miss Betty, the only female in the band with her saxophone in hand. She was one of only six females of the ten member staff. I guess she was there to keep us all in control as the bandleader came from Worcester once a week. David Harrow holds the tuba and I am beside him with a French Horn that I really could not play. John Dick is the second boy to my left and is the only one I am still in touch with as we are about the same age. Harrow, with the tuba, became a high school teacher and John Dick ran a plumbing business. His Dad was a well known weather scientist notably at the top of Mt. Washington, New Hampshire. Of course all the instruments were given to us. Miss Betty had the Matthies Cottage which eight to ten kids used as a dorm, but she, as the nurse, kept the sick kids there.

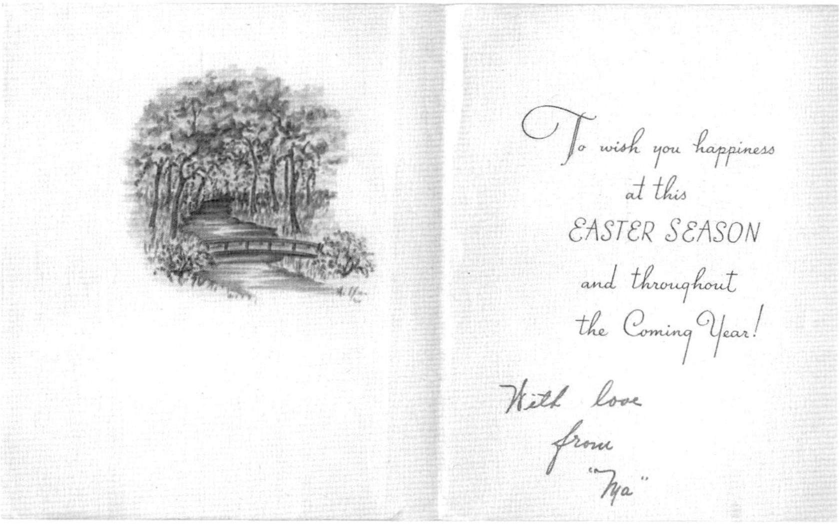

Picture 16. The Easter card signed with "Love, Ma" came from Ma Klehm while I was in the service. She was the one who welcomed me to Hillside as a seven year old and what little I could bring with me to Hillside. She put it in an upper cupboard, but I sneaked it back out the first night. One of the twenty boys in the Dormitory squealed on me and Ma took it all back, but she hugged me to stop my crying. I lived.

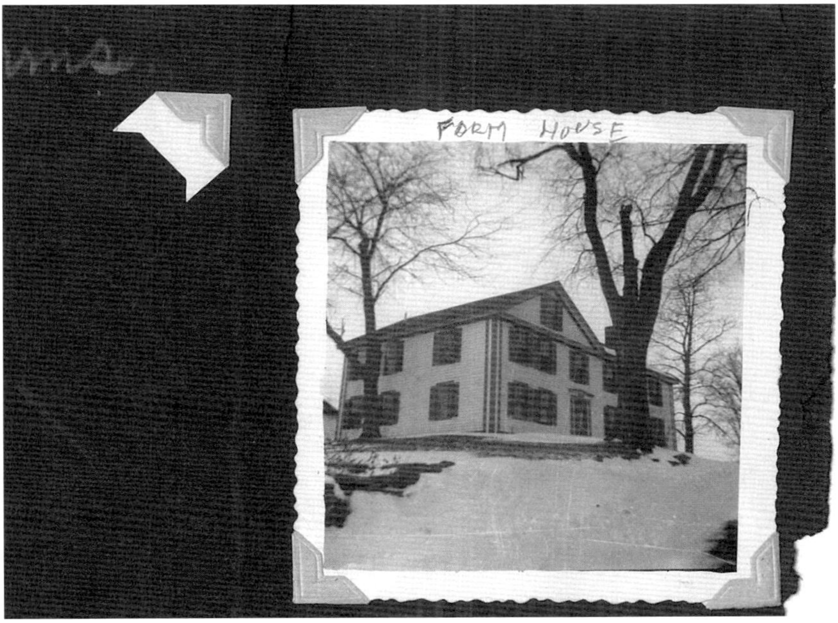

Picture 17. This is the farm house. I had a room by myself when I was one of the older kids that stayed on at Hillside after eighth grade. Almost all others left after the eighth grade. It was a tiny room, but mine. Pop Sanford, the boss of the whole school, lived downstairs although Mrs. Sanford had her own cottage nearer the brick administration building and first dorm for the youngest kids.

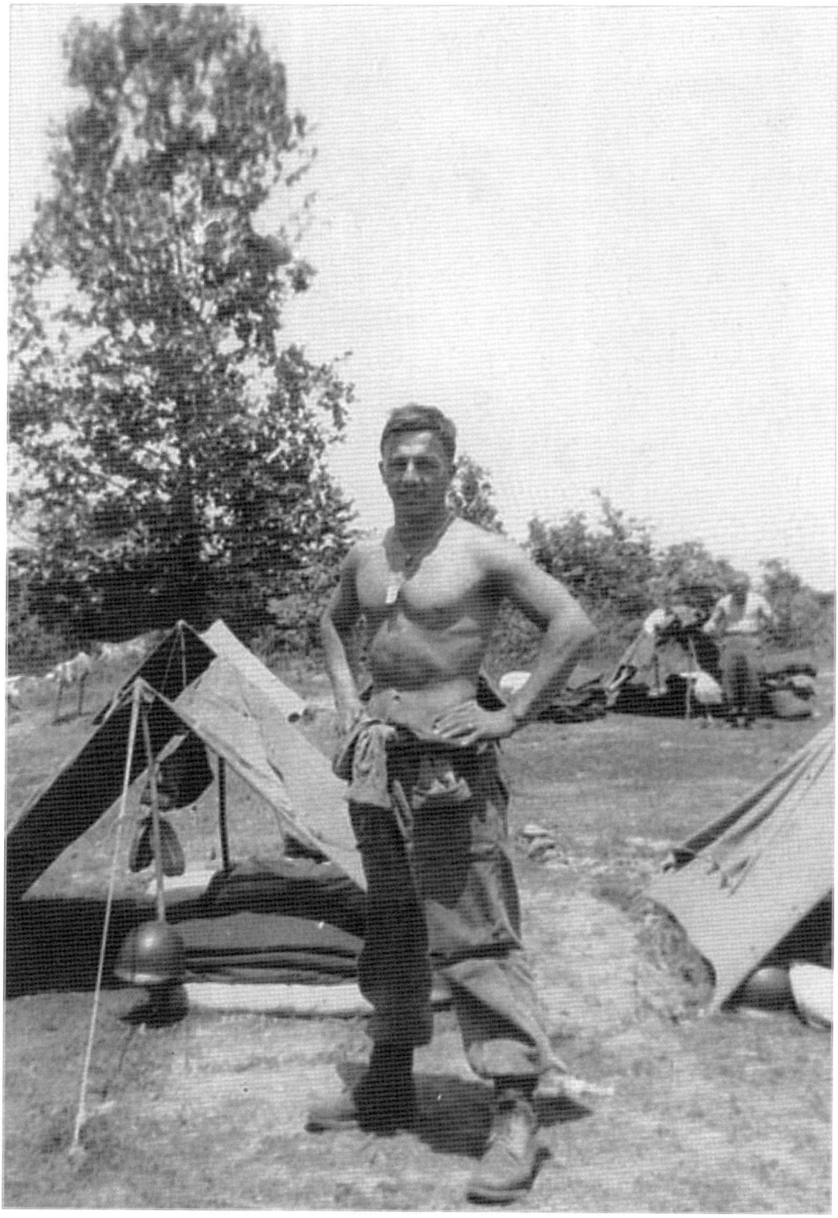

Picture 18. On maneuvers in the Bavarian Mountains in Austria and the Seigfried Line with lots of pillboxes to blow up.

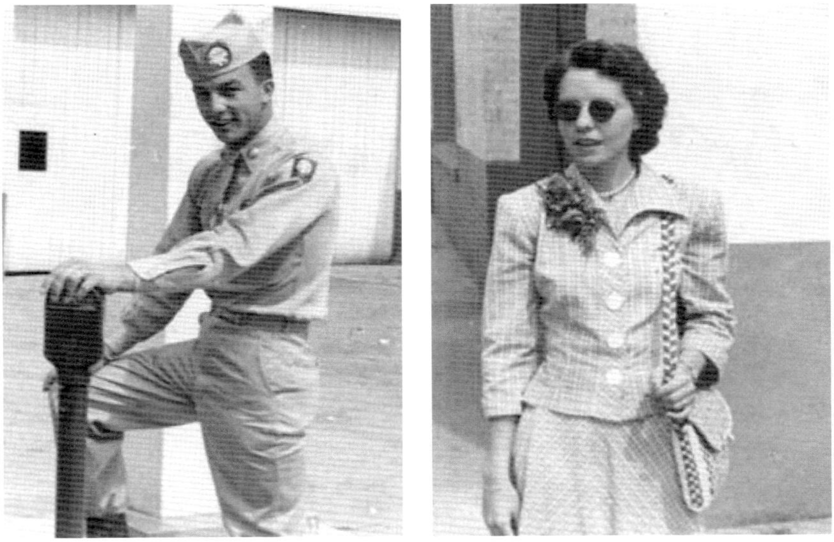

Picture 19. Marie and I on our late honeymoon day in 1948. Of course I'm the 82nd Air borne guy with the paratrooper hat patch.

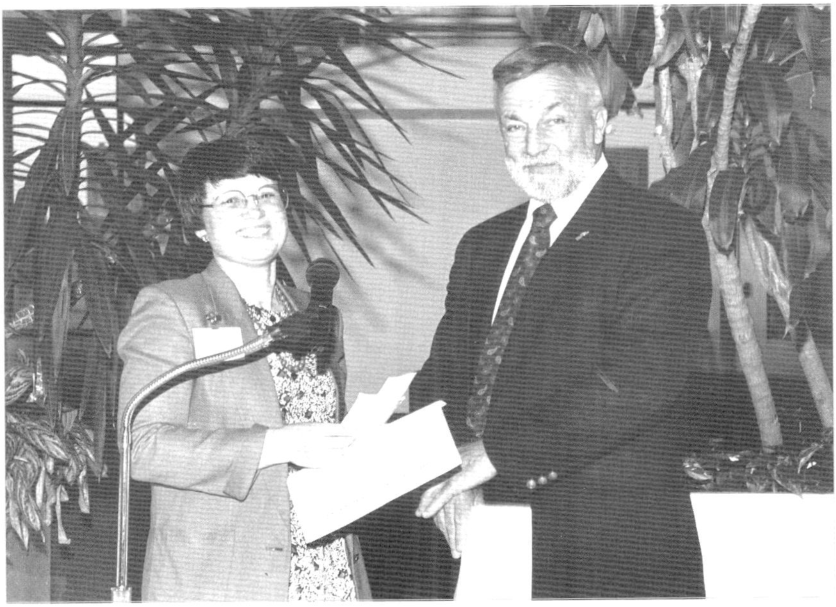

Picture 20. Dr. Wanda Haschek and J.M. King, 1991 in Illinois for a C.L. Davis talk. Wanda is the head of the Pathology Dept. there.

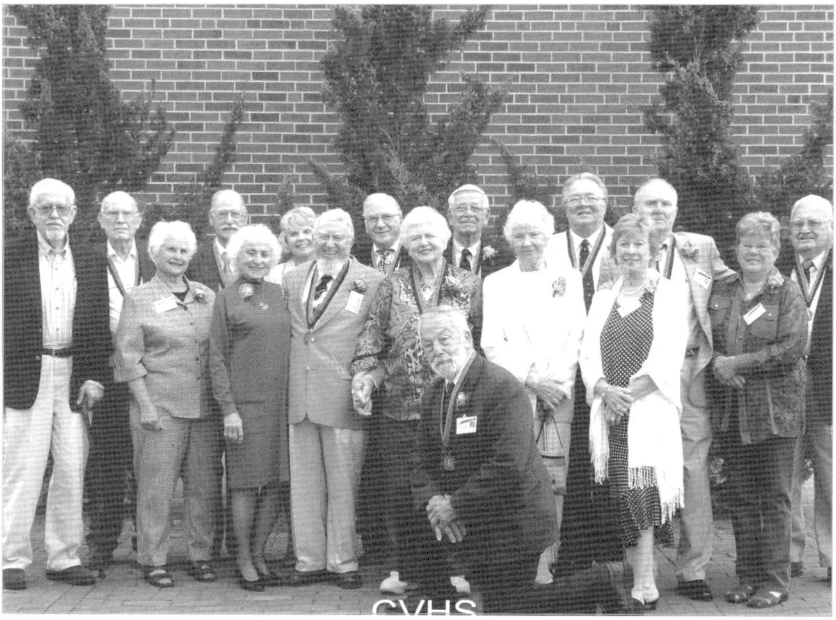

Picture 21. The fifty year reunion of our Veterinary Class of 1955 in Stillwater, at the Oklahoma State College of Veterinary Medicine. At the time of our graduation the university was called the Oklahoma Agriculture and Mechanical College. I am kneeling in front with Marie at my back, Dr. June Iben, our only girl in the class, is behind my head. We had thirty-two at our graduation.

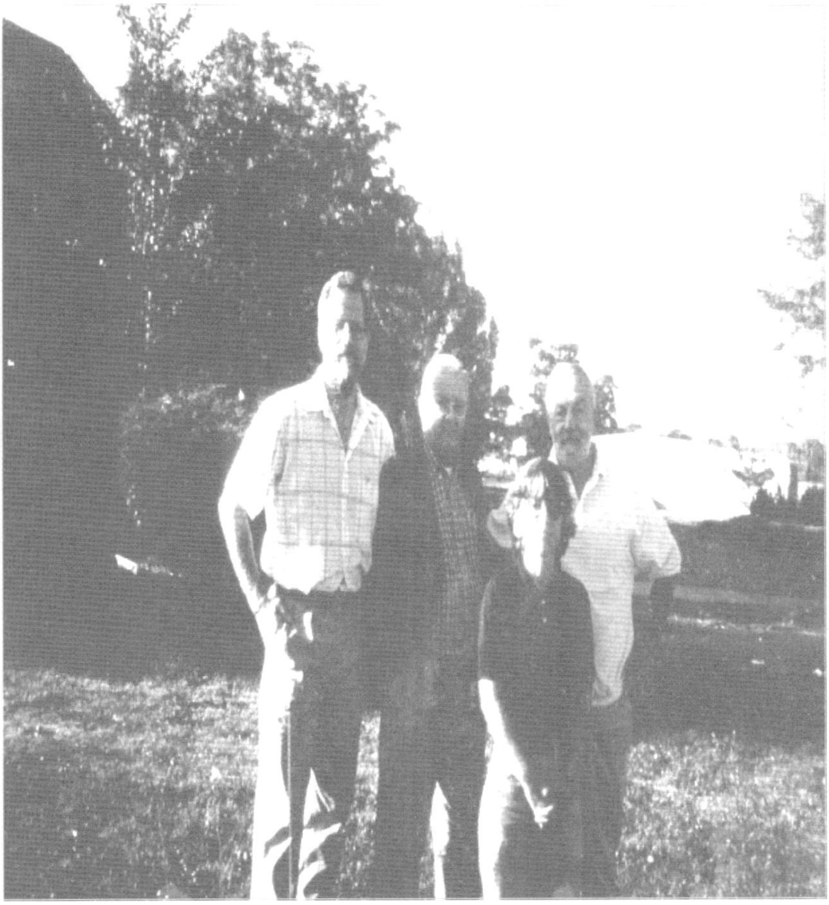

Picture 22. The tallest is Dr. John Edwards, Texas A&M, Ohio State DVM, a very good pathologist and resident for us at Cornell. The shortest is Dr. Lois Roth, Cornell 1979, and another very good pathologist and clinical pathologist. Dr. Roger Panciera, Okla 53, is mostly in shadow and from Oklahoma State Vet College. Of course I had to be in there someplace. All of us have done our graduate work at Cornell under Olafson, Rickard and McEntee and very proud of it.

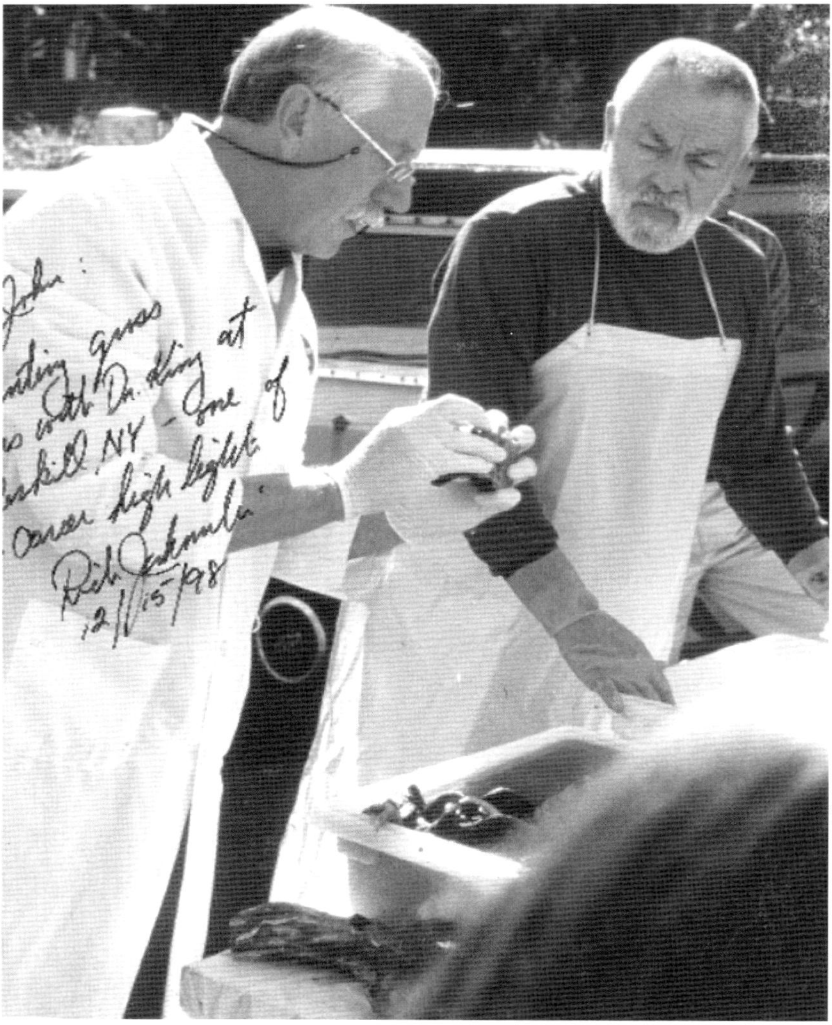

Picture 23. Dr. Richard Jakowski and I, Dec 15, 1998 at the Cobleskill pathology meeting during the Gross Pathology session. Dick is explaining a small lesion as I patiently listen. Actually it was the last "Show and Tell" given at that location.

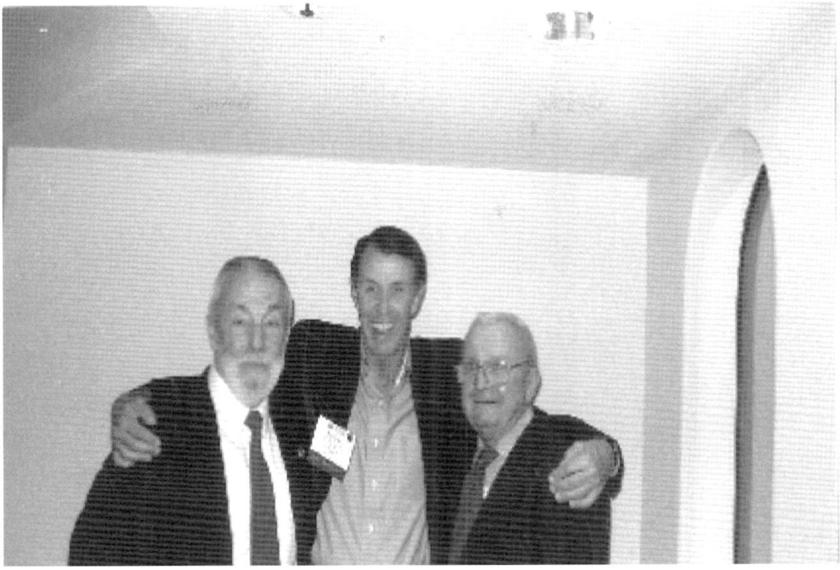

Picture 24. Here I am with Dr. Talmadge Brown, Okla DVM, Cornell PhD, who was my first resident and now is the head of Pathology at North Carolina and with Dr. Roger Panciera, also Okla DVM and Cornell PhD, who was my mentor and taught me for two years and got me to go to Cornell.

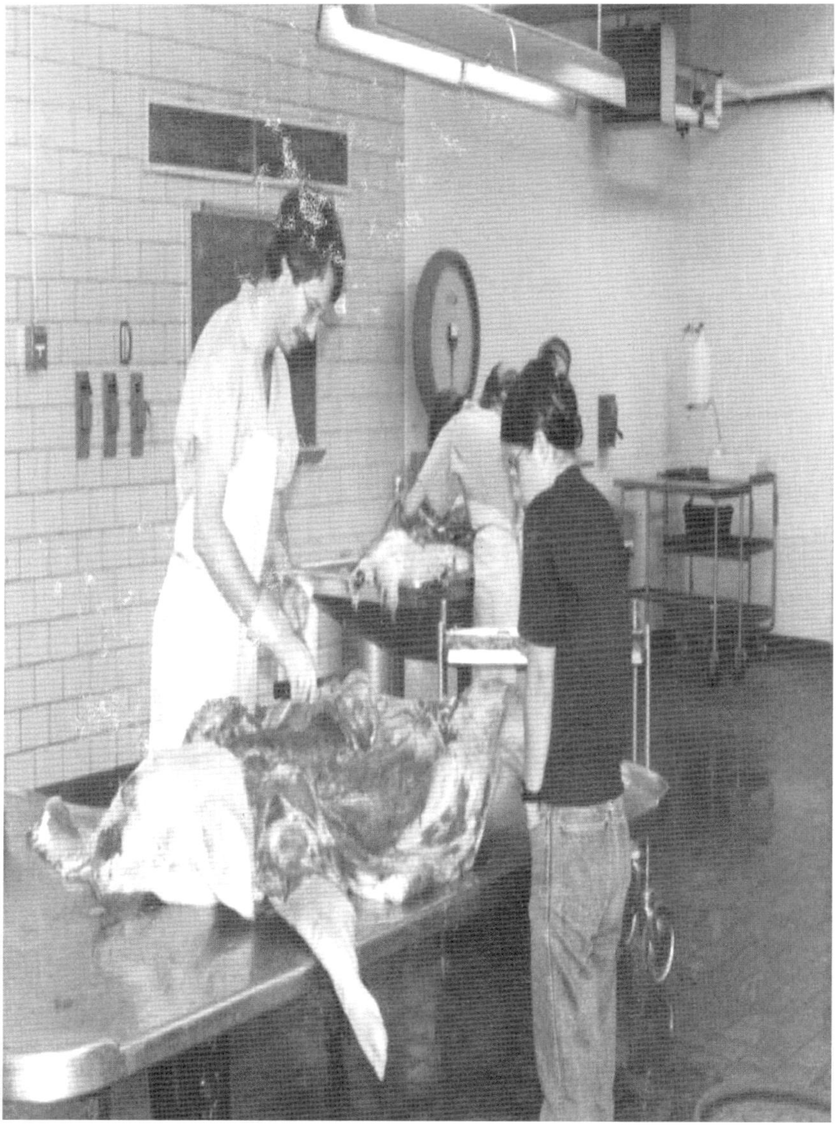

Picture 25. Dr. David Kenney, PA 1995, doing the necropsy with Dr. Lois Roth, Cornell 1979, doing the heavy looking on. Dr. Roth is one of the sharpest people I know. Superbly organized, willing and able. I am proud of her and consider her one of the best pathologists I know.

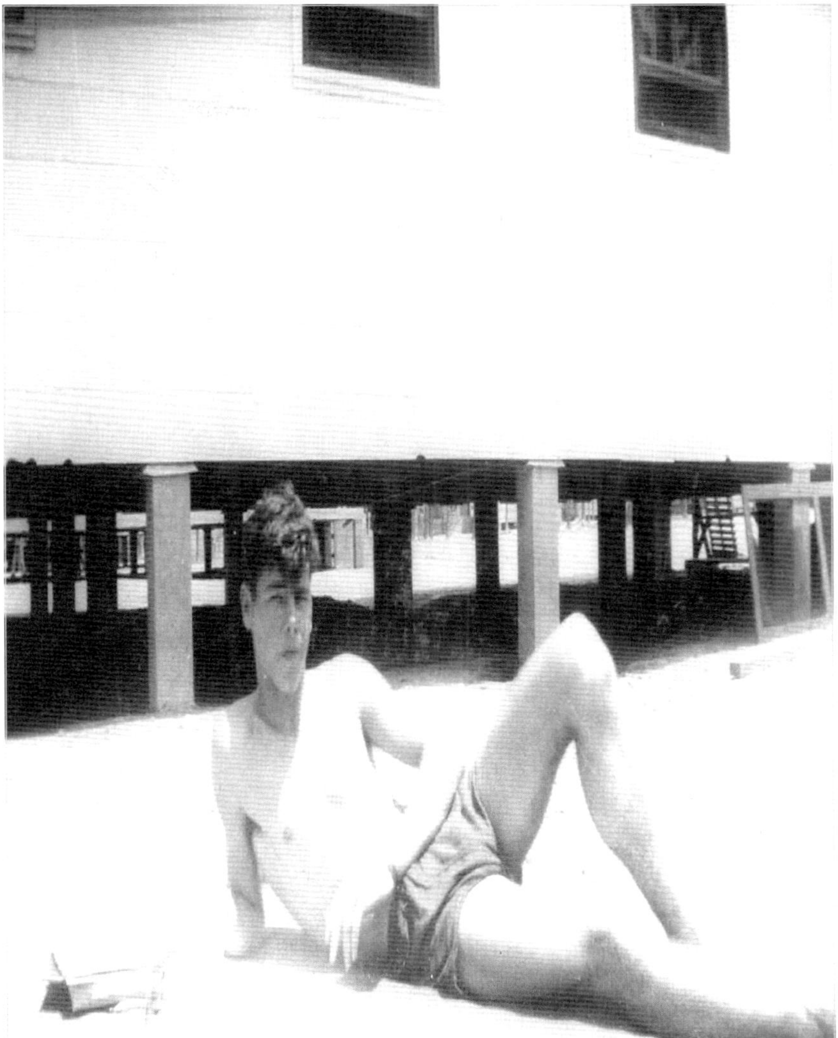

Picture 26. You asked for a ri val, but I don't know why, anyhow I found one when looking through a stack of photos from our past. Heck now I realize I had nothing to worry about.

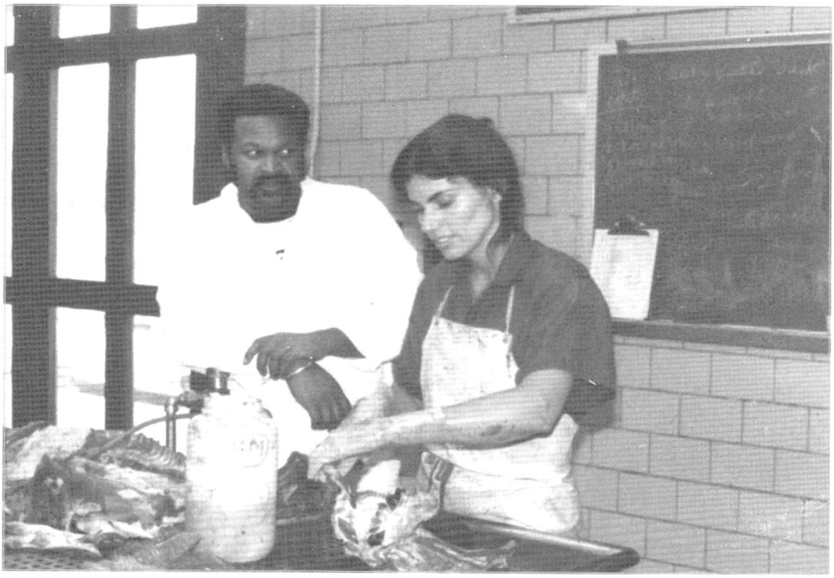

Picture 27. Dr. Melvin Chamblis is watching over a senior veterinary student do a necropsy. Dr. Melvin now runs a most successful veterinary technical school at Delhi, NY.

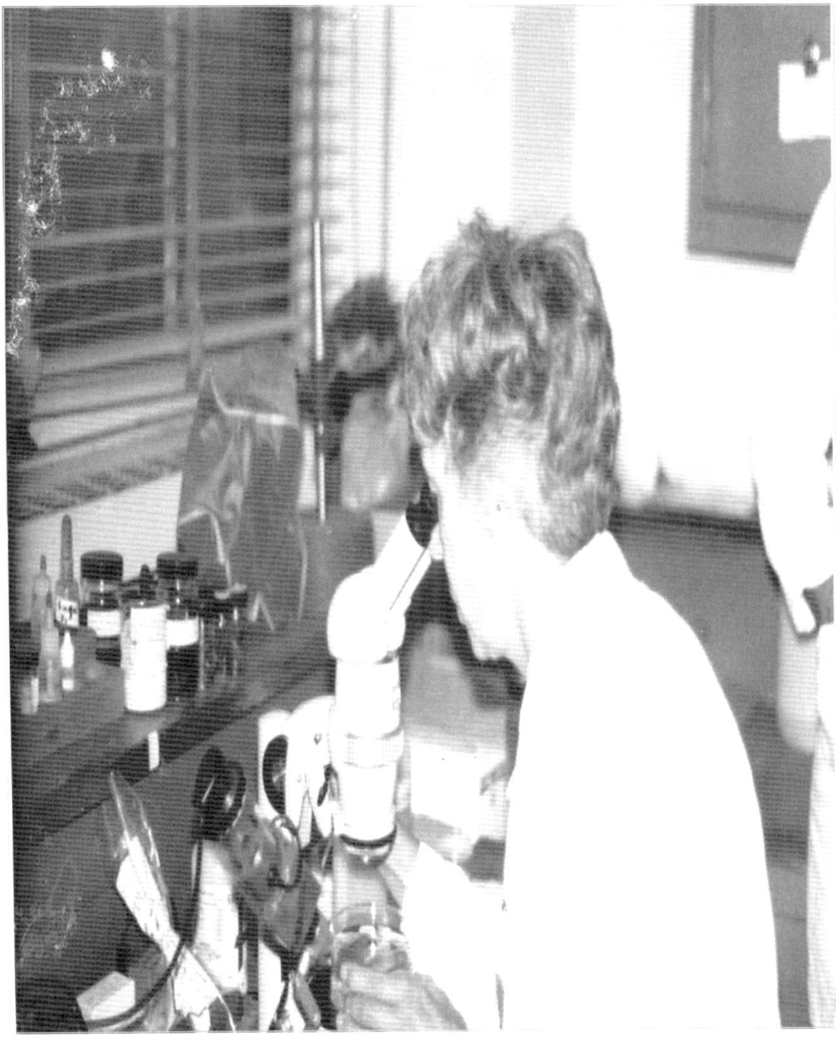

Picture 28. Many people have been helpful in the necropsy room, but one of the best and most capable has been Dr. Marion Georgi the wife of Dr. Jay Georgi, our eminent parasitologist. Marion can identify almost anything of significance we ask for help with. People like her make a fantastic difference between a fair lab and a great one.

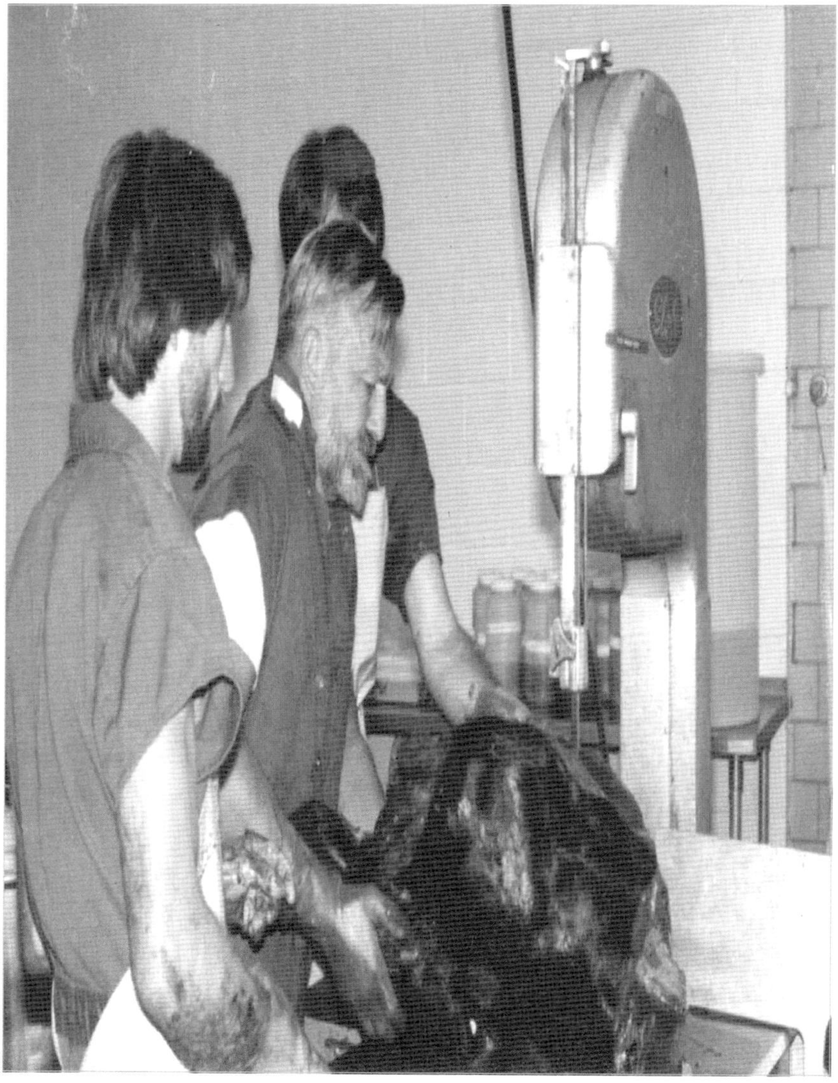

Picture 29. Dr. John Perdrizet, trying to help the old man, is one of the better clinicians we've helped to produce with an interest in necropsy answers. He even got a PhD with it.

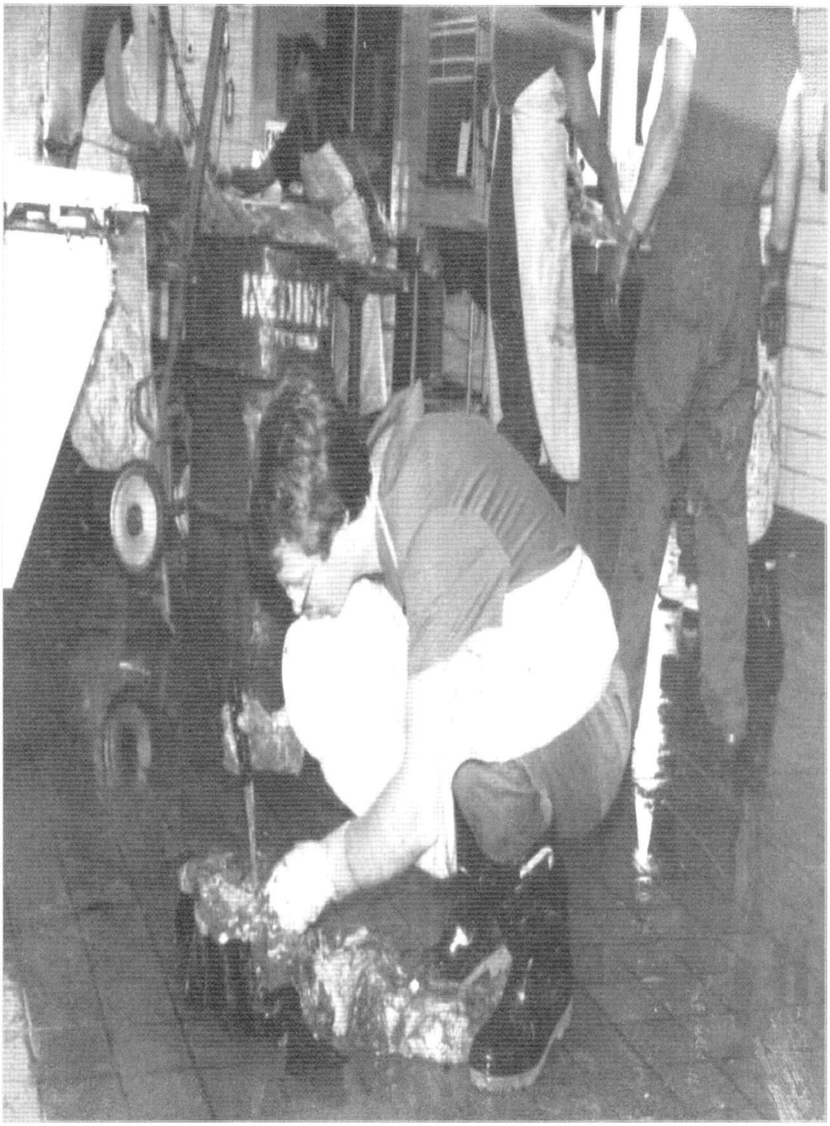

Picture 30. Another picture of Dr. David Kenney, a son of Dr. Robert Kenney, Okla 54. Boots, apron and gloves with barrels for carcass disposal and rendering. David received his VMD from PA and is a resident for pathology working toward a PhD here.

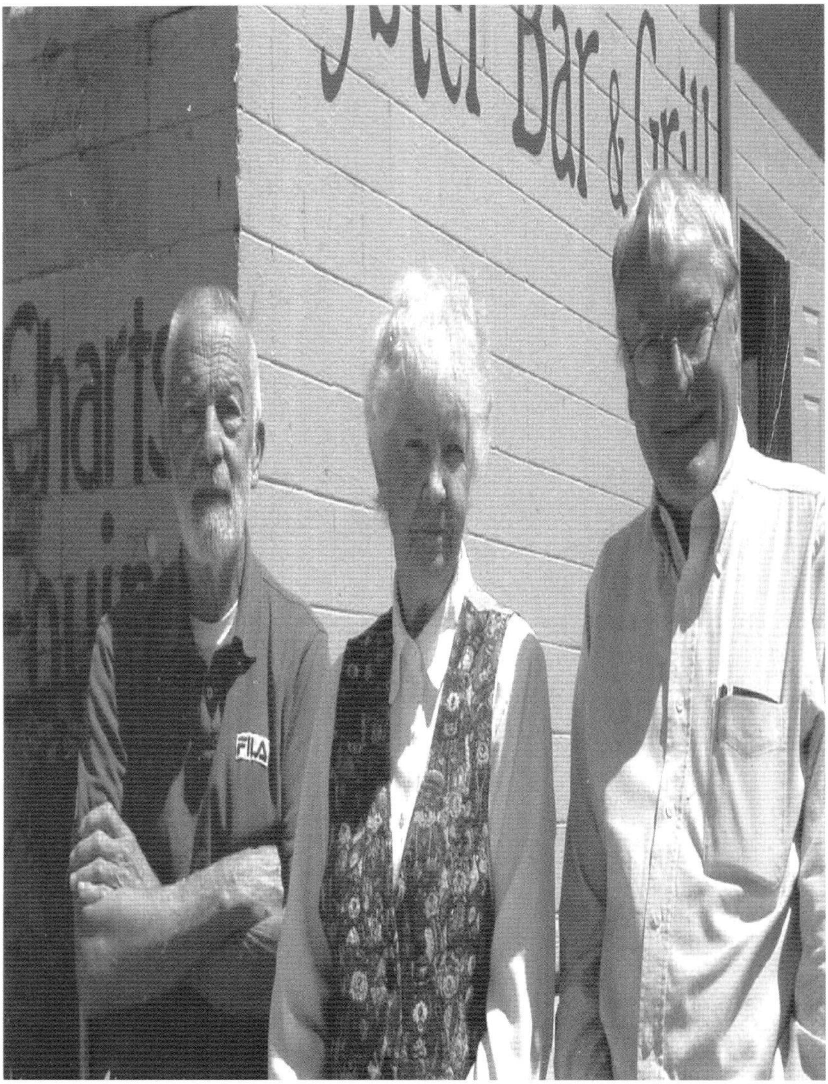

Picture 31. Marie King and I with Dr. Claus Buergelt who is now head of Pathology at Florida, Gainesville, meeting in Apalachicola, Florida in 2006.

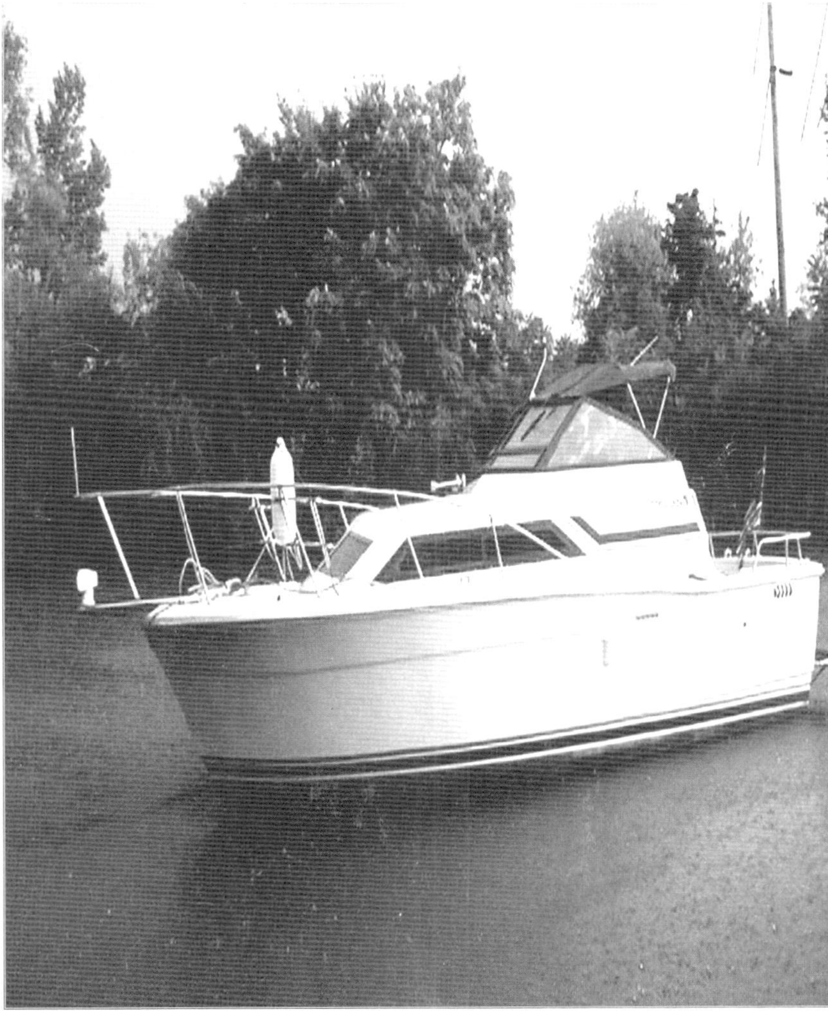

Picture 32. I admit it is a "STINK POT" running on gasoline, but that is better than one of us old codgers breaking our necks to handle the sails and roasting when there is no wind to pull (correct term) "Almost" along on Cayuga Lake in Ithaca, NY 1998.

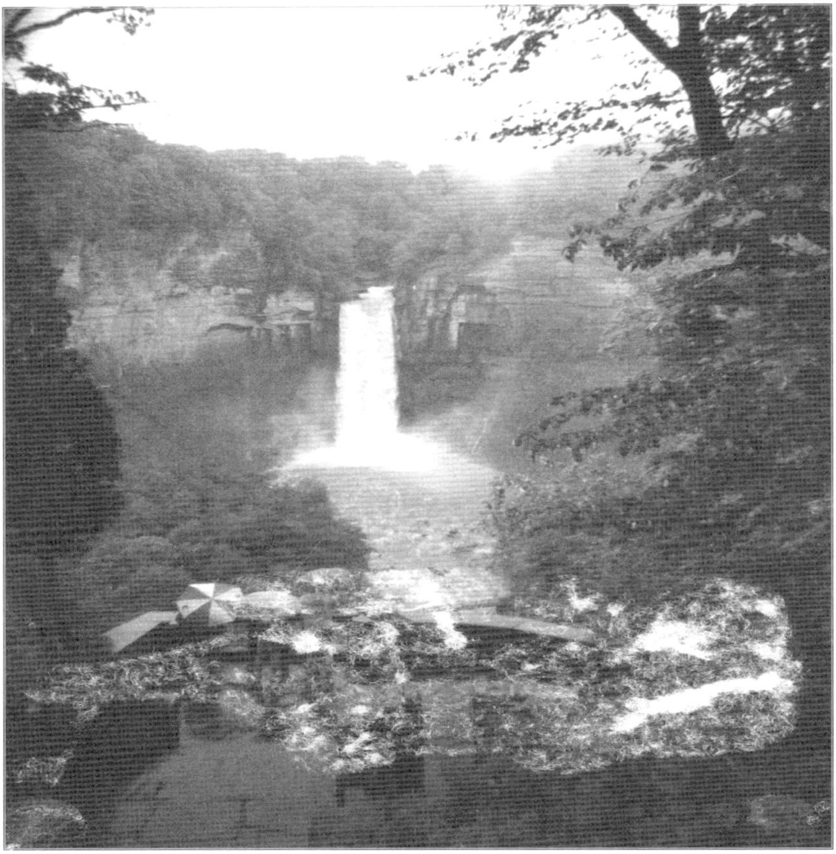

Picture 33. Taughannock Falls, partway up Cayuga Lake on the west side. At least it's possible a couple of real Indians did jump into them when Dad said NO, in 1006. The falls have not stopped crying in over 1,000 years.

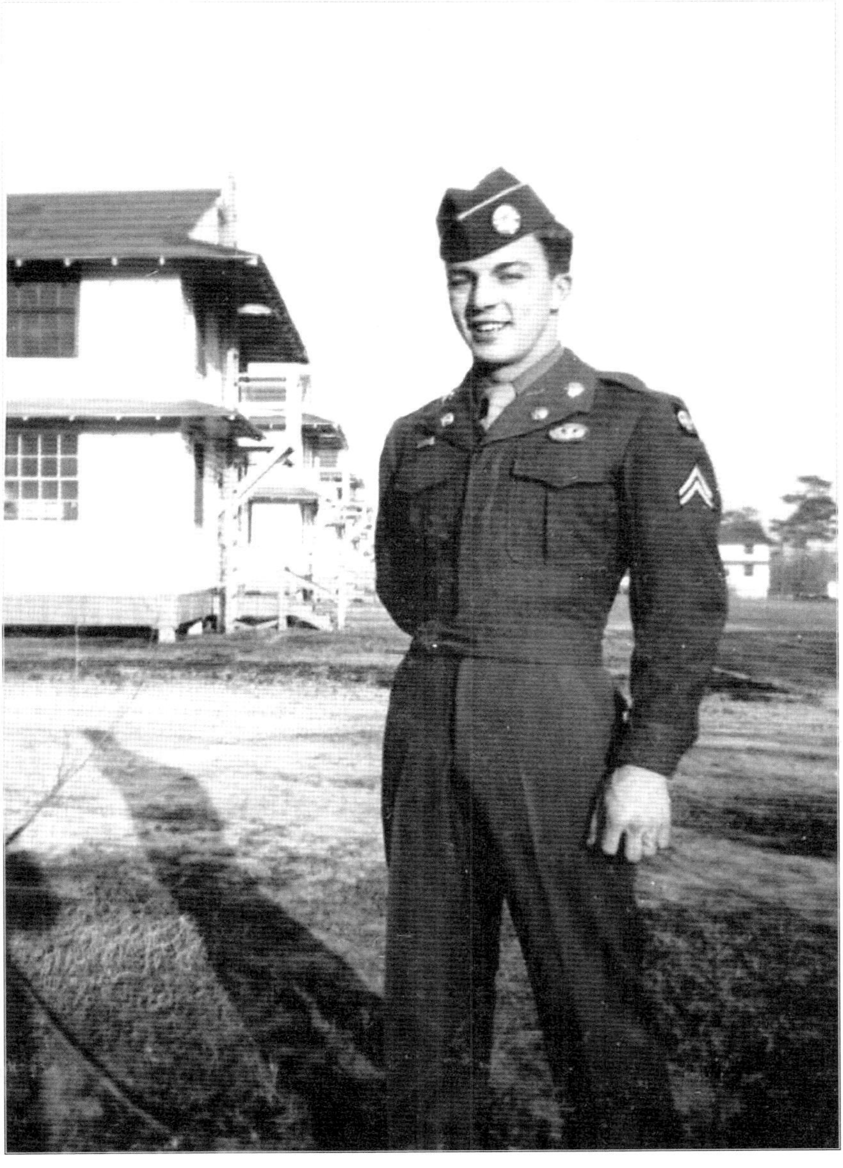

Picture 34. I actually made it to the old army grade of T4.

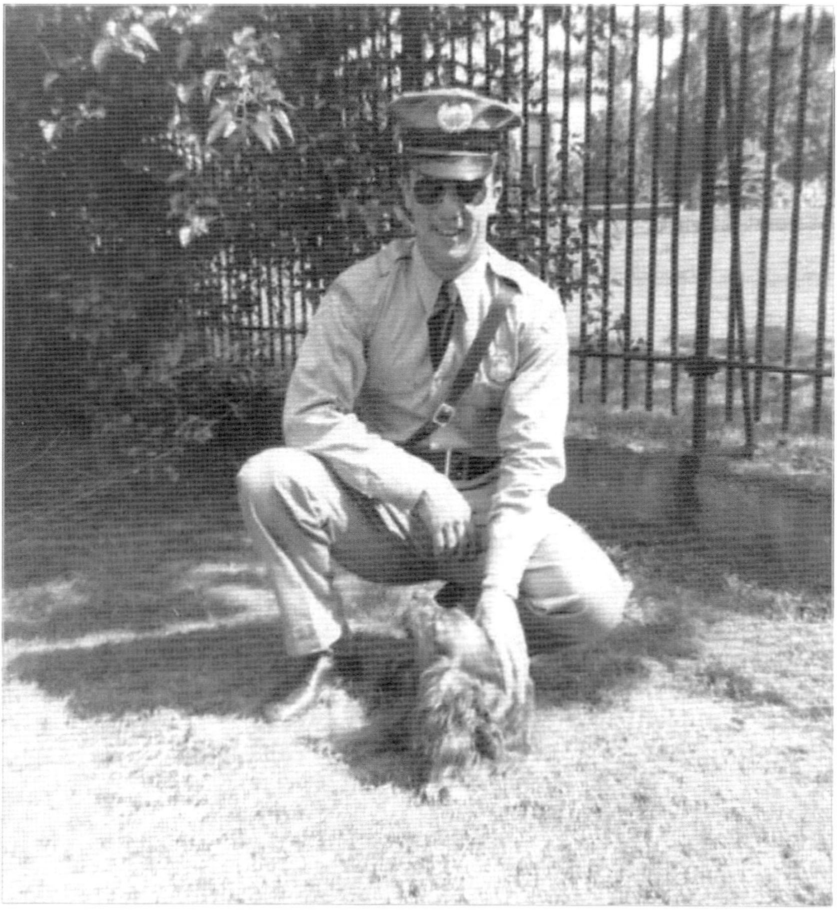

Picture 35. Now do I look like a horse track policeman? At Delaware Park, Wilmington, DE, 1948. Summer job.

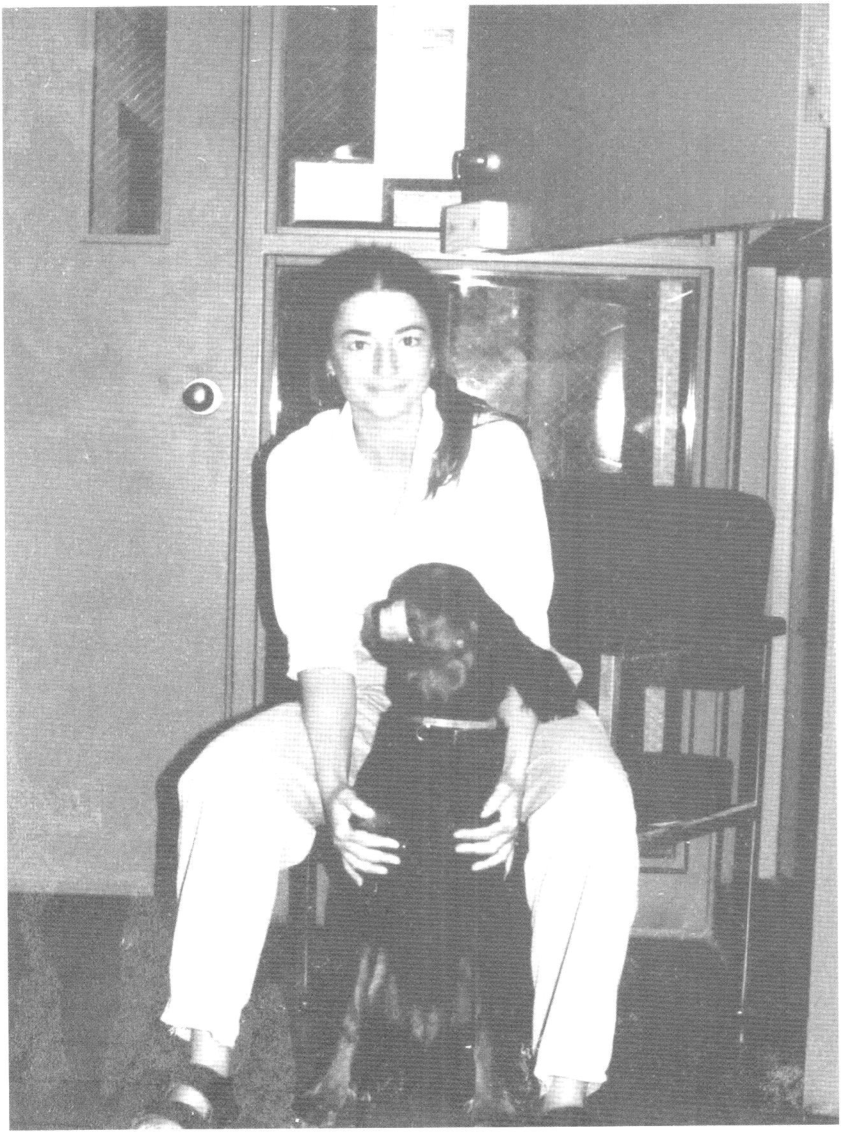

Picture 36. Dr. Linda Munson, one of Cornell's finest, now the head of Pathology in Davis, California 1985

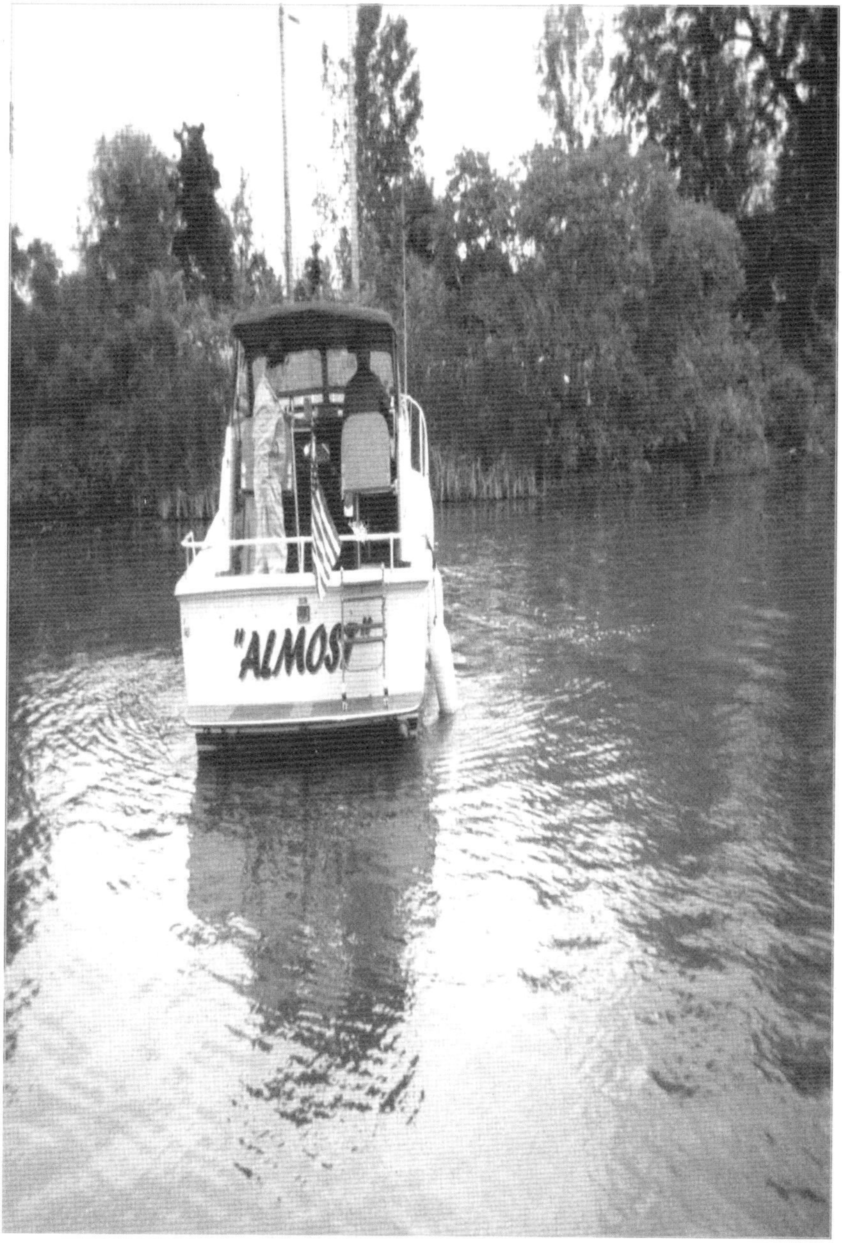

Picture 37. You've seen "Almost" in #29, but here she is trying to back into her boat slip, 2008

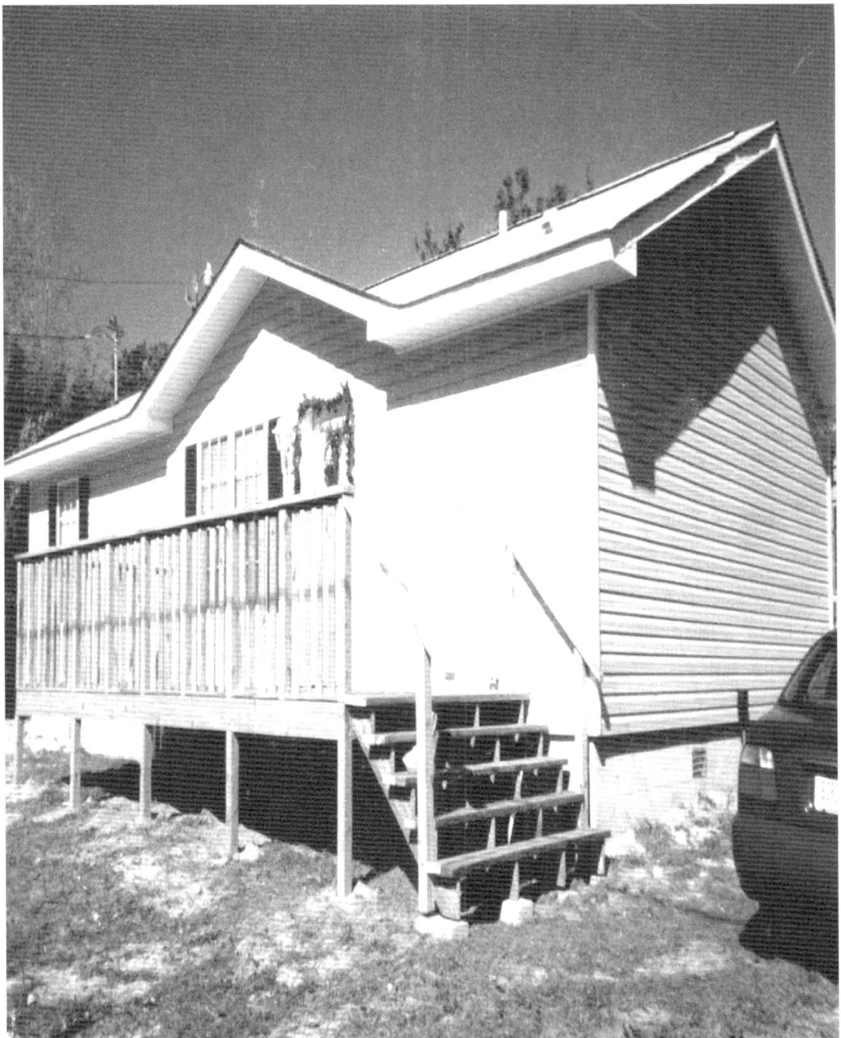

Picture 38. We finally retired and, like so many, moved to Florida for several months a year. We bought this modular home in Georgia, moved it to Florida on a beautiful river. Had it for a few years, but far too isolated. Son and I put a deck on front and back in 1999.

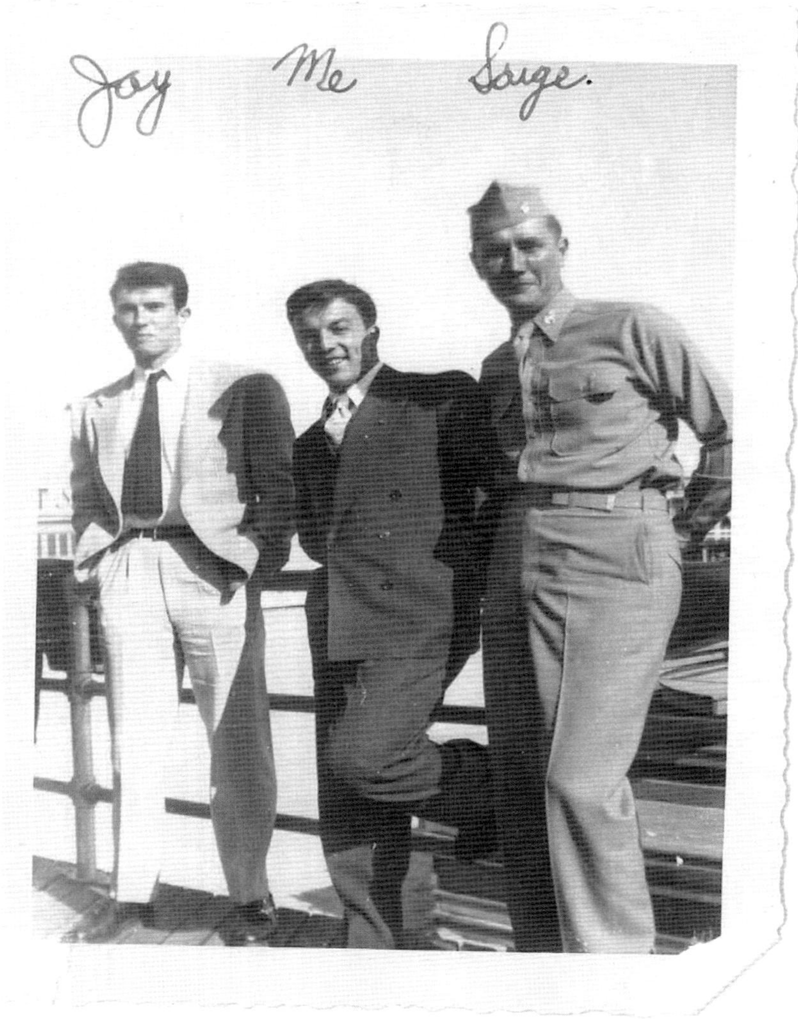

Picture 39. Went to Atlantic City boardwalk and all in 1949 with our best man Sarge Lindamood. Jay Clark, Myself, Marie, her aunt and Re's girlfriend. Gas was not too expensive in those days between the shore and Wilmington.

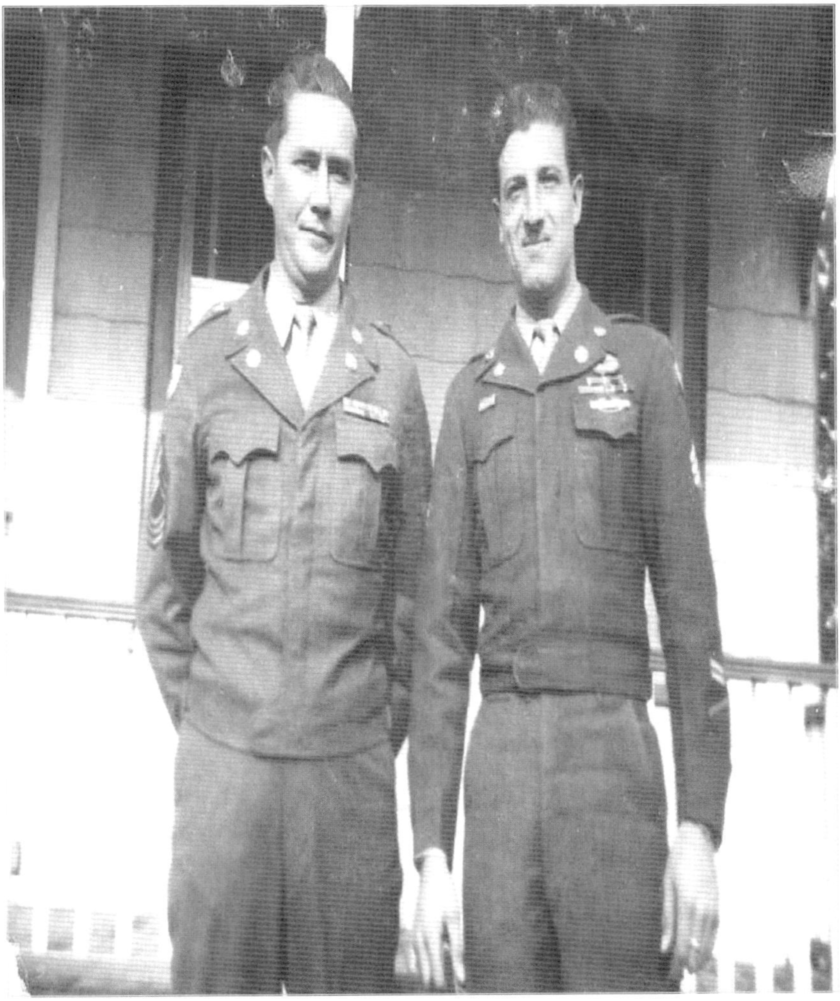

Picture 40. Sarge Lindamood was a warrant officer during the war, but took a demotion to Top Sergeant to stay in the Army. Mike Parendo jumped as a paratrooper into Bataan, Philippines in 1945. Both at our wedding in 1947.

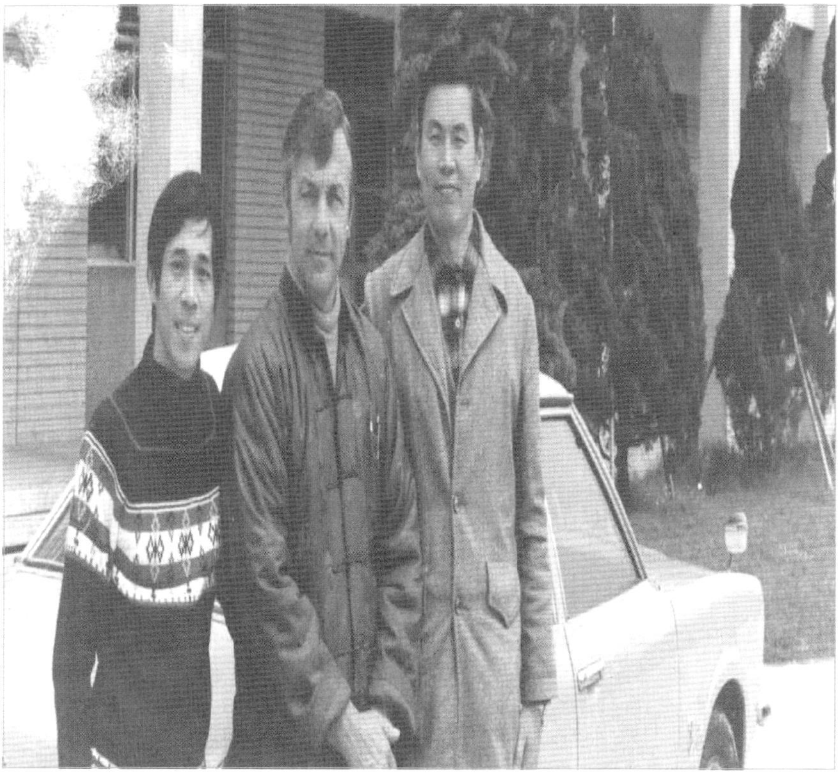

Picture 41. Marty Chang on my right and colleague on my left in Taiwan at P.R.I.T 1975

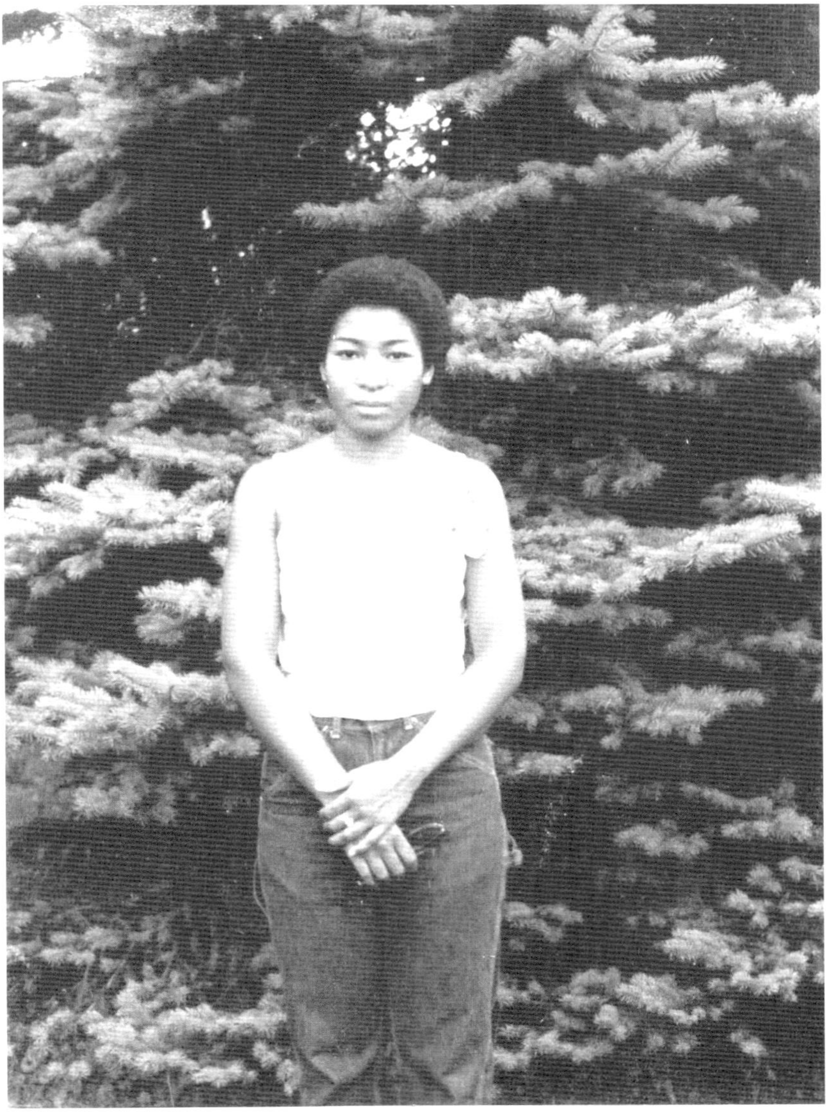

Picture 42. Dr. Theresa McCoy, one of the most interested and capable students I had while at Cornell, 1970.

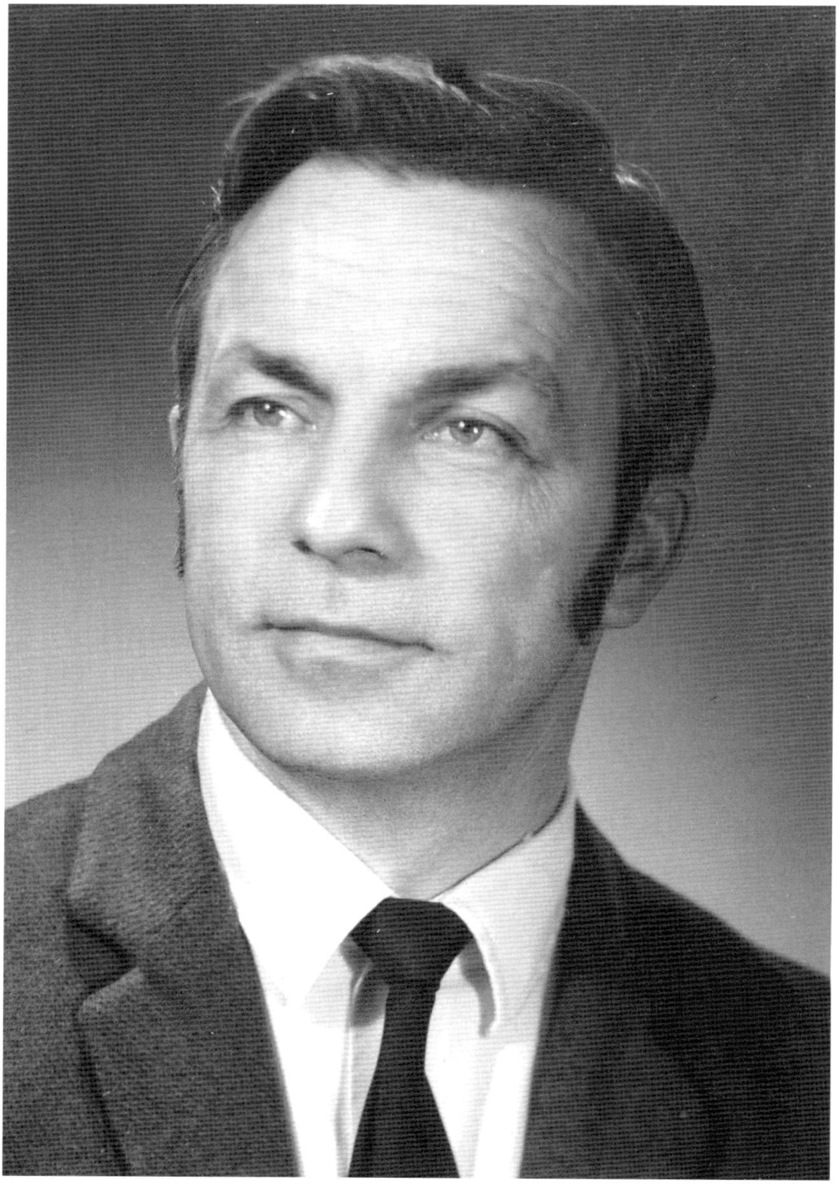

Picture 43. Graduation form Okla A&M, 1955

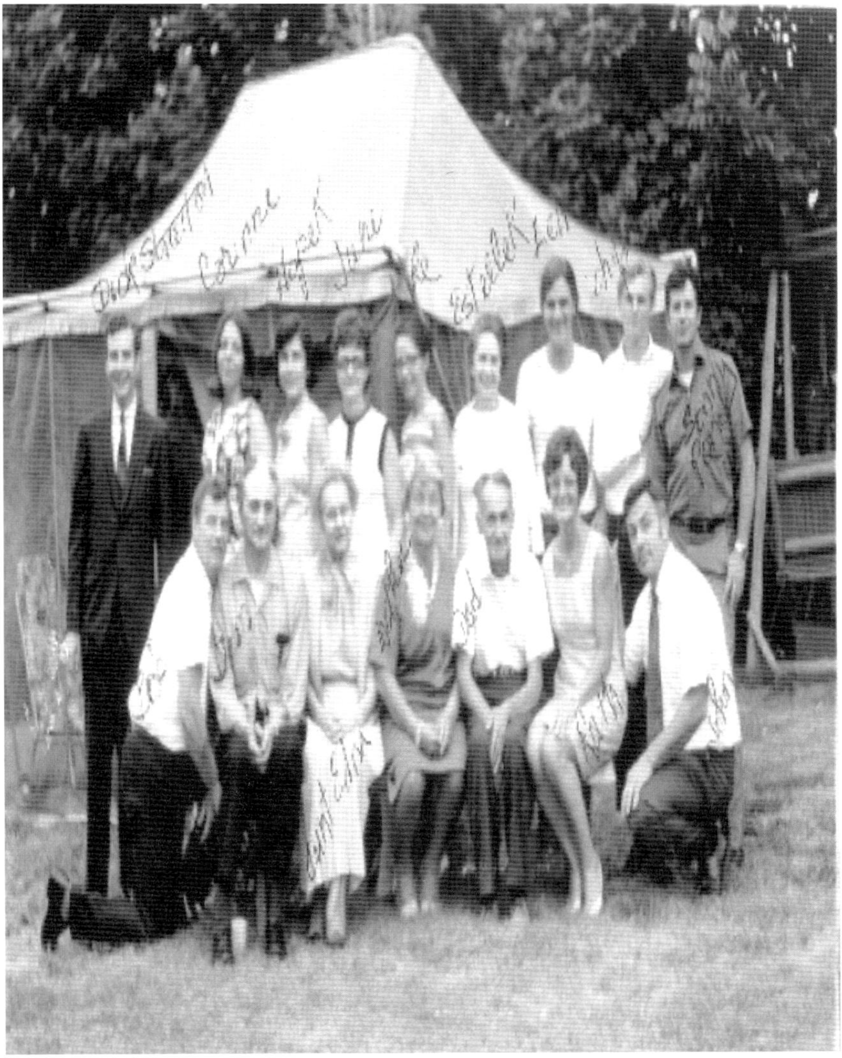

Picture 44. Almost my whole family in this picture at Judy's wedding 1975, I am on the right side with my hand on my sister Ruth's back. My Dad and Mom next to Ruth and Aunt Edna next to my Mom. Re is behind my Mom with my sister June next to her.

Legends of Veterinary Pathology
Interview with Dr. Donald Meuten

July 16 1996.

Refer to Davis-Thompson Homepage's Portal

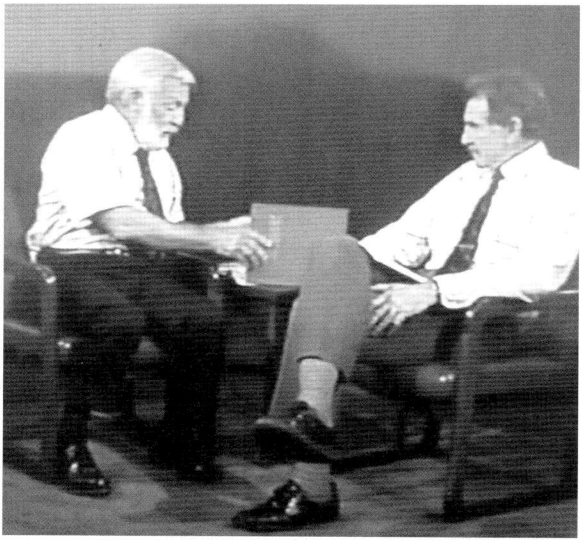

Meuten *Everyone will certainly recognize dr. King when the interview starts, but my name is Donald Meuten and I'm a former resident. Of dr. King's back at the Cornell days, presently I'm at North Carolina state university, and it was my good fortune to have worked with him for years. And I feel very lucky today and honored that they've asked me to interview you for apparently the first in the series for the Charles L.Davis foundation for the legends of veterinary pathology. And I think it's a very fitting beginning that they should have you up here first. So good day.*

King Thank you, Donald.

Meuten *how's it feel from your perspective to event invited you?*

King Uh, as a legend? Hi, I don't know where they ever got that idea about me. Cause I don't have that feeling about myself. I still enjoy what I do and I haven't left it. So. I'm still active. So that's great. And I'm glad for that opportunity, but I think you're a little bit, uh, too kind and all the limitations you've just given me by saying I've been that nice to some of you. Cause I think I treated all of you with a, with a tough, uh, I wanted to be proud of you. So I was tough and I expected a heck of a lot out of all of you. And in most instances, I got it. And I'm grateful for that.

Meuten *I think because you set that hurdle so high and you did, and you pushed us that, um, maybe when we were going through it, that there are times that we didn't enjoy it, but the fact that we survived, you made us a better.*

King Well, the alternative. You could have been truck drivers as I've told many. And they don't like that, but they should understand that, that I'm proud of it. And every pathology and all of the people have been in it before me who made it, uh, so darn good for all of us who followed them.

Meuten *Well, we're going to have the opportunity to talk a lot about it. Veterinary pathology. We hope. Uh, but tell us something about, uh, you and, uh, your beginning, because I think as part of the historical perspective, they're gonna want to know some of the personal sides of dr. King. So tell us something about the roots.*

King Uh, I was born a long time ago. That starts way back. And I remember during a depression, eaten beans were sugar and I loved it. And I also remember going to Mrs. Crow's home in Massachusetts with my, my younger sister two years old. And I was. And, uh, we lived in this home and we had actual flour sacks with holes for our neck and our two arms. And I loved it. Uh, and I'm surprised I loved it. And I don't remember anything bad about it because we had rice three times a day and I still love rice. But then at that voice, I went to a boy's school. Cause my parents went to splits. And my three sisters went with aunts, aunts, and I didn't know who to go to, or they didn't know where to put me. So I went to a boys' school for seven years and I remember crying the first night. And, uh, but at that boy's school, I learned something about the animals. Cause we had cows and pigs and chickens. It ended up, I stayed there for 10 years.

Meuten *How old were you when you went there?*

King Seven. And I stayed there for 10 years, maybe 11. I quite remember. And, uh, until I joined the army and that was a fantastic experience, the army, it was his first time. I was way away, away from home, or away from any, anything. And I had a great time in the army for four years, but at that boys' school, there was a veterinarian who came down from, uh, Wellesley or Natick, Massachusetts, who was our veterinarian. And he ended up writing a book called the horse doctor. And I was the one who was, uh, never remember the boys' school, went up to the eighth grade, but I didn't even have a home to, to go to when I was, uh, got ready to go to high school. So I stayed at that school. And went to high school, walked every morning, a couple of miles to get the school bus. I had typed the first class and my hands wouldn't think out. Until 10 in the morning. So, of course, I didn't pass a typing course, but I had a good memory in those days in my, I guess it's okay. Now I don't forget too much, especially the things I'm trying to teach. Well, maybe I do. And nobody's, everybody's too kind to tell me I've forgotten. I don't know. And that was all a pretty good experience with that old-time veterinarian. And he taught us or taught me such things as a. He saved all of his, his, uh, cigar stubs.

And he used those to keep the insects off of the, uh, his row, his wife's rose bushes. And that was pretty neat. And then when I finally learned about nicotine sulfate is in vet school. Another thing, another little thing, uh, clicked forever in my mind under those conditions.

Meuten *What was his name again? Lisa?*

King It began with an H, but I'll be darned if I can wasn't Harriet, but I can't remember the name right now, but I just remember Hirsch Hirsch something, but I don't know. He went to Harvard. Then, when Harvard had a veterinary school in, uh, 1907 or something like that. Goodman. I didn't realize they had a vet school. They had one of the first ones, but it didn't last very long. And then he also, uh, he had something to do with Middlesex. That was a, a school or some veterinarians still alive, who probably went there, a net that faded out early. So here just after the war. Yeah.

He's the one that got you interested in veterinary medicine and animals. Cause I took care of all the cows that needed. He would tell me what to do. I didn't know what I was doing. I was a fault on my, in my youth. I, at that boy's school, I was, they didn't tell you. How much milk this cow gave, or how much fertilizer you put on his field, or how many bushels of potatoes, uh, kids, uh, would have to pick, uh, from this, this field is so much acreage. I had no idea about that. And I think that was a mistake, but it was 80 boys at that school and one adult man who taught everything. So he couldn't do everything. And I. To this day, I idolize him, but that's okay. That's what started me. And I always wanted to be a veterinarian. The daughters of the American revolution took care of the school a lot on the side. They gave us a few bucks and every winter they gave us a mitten that they had knitted for us and stuff like that. Cause I had gone to high school with. With rubber boots. Cause I couldn't walk in the snow with a regular night. I have to go through school, rubber boots, and up to my knees. And uh, so I didn't, we didn't learn anything about women in those days.

Meuten *Haven't learned a lot since either I was gonna comment that explained some of the roots as well of you.*

King So we didn't know anything about the women and the rubber boots. I don't think that endeared me to any of the high school kids, but uh, I had a good time there too. I enjoy it.

Meuten *As the army would be plush after that, the beginning?*

King it was, and they paid me to be in the army. You know, I got $50. Uh, I became a paratrooper there and I had a fabulous time with my extra 50 bucks. I sent it to my mother and a good, yeah. I enjoyed the army too.

Meuten *And then when you finish the army, Then it was undergrad or..*

King I'm married. I met my wife. She was in the, uh, Marie. She was in Wilmington, Delaware, and she was in Hawaii YWCA. And she came down to Aberdeen proving grounds every once a week with the gals, from the, uh, YWCA from Wilmington. And I met her there. And I remember the first thing I said, dance ma'am and she didn't like me. Well, that was okay. I, my shiny boots and my patch and my cocky hat, probably my cocky attitude, I guess I swept her off her feet and that was in 1947. I just returned from Germany and, uh, we got married in November and that was very good.

Meuten *So your 50th anniversary will be next year?*

King Yes.

Meuten *it's like your dad gets anything big plan for,*

King No, we're going to be, we're going to be overseas. Uh, I guess, no, in December we won't be now. We'll be back from, uh, South America then by next June. No, nothing planned. I'm not sure I want anything. Maybe we'll buy a big new boat by then, but yeah. We'll see, I'll still be working so good. Don't want to retire too early. Cause as soon as you retired too early, you cannot be a bone of contention to anybody.

Meuten *I can't imagine you ever retiring, not entirely. And I know I'll have to adjust to it at some point. I can't call you up and ask you about things, but I can't ever imagine it will happen.*

King Hey, a bill at school says, if you care for Cornell, you won't retire. Unless you want to die in a saddle because it'll probably kill you to continue the political fighting and all that kind of stuff. While I, I stay out of some of it. Cause I try to hide in the necropsy room. As you know,

Meuten *you don't back down from many battles though.*

King No, but I don't leave the D Cropsey room to battle very often. So I'm pretty lucky in that job too. Let's see. Uh, after we, yeah, we got married a year later. I had. I had to have my mother's permission cause I wasn't 21, but, uh, she was over 18. She was 20 also. So, um, she didn't have to have permission and that was kind of a put down for me, you know? Cause here I have a pretty big strapping army guy. Yeah. Paratrooper, not just army. I mean the army, those guys walked, we jumped, I stand corrected. No. I said cocky little devil into, I enjoyed that.

Meuten *And then it's undergrad?*

King Yes. We went to university of Delaware. I wrote to Oklahoma and trying to get, all the vet schools. They wouldn't take me in Cornell or Penn because they had a quota from Delaware and New Jersey that hurt my pride a little bit, but I flunked high school. Well, I didn't flunk it. I didn't finish it too well because, uh, yeah. I never did homework, never, and I'm not proud of it, but there are several courses that gave me a hard time that I just didn't study. So when I got in the army and wanted to go to vet school, cause I knew I wanted to go to vet school. Uh, I had to take all these army qualification tests and I did pretty well. And they said, well, first you should be a lawyer. And that explains why that explains why I'll argue with. Yeah, Peter at the gate, you know, uh, and then the second thing you probably are best aptitude as far as veterinary medicine. Hmm. So that was, that was neat. And, uh, we got a GI bill for $105 a month cause I was married and I was in the army for four years and I got 48 months of school, but I always would, uh, enroll about six weeks late. And so I didn't get my, uh, My $105 for the first six weeks, but that gave me an extra six weeks. So I went all through school, undergraduate and vet school under the GI bill. And that was a fabulous opportunity that I took advantage of. And, and, uh, we went both to university of Delaware for undergraduate, excuse me. And, uh, Then we went to Oklahoma and M now Oklahoma state university, the education there was fantastic. You could do anything you wanted. There was no strings attached. We didn't have much faculty. So that means, uh, you did a lot at the veterinary school on a practical basis. And. That just wasn't enough faculty to do it, but they were dedicated teachers. And gee, I had a great time with all of them. Couple of them gave me heck one of them even gave me a, a D in clinic attitude. Yes. Cocky attitude. And I don't know where he got that from, but I remember doing things like, uh, Walking the needle off the bodies of the vertebra and going into the aorta, injecting the radiopaque material and see where, how my surgery on AOTA worked or on the femoral artery or some vessel. And it worked great. And, uh, but because I didn't have his permission to use his radiograph, uh, the X Ray machines or the, what do they call them? The X Ray machines. Anyhow. Yeah. So, uh, to use those things. He gave me a D and also because, I mean, I knew how to do it. He had taught me well, and, but just supposed to have permission, I didn't use it. So he gave me a D and afterwards I found out why did you give me a D I says, you've said, good things about me. You would recommend me to any veterinarian who wanted a good, energetic young man to do something, but you gave me a DCE as well. Your attitude. You're too cocky. I didn't appreciate that, Dan. And I'm not sure. I appreciate even now, because I was willing to do something. If the other kids didn't want to do it, I'll do it.

Meuten *Well, he think you've nailed since those days?*

King Uh, no. Cause early days, not really pan Sierra, he went back to Oklahoma and he was there all the time and I'd write him letter and I'd tell him to tell that professor. So and so. I'd probably cussed a nose. A nose times probably told him to tell him off, but maybe I should have listened because you know, who knows I could have been president of Cornell or North Carolina or someplace like that. If I'd kept my returned mouth shut. But at that boy school, that old man who taught us, he was pop Sanford. He said, would you stop getting the last word? Yes, sir. Didn't you hear me? Yes, sir. And that started it. That started it, but I was about nine years old when he said that. I remember it so well, because he did get up tight with me for doing that. Yes, sir. No, sir. And worse yet today is yes. Ma'am and no ma'am. Do you realize the number of women who hate that in ma'am stuff? But if I didn't say yes ma'am and no ma'am to somebody, I wouldn't get any dessert. So I had 10 years training in it. It's sunk in after awhile. I want dessert. Yes. Ma'am no ma'am yes, sir. No, sir. Not going to change that. The pattern, uh, Oh, things are changing today and maybe I better change.

Meuten *That's what I want to get into at some point is some of the changes, but let's finish some of the background. Okay. Uh, how many students in your, that class and any classmates that we should know about?*

King Uh, we graduated with 32, one girl, uh, not one too many young ladies. If you ever listened to this, we should have more of you, uh,

Meuten *more than one or more than what we have today.*

King Uh, well this is kind of political, so probably we will continue that. We'll drop that line. Yeah, we'll drop that line. Uh, no, actually the women are just as good as the men and they'll do just as fine as all I'm in there. They're nice to, to teach. One reason is they do smell better and they just smell good. And then when you hear a little click click down the hall, you have to wait until they go by your door to see who's making it literally clickety click. I've always appreciated that, but now I can't make any comments on that, you know, uh, gotta be really careful now.

Meuten *Had any troubles?*

King Uh, twice I've been to the Dean I've been to, well, I've been to my chairman. I've been to the Dean and I've been to the president of the university. But, uh, in talking about such things as uni, lateral shut down and atrophy of the kidney, for instance, you know, when you. Have to tie off or if accidentally, for instance, tie off the . Yeah. Tell us that story. Uh, I'm may to here. Uh, well, you know, when you're, uh, you're a prisoner and you're captured and somebody, they want the inflammation out of you and they're gonna punish you or torture you and how they do that is they tie off your, uh, we week. Well, I use the other word and, uh, That went in the letter to the president that I was being, uh, I don't know, well vulgar or something. Well, actually that did come up that it was being vulgar. And, but it's a good thing because in cats where it's so common, they'll get calculi in the penile urethra. And, uh, it'll block, both kidneys, one will shrink and one will stay normal and stuff like that. Everybody calls it hypoplasia but that kidney was normal beforehand. And the reason I know is several veterinarians said, that's what we, what we, uh, the cat was blocked and we washed him out and we opened his belly. His kidneys were good, everything was good. But now here he is six months later and look one kidney, small ones big. That was the first clue. I mean, veterinarian said it. But I needed that proof to say that it wasn't hypoplasia cause how many times you see hypoplasia and little and young animals? Uh, not very often,

Meuten *Especially in one side.*

King Yeah. So anyhow, so this is something different. And then when I proceeded to tell everybody that everybody usually laughs and giggles, unless they have an ax to grind with you for some reason, my cocky attitude. So, uh, Then they, somebody said, well, why did you use that example? I said, Hey, it's a good one. And anyhow, I thought I was teaching in a veterinary school, not Sunday school. Well, that went to the top, but they understood it. And, uh, how did he get unilateral renal shut down from that? God said. So don't you realize you don't know why any of your animals die because I'll bet you, whatever, any animal you autopsy, you've seen another animal that had. More wrong with him than that. And you had to kill the other one and this one died. So that animal is just a wimp. You know, he died with these admins full of something, some disease and pestilence, and he died with it, but others have worse and you had to kill him. So there's no good explanation for a good general diagnostic pathologist to explain death recently, all these cows we had that school. Uh, 38 of them. And, uh, nine of them died including one great big Angus bull. I was glad died because he challenged me when I got in into pen with him. I didn't even know he was sick, but he kind of put his head down, was going to tell me to get out of that pen. Well, I got out, but this is recent. Yeah. About three months ago. Hmm. Anyhow, I got out of the pen. So what, so why would that a nine of them died? All with diarrhea. I beg your pardon. None of them would diarrhea, but they died suddenly we would die. So suddenly we thought of poisoning, uh, except the two of the nine had lesions one, a little North Carolina graduate found them first, actually Elizabeth Malden. Yeah. And that was pretty neat because you know, she's taught by you. And probably like us in some to look for everything. And she found these things in the esophagus and they didn't find anything in the gut until I got there, but that makes me, Hey, this job security for me. I want to teach them everything. Cause I wouldn't have a job if they knew all that. So anyhow, she found it and they, we isolated the virus and uh, on FAA and they asked her he got the virus, but they also found it immunohistochemistry and a F a.

Meuten *Hm, what is it?*

King BVD. Oh, but no diarrhea. Hmm. Pirate and patchy lesions. When you show yes. When I showed up, they had some, but come on these, these young people, it's not an easy job because everybody said poisoning, but she found those esophageal lesions and then Fox get in on the act and do Bovie and all of our hot shots at school or good naked in, on the act. And yeah, it's BBD. But why no diarrhea. So why do animals die with bovine virus? Diarrhea that gets tricky. If they don't have diarrhea. Now I've seen a lot of them die with diarrhea and no lesions, but then you say, Oh yeah, electrolyte imbalance. And they died, but that gets tricky. Anyhow, that was nice. So we don't know all the answers to everything and.

Meuten *And that's where we started unilateral renal shutdown. I got to chime in with one thing in there that, that I know that story has gotten you in trouble. And, uh, you on the road with your show and tell buckets and a black box and so forth when he came to Carolina, um, you told that story on the unilateral renal shutdown, and there are two people out in the audience that day one was my grad student. Uh, and I won't use the names, but she preferred to work. Uh, in the, uh, ultra structural lab, much less the gross necropsy floor, uh, but for the boards and other reasons she wanted to hear you. And I. I told her, I said, well, I want to make sure you hear this professor of mine. And then when you decided to tell the story and you chose whose penis was going to be tied off, you pointed to her husband and then went through all the details and all the explanations. And I thought Kathy was going to, well, there's part of the name. I thought she was going to come up out of the chair at some point in that story. And I know it's gotten you in trouble over the years.*

King Yeah, that's kinda, that's kind of a backlash, I guess a little bit. Yeah. Maybe. And we actually deserve it because we have no right to be crude and mean to anybody, but in a veterinary school, you should. I mean, I think we should be allowed a little bit like that.

Meuten *And if you whack your nail or finger was something you ought to be able to cuss a little bit. And that's the only reason I bet she'll always remember unilateral rentals shut down.*

King I hope so.

Meuten *Yeah, because it's real, the impact of that story helps.*

King Yeah. And, uh, but you can't, you can't be free anymore to say what you want in some of the classes, because the kids are a little more sensitive and they can take advantage of it. If you're their friend or you were their friend or something, if they want to, uh, They can take advantage of it. And, and they'll say, well, you took advantage of us for, you know, 400 years as men and maybe a turnabouts a little bit it's fair play, but when it falls on me, I don't, I didn't appreciate it. I don't appreciate it.

Meuten *You want to talk a little bit about how the classroom has changed over the years?*

King Uh, well, the women are more dedicated than most men. Hm, I think, and the women are sorry, certainly just as smart or maybe they're no smarter, but they're not as driven by their hormones, I guess as men are because men are always looking for something a little exciting, a little different, and women are, are not quite that blatant, but that's not veteran in medicine. So I think that's just school. Our curriculum is changing. And it's going to case based learning. And a lot of the two tours are not veterinarians. And I find that as a kind of a shame because the students don't have. The veterinary students do not have veterinarians as role models, good ones or bad ones, but at least you ask a veterinarian, something on dogs or cats or cows or horses, they will give you something in a research type PhD fellow. He's there the best citizens in the world, the best husbands, the best, uh, whatever in the world, the best teachers on the CNB or the T and B cells, uh, something like that. They're they know that very detailed. But I'm not sure our veterinary students should have so much of that even available to them because these, these fellows women, they will teach that because that's what they know best. And some of our faculty, you know, in some departments, uh, we, we have some in different areas and they're, they're, they're not veterinarians. And so they'll not be teaching veterinary subjects. And when they get graduate students, The biggest, almost the biggest gripe to me is that they, they don't get, DVMs just a simple young DVM, 23 or four years old to teach, to get a PhD in their subject. And, and, uh, and why, because it costs too much to. The veterinarian already has to pay his, uh, his school loans off, whereas a master's degree in biological science and on some other campus, you know, you don't have to pay him so much cause he didn't owe so much money like the veterinarians veterinary students. So that's a fault for the thing, but maybe it's not a fault. And um, I'm holding my final opinion on it because when a Cornell went to full time, um, Students, I mean all year students with the seniors, I guess we wanted warm bodies and sped it. Instead of paying summer cruise, we went to warm bodies. And so we use seniors all year round. So now this, and I knew everybody was going to complain about it because the students who are going to be in school, the seniors all year, and the faculty is going to be uptight because you don't get a break from students for a little bit of time. I know Texas has always done it all year or something like that. Or maybe some schools have,

Meuten *it's just senior year, just a senior?*

King Yes. And I knew everybody was gonna really hate it. I knew they were all going to gripe and moan because of this. And the outcome is I haven't heard one gripe from anybody, the students, the faculty. Or myself, for instance, I think it's fabulous. Instead of having four students or five each rotation, we only have three because they have to divide up their year from, for the 80 students. And, uh, the students can leave town anytime they want to, you know, for their externship blocks, you know, stuff like that. I haven't heard anybody gripe and we know every for every two weeks we're going to get three new students and you can plan on that and it's not bad. So if I was so wrong there on such a major change in, uh, academia, maybe I'm wrong in this other way too. I don't think I am because I don't think I am, but who's to say I'm not because. As an old, older, uh, instructor, gee whiz, I think I've got lots to offer them, but you don't see them. And therefore, uh, and other teachers, great teachers have the same kind of, uh, uh, uh, feeling that something's missing for these young people in these case studies,

Meuten *Have they sought you out to help solve some of these? Cause that's how they theoretically get exposed to these people.*

King Um, maybe that's one reason. I'm a little disheartened. They haven't done it as much as I think they should have. And therefore, maybe, maybe I'm I'm tender and, uh, my feelings are hurt or something like that. So maybe that's a fault, but I've heard it from too many others who have the same opinion and who aren't as old as I am. So you have to give them a break and you can't condemn you can't. Kill the messenger shoot the messenger. And that's what these young people are. They're the ones who are bringing, you know, the fact that they don't, they don't know something. You can't shoot him for not knowing it cause they probably didn't teach him. But I honestly don't know. So I just, the proof of the pudding, it. In a, when they get out and when they have to compete with everybody else, when they come into postmortem room, you know, you know that large animal that they do, cows, they do horses, but large animal anatomy is only an elective. Now at school, they don't even have a peristaltic course. So if I ask them, well, name the, uh, what's the tongue worm, what's your soft GL worm. Uh, they don't have a clue and I feel that is wrong and they'll never have opportunity to. To speak up. Maybe I have been like, I treat some of them like adults, like you residents. I would treat you like adults and give you heck if you miss something and constantly give you heck, and this is how

I like to teach when you're, when you're in school. Uh, I don't let you make a final decision. If you're a student on anything, I check everything you do. I think I should. I think some schools don't do that. They have the resident, I'm talking about a residence, I guess, as a resident, you go out to the postmortem room and, uh, if you need help call me, I'll come out and look. Well, that's kind of bologna in the sense that how do you know you need help or you don't need help that list of things I gave you. A lot of those things are, are, um, If you've never known it, you'll never think to look, uh, if you do a complete post, you'll do a pretty good job on most. You won't miss a lot, but you're not looking for all the little things as a senior. So you could, you can miss some of it. That's why we have a job guys like me. I think it's great.

Meuten *Somehow, as a resident, you taught me to look. And part of that may have been fear cause you were going to come in or you were over there in the corner working on something else and you'd be over there. Uh, today, sometimes it seems the residents look for the disease that they were told about in the history. And I don't know how to overcome that..*

King Oh I do, uh, do it the way I do it. Of course. That's why I do it my way. Of course, I'm just the straight man and this other boy, uh, Don't read the history. So I don't read histories ahead of time that pardon? They hate it. Oh. And I don't blame them. I, especially, I don't blame the seniors because they want to, they want all the help and they need all the help they can get. And I don't blame them for that, but the residents, I kind of bumped him a little bit hard. Uh, and when I come up to them and say, well, what do you think that is? The other day, a good little story. Uh, I threw an ear tag. It was in a bucket, uh, an ear with an ear tag in it from a cow. Yeah. I said, okay, what's your diagnosis? Well, that slowed everybody down. And I says, well, is it a new air tag? Yes. And this is a educational thing for everybody listening. Uh, sure. Is it a new air tank Sheryl? Well, why would a cow have a new air tag? I'll even my is me. Sure. I got a, I got a new ear tag and this cow, Donald, uh, when his cows here, what the die from,

Meuten *uh, must be sudden death lightening, or could have been one of those things, but why a new ear tag anaphylaxis a new air tag.*

King Okay. So it's not all that easy, but why would you put a new ear tag in an old cow on a farm, right? You probably wouldn't. Yeah. So you'd probably want a sick cow. Yeah, you wouldn't put it in a sick cows area. And, but, uh, how about a new cow on a farm? Would you have that? Would you put a new air tag and a new cow on the farm? You bought it the slot at the auction. Sure. Right now where's that auction next door or did it might be in Albany Cornell. How'd you get it to Cornell? Did you, the farmer walk that cow and feed her a piece of hay every now and then all the way to it's a COSO. No, you'll probably shipped it now. What. Disease you get when you ship cows shipping theater. Very good. So I make them think like that. I don't want it. I never asked him a question. That's, you know, everybody knows the answer to this. There's no teaching value on that. So this is how I really teach now. Some students, especially as new curriculum, I've just had a little problem with a young lady that. I would pick on her for that. Cause we had been friends before and she'd do this and I expected this out of her because she had been to many show and tells was the other two fellows in the class had never been, I don't remember ever seeing him at a show and tell it, well, they might've been there. And, uh, so I picked on her and that really got to her and she got to her again that I had to. I didn't have to go see the Dean. I had to go see the Dean of students, but that's something else. And that's kind of embarrassing in a way, but it takes the spontaneity and the fun out of teaching. Yeah. As you get older because you can't get away with grinding it all the way, but they can all they can while that's something else, that's their new freedom. And they can take advantage of that. And, uh, and complain that I don't think is necessary now. I can, uh, and I expected more out of her, so I didn't give her the top grade. And, uh, but it's my, my, she has, she has 25 classes like this all year and mine is just gonna average in there and it won't hurt it very much, but if it's early on in her training and she better think that some of us old geezers are not gonna put up with that, but that's okay. Well, let's see. And all of a sudden did this. All of a sudden would sit there and all the old timers on Minola students who graduated before 60, 1960 something, all of a sudden would ask this question, okay, what is it? Then he'd stand there like this and those students, they don't have a clue what this Brown piece of dumpling is in the bottle of formaldehyde or something like that. And, uh, they had look at it and he's waiting and he's waiting and it'd be three minutes, complete silence, everybody standing on a feet, he's sitting on a stool, moving back and forth and he would be gruff. And then he would, uh, they had to answer him politely and properly, and they did, uh, But, or they couldn't answer and no, he had the, he had fry them like that. He fried them cause they stood in place and sizzled, I think all of sudden the grand old man and he's for years afterwards, you know, when he stopped teaching, I'd visit him every week or so. And we talk and I said, Hey boss, you scared the heck out of everybody. And no, I didn't. I said, yes, you did. And then all come back and I'll tell him how much he scared him. Like you did this morning. You said, well, you scared me. I never scared you.

Meuten *Oh, without a doubt. You did you remember the time you sent me back to the buckets to pull out the legs?*

King I would do that. I would do that just to, cause I don't believe anybody. Yeah. I have good reason not to believe anybody. Not that I'm smart. But come on, I've seen it. And that's what makes a little difference between, uh, an academic, an academic, uh, than somebody outside doing diagnostic stuff outside. There's a tendency, I think, cause I was outside for six years. Uh, there's a tendency to start believing yourself. Whereas at school, I don't think I've ever asked a question that residents or undergraduates wouldn't jump me about. And try to tell me I'm wrong or a new resident, because if you came from, well, you came from Ohio, I mean, you were from Cornell, but then you went away and you get some education, Ohio and other places. And then when you come back, it's put you down. It's put dr. meuten down to, to make him think real hard. And don't give me that things. You think you learn someplace else, but except I would ask you and you would give it to me and yeah. And the way to teach is I said, well, you don't know what it is. I signed deal. You don't know what it is. Otherwise, I wouldn't have asked you that question. Cause I know you don't know, but I want you to think about it. Well, I don't know what to do. I said, well, do you think it's a brain? You know, you're looking at a elbow of a yeah. Of something is what do you think is the brain know while at least, you know, the anatomy. So do you think it's tumor, do you think it's infection? Do you think it's parasitic? You must be thinking something because why do I ask you like that? Because there's 14 other or 40 others or 80 others right there. They don't know. They don't know either. And they're so glad you're under, you're under these diff Klieg lights. And so they want you to get stuck. And, uh, so I'm trying to make you think a little bit.

Meuten *What about the resonant today or the vet student today? Do they take the heat as well as we did or the generation before that? Of that type of questioning and being put on* *the spot.*

King Uh, that's why I think the new student is, um, the up and coming student. Doesn't like it as much. Uh, and, but I don't. I don't care if they don't like it. I mean, it doesn't bother me that much, although I understand their, their reluctance and if they don't show up, then I can't teach them anything. So I think I either have to mellow a little bit, cause I want more of them to show up even just to listen to me knowing I won't question them too hard. Uh, some students don't mind and those students are the better students. They're wonderful to teach. They don't mind being wrong. They want me to. To correct whatever they think, and it doesn't hurt their feelings, but if you get some little prima donnas men or women, you can hurt their feelings. But I don't know I'm hurting their feelings because I think, well, gee, I know me pretty well. I've lived with me for what? 52 years, you know, maybe a little bit longer give or take a little bit. Yeah. And, uh, so I know how I am, but they don't might know it. So maybe I got a mellow for that reason. Or maybe apologized. But then when I find a couple who are pretty good, man, is that great because they answer the questions. They don't wait. And remember, I only have an hour on my show and tell periods I used to have almost every day and now it's cut down a bit. Uh, I don't have time to wait like Oleson did, but he only did during a quiz and that student had his four minutes or five minutes. And if he stood there, Okay. Mute, mute for five. I get five minutes, you know? Mmm. Okay. That was it. Yeah. That was it. That was bad. Bad news for that young person. Young man usually. Cause he didn't have too many women. Uh, yeah.

Meuten *How often do you run your show and tell now he eventually made it to be a double header on Fridays then?*

King Yes, but there's not that much interest in it right now. I don't know why. So we just have it Friday. But we still have, uh, during the summer we have lots of Spaniards here this summer, and they're wonderful to teach because there's five of them and we're going to have six one coming up and all they're wonderful of teach cause they all want to know. And they're not used to my w I don't know what is it? My style, my style. They're not used to it. But they don't understand that I'm really giving them heck if they don't answer it, you know, in a hurry. And if I go on to somebody else, they don't understand that. I really expect them to say something and I sometimes speak in Spanish a little bit, you know, some words cause I'm learning Spanish slowly, but anyhow, they're there and they're wonderful to teach because they're always interested. And they want to get it cause in their countries, you know, other countries, they don't have this discourse between a professor and one, it's not that it's not good or they don't recognize that it's, that they have 450 students in a class. And if every student has a question, yes. And if every student or 250, I'm sorry, and all four German schools to 150 and other schools, they got, you know, 150 or 200, 300 and. If every student asked a question who would ever have time to teach, if all the students asked one question, you answer it while you'd never get anything taught that way. I guess. So the Spaniards, well, all of the foreign kids are nice. And when we get, you know, you're like you're young Elizabeth from North Carolina, she's learned lots of things, but she speaks up just like that. She's a being a sexist. She's a cute little Southern. Uh, w Tanny, I mean, she's nice gal, but she goes right along with it and she'll answer immediately and roll on her. Right. She'll answer. And it's nice because she's going and she's joining the game and she was pretty quiet when she showed up. Right. And she answers more questions correctly by far, and it's a pleasure to teach them. Yeah. Yeah. But I'm lucky to have residents. If all I had was undergraduates, I'd find that a little more difficult because you can't expect that much out of them.

And so I liked the residents. Uh, I teach both every morning at eight o'clock. We have a histopathology seminar. It used to be that I'd make them read them ahead of time. Yeah. That gets, and I don't get many history.

Meuten *How many slides?*

King 15, 20, 20, 25 yet just a little boxes. And so now I just show 15 to 25 slides and I show the lesions on a scopes, multi, multi head scope or something like that. And then I'll, I don't ask them questions about the slide. Cause as I'm showing it, you know, they'll see the, every time you have my Kotick enteritis, you expect thrombosis. Otherwise you probably don't have my cottage from, you know, in the rightest. And if I, so if I show thrombosis, I would expect Elizabeth or anybody. Yeah, that's mold, but then I'd say, well, why did they get it? Cause that's not in that slide, why they got it or didn't get it. And they don't have the history and they better say, Hey, it was given too much antibiotics or it's overeating. If it was in the Apple Mason or something like that, I'd expect them to know that. And uh, so that's every morning you do those every morning for an hour at eight to nine and every morning at 10 to 11 it's Kodachromes how many residents. Would attend. Those does eight and all those, the Spanish and about 10 or 15 every morning. And it's okay. It gets a little too much for our regular residents that we pay the Spanish. Of course, they're all freebies for the summer. And a lot of other guests come in or some of the guests come in. It's a, it's a pretty good way of teaching, but then I ad lib the stuff that they should know about these. About these here's mineralization along one. Yeah. I'd expect them to know that it's hypercalcemia malignancy, vitamin high vitamin D low vitamin a stuff like this. They should know that and they'll get it. And if they don't take notes, they're the one. That's how I find other are the ones that don't do the best are those who don't take notes. If you just said lung mineralization. Uremia I mean, Uh, or hypercalcemia of malignancy or something like that, you know what you wrote up. Thank you so well, cause it's really proved to boon in our place.

Meuten *Oh, has it?*

King Oh, it's a good thing that you, uh, pick that up. Cause I had seen it. I never recognized it. I had seen it and I never gave it a name, you know,

Meuten *In cattle with Yoni disease. You'll see that mineralization sometimes up in the aorta,*

King And aorta. Thank goodness we had a Buffalo last week. And it was probably Elizabeth Case again, but it could have been anybody's and darned it didn't have good lesions anywhere. No good lesions anywhere, but it had a history of two months diarrhea, but no lesions of unis that's okay. So you don't see them? No. Lymphatic lymphangitis no dilated lymphatics. Um, you couldn't say Yonas except when you get to the order. You know, posture, AOD audience, usually behind a diaphragm or sometime in front. Beautiful mineralization, just like any cow with unis and just cause we did the cow, the bison last week. I didn't see the acid fast yet, but I bet it's there. Thank goodness.

Meuten *I, since I know the answer to this question, but I'll ask it anyways. Why, why does it have that mineralization,*

King What's that site ask God? Yep. We all ask God, just figured I'd check. Okay, sir. It hasn't changed. Ask God. And I don't like really doing that too much. Cause I'm too close to, to ask it him person compared to a young whippersnapper, like you,

Meuten *I suspect you'll straighten them out, but some things as well, knowing you, uh, Jeez, we've covered a lot of territory here and we started way back when in a vet school, classmates*

now we've uh, yes. Fast-forwarded. So you let's finish this for the first 50 minutes, right? The, uh, after the vet school,

King it was after the vet school, when the fellow said that while you're, uh, Yeah, the best student in the class or one of the best students in the class. I don't think you would have said the best. Uh, your, your attitude has to change. Anyhow, I go to Cornell and gee, it's a nice school jump had just left. So I replaced job at Cornell and Penn, Sarah. I was still used to staying up all night every night. Uh, Duke Cornell. He was at Cornell. So I took job's place. Carmichael was upset because Carmichael went to Cornell thinking it was going to work with Alison, but then he went on to Carmichael virus, herpes one, and now the petite virus or herpes of puppies and stuff. And he's just retiring this year. Yeah. And, uh, so then I got in there with all of sudden McEntee and record and bending Smith. Ernie Burstein was there, uh, taking care of bending Smith's job for a year while John was on sabbatical and John and Mac and, uh, Ken McEntee both come back every summer to Cornell and stay around. But with, uh, I would always take specimens and, uh, I would take this wheel barrel, honestly, the wheel barrel from the, uh, From the necropsy room, I'd take it over to Fox's class in Roberts's class and finches class. They all wanted me to bring the guts over, to show the students. So I'd bring the buck and they would, let me just walk in the door was a hallway wheeled down a hallway. It didn't leak. Uh, and I'd go over to. The old, the old vet school. Cause we were down a lower campus. When I first got there in 55, we didn't move up to the new building till 57. And now just this year, a 40, 39 years later, we've now moved to the new newer hospital path is still in the old and the old place that's going to be remodeled and. Modernized. I don't think they need it. I think all they need is somebody out there who's interested, keenly interested in necropsies you don't have to worry about the buildings and, uh, one more minute.

Is that it? Five Oh five. Okay. And then, um, I'd wheel them over there. To, uh, to the different classes and just show him what yesterday's cases were and then Fox or Fincher Roberts, whoever would Hillmann even, uh, cause he was a resume know a resident. Yeah. Uh, could he graduated in 55 to, I think anyhow he's retired. I think they're all telling me, actually, my job, my job, you know, is already, uh, advertised. And, uh, the chairman came and he said, John, it's not that we want you to go, but it's already being advertised. And I haven't even said I'm going to retire. So that's kind of cute too. Anyhow, I would show the wheel barrel of stuff to him and then I'd bring it. I'd bring it back to me. I'll just turn around, come back. And then Fox would go and tell the students, well, you know, that was a case you all saw yesterday or three days ago. It was so such and such. Then I'd bring this stuff to all of sudden or cause all of a sudden was kind of of a little different school. He wasn't out there for everything. He would expect me to bring stuff into them or Roger Penn, Sarah. And, uh, and we did cause Roger and I had a good, good, uh, association. And uh, he was willing to teach me, uh, almost anything. And we did that. But all of a sudden, every time I had a good specimen, I'd usually show it to Matt Gundy record and Oleson cause they're all right around. And uh, all of a sudden last, and he said, what McKinsey say? And he said, well, what did Rickard say? Cause he was always getting those two like this and I'll get different opinions sometimes because I'm always showing him lesions. I'll tell you about some of them. How's he gonna say? That'd be it. Good point to pick up with after the break. Fine. That'd be good. And get in with, Oh, listen. I think we're hitting the high points. I hope you're happy with my answers. Oh, I am. Yeah. So everybody else out there is I haven't insulted anybody too badly. Can we take a break then? Absolutely that. Okay. Thanks. Good.

Meuten *I like it. You had started into some. Observations when you were with, Oh, listen, pan Sierra, and then playing record and McEntee against the pickup with that. And tell us more about those days.*

King Uh, it was pretty, let's see how to say it the best it was Al it was always, I think it was always confrontational. Nobody. Uh, nobody was just willing to accept what anybody said and we, uh, It was great to ask them and get these different opinions for guys like me. Now you had to be careful, or I had to be careful that I always introduced what I thought first, the main reason is then they know what I think. And I'm not a yes man to them because whatever I thought when I first brought it into him, like I remember walking into Charlie, Rick had one time when he became the associate Dean. Cause of all the people. I'm sorry to say this. I hope I'm not hurting anybody's feelings. Uh, but of all the people who have died in my life, you know, they've, they've met their time, but I feel sorry that dr. Rickard died. And he's the only one who has died that I would. Love to welcome back because he meant that much. To me, he was such a wonderful teacher in a man in every way. Uh, all of a sudden too was, was nice, but he was a grand old man and he had passed. Uh, but I miss Rickard. He just died a little too darn early. Uh, and I'm S I'm so sorry for that.

Meuten *Was he kinder?*

King Oh, he was always kind to everybody. But I remember bringing this, the first cases that I think had been described ALO a Wayne crowd at Georgia several years later gave me some cases, uh, that he had. Uh, but these cases were, uh, kidneys from a pig that had chronic diarrhea and Johnny, if it didn't have. When I brought it down to Charlie on a tray, I said, Charlie, cause he's about doing a guy. I'd never call Peter Olson, Peter, but Charlie, Rick would, I'd say Charlie said, what do you think of these?

These are thrown by in the renal veins. And how do you think they got there? And he said something effect, Oh, well, um, and I said, remember, they're in the veins. And then he kept looking, kept working. And then he said, well, embolize embolized embolization. So no, no, Charlie. I said, uh, in the veins. And how do you explain those? Well, ordinarily he never made mistakes like that. I mean, cause he and I, and I never knew when the heck he studied cause he was the hardly ever in the post-mortem room. I mean, he'd come out if I asked him, you know, when the year pinch your eye pen, Sarah and I were on together after John had left and we were alone. We'd stay there until one and two in the morning, every night. And actually for all you young people listening, I don't think it's worth it to hurt your family that much. Maybe I benefited my family by not being home and given the kids about something. Uh, cause I have all these 42 years old now, but can I build houses on the side at night weekends, but that's an aside. It's something to do that we're not all in pathology all the time. You have a good relationship then. When he was growing up, I was in a post one room until two o'clock in the morning reading slides. So in the last four years, we build houses at night and weekends, and we have a blast. We can tell each other the nastiest jokes we can, we stop and have coffee anytime we want to. Uh, I'm kind of the bank, uh, He works at up, he went to Cornell hotel school, but he learned business and that's wonderful, but he's a nice guy. He'll give you the shirt off it. Oh, John Mune. How about a beer Don? You know, and he will, he's a nice guy. I'm not, I won't do that. I, I never had money as a kid. I never had money until I got in the army a hundred, you know, I made. What, $50 a month or whatever it was you made, man, that was a gold mine. So that's why I liked the army. But until recently I never had extra bucks that I could, you know, spend for beer for everybody around for everybody. I mean, that would be so foreign. I don't drink anyhow, but it's so foreign to me. So I wouldn't have done that, but he does now. I didn't, he doesn't have that much money either. Cause he works at the hotel when he's not building houses. With me because he wants to be ethical slum Lord, and that's kind of cute, but we work together. We have a good time. Good. But don't stay in a postmortem room. Uh, quite as much as we did. I don't know why we did. I mean, maybe it was John who lived in a postmortem room and then Penn Sierra and then King incidentally, we've been talking a little bit off stage and all about. The young people, young residents as being, you know, they're not driven like we are, you might kind of believe it. I might kind of believe it, but maybe there's some doubt in even our minds because there's some guy a number of years ago who said the young people, they don't want to work too hard. They want to know what's in it for them. How much time off they get. Uh, they have no re really respect for their elders. You know, that little veterinary student who told me to. Hmm, do something, you know? Yeah. Politely. And, uh, she asked permission. No, but, uh, things like this, uh, this, this person years ago said that, and you know, the kids aren't up to snuff, but that was Socrates about 3,200 BC. So maybe it says we get older, we feel this about the young people and maybe there's a little more hope for them than what you and I have now. You're saying Darren King he's mellowing too much. That's right. I know. You're thinking that. Well, maybe solve a heck. I don't want to go see the chairman of Dean and the president of the game. I better be careful. Uh, let's see. Where were we? Yeah, it was,

Meuten *Oh, the hours in the postmortem room and.,*

King I'm not sure I'd do, I would do that again. I don't recommend that for other people, but you need somebody who's critical of everything you do. And I'm critical of everything that residents do. And I love to sit down with a scope with them. Cause I read, I used to read over half of the slides and do more than half the case. I'm getting out of that a little bit and. You take any student trained in Europe, for instance, if they culture an organism, what killed that cow? That organism and that's absolutely bunkers. It's the only organism that'll grow into the media, the media conditions, their change of venue from the carcass to the Petri dish and airfoil that's causative. You know, I think that's full of beings. Uh, if it looks like it's a good. Uh, fibrous pneumonia. Don't tell me you culture, the coal out of it, or actinomycetes that's baloney. I really still think it is. And then somebody say, wow, that's all we culture. And I said, sure. Cause when the animal's sick for five days, you pop them with antibiotics and it might stop the growth of that organism and a Petri dish, but not in a carcass or something, whatever. And that's a, that's a mistake. That's a mistake. So I like to. You can always make them all think of what they're, what they're doing.

Meuten *You know, you told the residents today, not to do that. If you're going to tell the residents today that wanted to end a career in veterinary pathology, the DVM student one ended a career in veterinary pathology. What would be the one piece of advice you would give them?*

King Uh, Hmm, give me a hint. I need, I don't know what I would tell them. I think there's no better. Uh, well actually I do have a problem with that because we have several experts at our school who sees the animals alive, for instance, on eyeballs. We who see the animals alive with central nervous CNS diseases who sees them with skin diseases. And then they also follow them into the necropsy room with certainly biopsy stuff and they get the whole picture. Whereas you and I, as general diagnostics in general diagnostics, um, We don't get the whole picture and we can't follow it as deeply as those fellows can. Cause we don't see it ahead of time on some things, certainly, but not. Uh, I would, maybe I would go into a specialty if it was me. Cause I feel that many schools, uh, I consider veterinary pathology or veterinary pathology kind of radios going off, they represent a subject. John King. I can probably take 85%. I can go from the middle all the way out. I know 85% of the stuff coming through the door without history and stuff. I can recognize the lesions on 85% pan Sierra. Kind of my mentor, Richard or McEntee, they're all a little bit smarter than I am. Uh, they'll get 87% individually, 87%. I will know a 2% difference that Roger doesn't know a Rajan, you know, stuff like that. So I can add if Roger hired me at Oklahoma, I could go to Oklahoma and add up to 89%. Cause he knows 87 being a little smarter. I can add 2% that he doesn't know about. Up to 89% and CNS, you get a guy like Delahunty, who's kind of a genius in the CNS. He can take care of 85% of every neuro case that comes in. Uh, that's what makes the schools better? I think then, uh, David Dodd, he's another 85 or 87% in general diagnostics. Yeah. Do you think it would be a better school with kinky? Well pants, Sarah and Dodd? I don't think so. What would be better school would have any one of the three guys? Maybe King's the lowest that's okay. I'm not proud. Uh, and then you'd have a guy who's 85% skin, 85% brain, 85% ovaries, and testicles. If you were going to reproduction 85% in muscles, like Cooper. I don't care for Cooper tall personally. Uh, but I respect his brains cause he's really sharp. And uh,

Meuten *we started together out on the necropsy floor.*

King You and he, yeah. Oh. Cause I remember telling him off than even then, but he's faculty now, so I gotta behave myself, but it's uh, Helen joy hearing the fact, at least he made it.

Meuten *Oh, he'll hear this.*

King I hope but no, he is smart, but most of the Australians are for instance, or the British. Because they come off the top of the heap academically to get into their veterinary schools. Whereas you and I had to compete with the other farm kids who are, who are interested in being a veterinarian and had a fair grade. They weren't dodos. But, uh, cause I was a farm kid too. So I had to compete with other young men, you know,

Meuten *did you ever get tired of coops, tick paralysis stories?*

King I get tired of the coop. Early on. And I probably didn't, if he's given a seminar now I probably wouldn't attend it unless he's talking on muscles. I mean, if he's going to because he's into it. He's Oh, he's that good? Yes. Yeah. And his wife is good on the muscles too, but all that, that's what the schools need. They need more experts, uh, and you don't need depth. And these other things, if you have a good diagnostic diagnostician, you don't need the others. However, who can afford? The others, unless you have a clinician who's really interested in CNS, he sees them clinically, and then he follows the cases. And that that's wonderful. So maybe the pathologist should do that. Cause it's not much respect for general diagnostic pathologists anymore though. They all give me lip service. Oh yeah, you can do that, but I'm not sure you get the respect and thus the bucks and that's the, uh, Whatever prestige or something like that, but I'm not doing too bad. Cause you know, I've got a sabbatical coming up and I'm going to every place I want to, everybody wants me. Cause I'm willing to, I don't insult too many people. If you go places you're widely traveled just about everywhere except Russia. And I enjoy it and I've learned. Cause all I do when I go anywhere really is um, I do the autopsies in the morning. Or for three or four hours, or I give Kodachromes three or four hours a day.And, uh, I show the Kodachrome and I discuss it. That's what I'm down here for too, in a sense. And they liked that because I will introduce the other person's opinion, even if I don't agree with it. But as the world says, well, gee whiz, you know, when you have pulpy, kidneys, what makes the, uh, kidney pulpy. Well, they say no toxemia. I said, no, no, no. This is a cow. I just gave glucose to last night. And she died during the night. Why? Well, the glucose is in there acting as a substrate. This is pathology, pure, not historical. Although I've seen it all my life, I showed it to Olsen and he said, well, it's endotoxemia. I say, boss, this is full. And it was just given glucose and a died, you know, shortly after. And then we didn't post it for six hours. The glucose acted as a substrate to cause the autolysis of the whole kidney. It looks like mush except for the medulla, the medulla, it looks perfect and histologically, that's what you see the same way.So it's really that glucose now in Entero, toxemia of sheep. That's why you put a dipstick in the urine because you know, you find sugar, but that's what makes the kidney early. Rapid, uh, enhanced I call. So it's kind of fun. And talking to the old guys, you show him the same thing. And, uh, with blackleg, all the new things, like 30 days postpartum, blackleg of the, of the paraniem, you know, and you wonder, well, gee, 30 days postpartum while these are new and different things, you know? But it's taken a long time to see these things. And if you're not in a postmortem room with a good caseload, you're not going to see these things.

Meuten *And you need somebody to put all the pieces of that pie together.*

King who is there all the time doing it. And that's why it's worthwhile. But, uh, so you need a generalist. Absolutely. But you don't need three of them. You, you need two of them. Cause one of you got to take a break, but you don't need three of them. And I know some schools have hired one good general diagnostic pathologist, or they've got one, they get another one, they get another one. They don't, they don't compliment each other very well because you know, you pass the boards and certainly, the boards are the minimal requirement for a dog, for a pathologist, absolute minimum. Because many of them, and I used a FIP a little bit as an example, many of them, all pass the boards and they do a darn good job at it. They're very organized. Uh, and they do a very good job at it. But if I got some of them in the postmortem room, including my host, uh, today, if I got him in a postmortem room and asked him what these things were without a square frame around him, I'd make him sweat a little bit more than. He thought he would sweat and even made us all sweat. Yeah. And, but that's, and it's fun, but it takes a lot of time. And if I'm not out there to collect these specimens, every senior will have a hamburger that liver or that, that kidney, we were talking about that, uh, yeah, a minute ago we were talking about the renal vein thrombosis with Charlie Rickard. Well, he had never seen that before and nobody else had. Except in humans, you see it. Anybody who has multiple, uh, or exceptional electrolyte therapy or diarrhea. So you see it in children and old people, a lot of electrolytes, old people, children with diarrhea. Well, these pigs all had diarrhea. Now we see it mostly in cows. Cause they're getting fluids out the Gazoo and we'll see it in them with Abba, Mesa displacements, or it doesn't matter anything like no, whatever they're getting lots of fluids with. Yeah. Now, this is renal vein thrombosis. Uh, with Apple Mason, displacement, you get a new lesion, and without thinking about it without having just off the, just off the top of your hat, I have massive throne by, in the portal. No, I have, yeah, massive thrown by in the, uh, uh, a port he paddocks portal veins, you know, I mean, in the liver themselves, in the liver itself, not in the portal, vein, none at the intestine. Why do they have those? Not many people describe them, then they make, they don't make good infarcts in the liver, although they're thrown by why not? Well, because these are from displaced, Abu Mason, and during displacement, you get stagnation thrown by or something, whatever. And then you replace that displacement and they become free and it's just right up the liver. So you've now had nice lesions there, but if you're not thinking about it, and this is why. If people want to do what I do as a general diagnostic pathologist, you have to do a lot of autopsies. You can't say I'm on duty. I'm sharing a necropsy load with 12 other pathologists. Cause that's pure bunkers. You're not learning a lick. If you do that. Cause you only get one 12th of the cases and the other one 12th, you're doing the other 11, 12th, 12th. You're forgetting that one 12th you saw actually you go backward. So you have to do it all of the time. And, uh,

Meuten *any idea how many cases you've seen over the years, you ever tried to tell it somehow,*

King 120,000, actually, if you consider, I have the largest private collection of COTA cools in the world. I'll bet you, I almost have as many as the AFI P S probably not, but better be careful. Yeah. But no, and I can find any one of them in 20 seconds or. Right now, if you asked me if that's why they want your collection, then yeah, I can do that in 20, 20 seconds. Now, if you want distemper, I have to go to the brain all every now and then I have cases for you. Pathologists start getting them organized early. Cause if you don't, you're going to have a heck of a time later, but you'll. I got Kodachromes all over the office. Mine are filed in there. I can find anyone I'm pretty quickly because of the filing system, the boxes on the shelf, briefly the boxes on the shelf say Apple Mason. So don't look anyplace else. They're only Apple Mason. And if the yellow it's a horse, if it's blue, it's a cow. If it's white if it's sheep. So all these folders are all labeled like that. And now if I have 12 folders, Apple, Mason, that are all colored while we can't be yellow, can't be orange or yellow versus don't have an Apple Mason, but they'll edit that out. I would see it there. And then I go down through Dwight, you want a parasite and I'll have, you know, the 20 Kota Kodachrome holders or DIA positives. If you're Spanish holers, there'll be 20 folders in there. And only two of them will have parasites, parasites. I've got two folders, 40. Kodachromes and there's all the parasites of the room, you know, like a glandula NEMA they're in the room instead of the esophagus or, or, um, um, grubs in the back, you know, so I can pull them out. I've got them right there. I mean, if you're talking about, uh, ruminal drinkers, I just go to metabolism and it's got, it would be cows. So there'd be. Blue or whatever the color is the cows, and they're all the same through all those boxes. So I got a box for the ovaries and the testicles and four boxes in the living room,

Meuten *bud tenant could ever retrieve his Kodachromes that quickly.*

Now it's kind of, it's a, you got to learn that too. Yeah.

Meuten *When you go to these countries, do these courses and the necropsies and so forth, is it all in English?*

King Not now it's in Spanish, but what good, what's good about English is half of what we teach and what half of what, you know, if I said all I go, what would you think of? You know, and if I said, uh, uh, uh, hyper, what would you think of and all that stuff. So that's Greek and Latin. You and I are absolutely lucky. That we know Greek and Latin, as far as medical terms go, we don't have to speak it. That's a dead language, went out, you know, uh, without, and so half the language we use it's universal. So there's 50% already. I already know English. Not too. Well, a lot of people say poorly, but anyhow, I know English. And then now I just have to learn a few Spanish words and all. And remember, as a teacher down there, down there, or in Spain, you ask questions, don't date you have to get an article that fits with the noun, you know? And, uh, so you say don't de a style. That is where is good. And your gut or Quando win and you learn some of these good ones like that, but I can go through and, uh, in Spain, they say either, go on someplace else, say, say it a little bit different for the liver and pull Monet's and stuff like the other day, it was even interesting. I'm writing a reporter, I'm correcting the report. And I said animals and I M a L E S S but then I'm thinking that's wrong. Why is that wrong? And I can't think why, because I'm studying Spanish to go for the sabbatical inside of America. There's no III and Anna it's Ani Molly's for Spanish. And I was so I'm making mistakes in my English favorite country, South Africa, because everything you want to do, uh, everything you want to study in South Africa, for instance, Uh, virology, parasitology, toxicology. It's all on under support. When I was down there in 75, 76, part of my sabbatical, uh, system sabbaticals are great. Everybody should use them, even if you don't know a lot of people take advantage of them, go goof off. Uh, we have faculty to do that, but if you don't go someplace else, Uh, you're not doing your profession well or yourself. Well, now, if you've got three kids and you gotta haul them with you when you're a young professor, that that's a little tough. I understand that. Uh, but South Africa, apartheid was real there. It's not there now. So, uh, but I enjoyed that country cause it looks more like ours. So, therefore I'm not, and they spoke English. Thank goodness and Afrikaans, but, uh, so that was nice. And they had very, very competent people in bread. Yes. Because I dunno why, but, uh, they're very sharp and all those veterinary students come off the top of the heap academically, too, just like the other English or some other countries. But I, I liked that the best. Um, see how its water all out the Gazoo heart, water out the Gazoo, uh Cowdry uh, I learned to make smears how they do it, and they were willing, there was a guy named PNR there and KOOS Ketso who was here, I guess, at the FIP. They've just got a book out or KOOS has, uh, Uh, on infectious diseases of South-South Africa, fabulous book, beautiful pictures. Well done. Um, now I would, I would go back there to study cause you know, come to Cornell for beef cows. I don't think I'd go to North Carolina for, for, um, beef cows. Oh. Yeah. Well see, and, and, uh, for the parasite where you have more than we have, it's too cold and New York for parasite to live over, you know? Yeah. So we don't have that many problems every now and then we get an import and he's loaded from North Carolina or some other place. What are the good diseases from South Africa that you enjoy? Or some people or hairy incidences. The wildlife down there is great. They do a lot of that and they were willing to share everything with me and every morning, peanut, uh, or coups or something we would, uh, cause I w uh, I would give two hours at COTA Combs and he would give two hours of Kodachromes and that was the most educational thing. And I've done that even in, when I was in Australia, I did that, uh, as there for a year. And you. You share your Kodachromes ELV. They'll let you copy anything. I let them copy all mine, whatever it was a very good give and take. I had a very poor time and in Switzerland, and I think it's the culture. It's really a culture shock to go to Switzerland. It was probably my fault but remember many. Countries European or foreign countries. The professors aren't used to being questioned critically. And I know remember one professor went, a friend of mine, went to Oklahoma to be an, a faculty. And, and, uh, my classmate was, uh, Louis Stratton was on a faculty and this guy went there for the job interview, uh, and he got the job. But they were interviewing some other people I forgot, which was first. Then he was on a committee to interview other new members, uh, potential faculty. And he jumped one of the speakers. I shouldn't play with that. Uh, he jumped one of the speakers, uh, pretty badly. Cause the fellow used pathological terms. He wasn't a pathologist. He was going to be something else. I didn't know what, and he jumped all over him in a way. And everybody in the audience was amazed that here's one of their faculty jumping this speaker. I thought it was wonderful. I wasn't there, but I thought the hero, well, he jumped all over him and I says, well, of course, he did. The guy was, he was a jerk and he should have been jumped on the hired them anyhow. And that was bad. They hired him anyhow, I guess. And, uh, It didn't turn out so well, but my classmate said, well, he had no, right. I said, yeah, but the guy saying something wrong. I mean, what, why shouldn't he be knocked for that? And, uh, that's why I guess a lot of people do Cornell without, you know, a lot of protection somehow, because they're going to get blasted by everybody, I think. And maybe it's, you don't have to be too bad, hard, but that's life. Cause I get blasted. Anytime I say something wrong and I'm quick to blast back.

Meuten *How about Taiwan and your book and Dr. Lee.*

King Lee's Lee. Uh, I first met him as a graduate student at Cornell in the early, in the late fifties. His brother was a Nobel prize winner in physics or something like that. And Bob was a, uh, say one of your books. That's okay. Uh, um, and Bob himself, Bob Lee, CT Lee. He was a minister without portfolio. He was a, uh, um, like the minister of the interior. What's that secretary of the interior for Taiwan. And he did a fabulous job, getting everybody to Taiwan to teach. And he asked me to go, and again, I just showed Kodachromes. Now they don't have many cows and they don't have one or two horses. And, but the rest, they have a lot of pigs. So I learned a lot about pig path and, uh, but he made the opportunity available for. Many Americans everywhere and also for the Chinese themselves to come to America. And that worked very well. It's fun to teach the Chinese, except there's a little bit of a problem with it. Do you understand what I'm saying? Yes. Uh, they'll say yes and smile and that's disconcerting because you think they do understand, but if you ask them a little bit of a question, they might not have learned it. Yeah. And that's kind of embarrassing for me in them. Cause I thought they all understood it when they said yes, because they don't want to insult anybody. And when I told them I stole a cup, a couple of them after I showed him a heart anomaly are the single most Carmine common heart anomalies of all animals put together is the incomplete symbiotic stenotic ring. So you tell him that the most common anomaly. It's the most common heart anomaly of all animals put together. Dr. Muetan is the incomplete symbiotic, static ring. And don't you forget it. And if you don't take notes on that, you're going to forget it because you forgot it last time. That's right. I better write that one. I think that was a new one, much less than it's the most common it's by far the most common one. Anyhow, you tell them that. And you're the only one here and your other classmates in Taiwan are doing something else. I said, make sure you tell them the next morning I asked Dr. Lee or another Lee or whatever. Hey, what'd you think of that harder normally, yes. To do that most common one. What? Heart, a normal heart. And what heart anomaly. And you didn't tell him that. I see you. Well, why didn't you tell him and you'll smile at me, but I won't get an answer out of you. I could strangle you. And I guess it's because of the higher, one of them said it was a hierarchy. They have a lot of people over there and there's only room for a few at the top. And if I don't tell you now, I don't know if that's how they think or if it's just natural or something.

Meuten *What is this incomplete? Subaortic right. It doesn't cause mega esophagus.*

King It's no, it's it is the single most common heart anomaly. That's not clinically evident in most cases. There's nothing. So you will overlook it

Meuten *And it's what I've done over the years?*

King Yeah. Cause it is in all species it's with cows. It's just, it looks like a start of a, you know, a stenotic ring, but it just only goes that far or it only goes one dot size, but it's right on the order. Maybe what animal it is. We just need some photos of that. Yeah. I think in that last batch you sent me and by the way, thanks. No, I don't know where I'd put that, but it's, it's, it's just a little thing to talk about then. The interesting thing is another, it's another thing in respect. Uh, several people at Cornell wrote a book and they wrote a book on anomalies. And the catch on that is did they come to anybody in the pathology department and ask them. About what the common higher anomalies are or something? No. And that bugged me a little bit. That's all. I don't know anything. Well, maybe I don't know much in great detail because we have all these experts and why should I go look up something on the CNS system when Della Hunter knows all of them, just at the top of his anywhere. Yeah. And he knows him in great detail. I could only go down about three. Three notches of information, whereas he would be very good and I love those guys, but it re it does take a little bit away from me in the sense that I don't take the time to do that because he's there. And if they've got Scott on the skin, but it makes our place a little bit stronger in many ways, because we have these extra experts. And when I do finally think of retiring because. I got into the system when I don't have to retire, I can go like this until I was about 105. I don't have to retire.

Meuten *I hope he keeps doing it?*

King Ah, yeah. Cornell has been blessed with some excellent people over the years. They've written a lot of the books and we've got some new ones coming along and doing the same thing.I mean, we're glad to have Scott with his 85% skin. Probably 90% skin and haunted with all his brains and Reese with his eyeballs and Schlaffer with his ovaries and testicles and Cooper again with his muscles, you know? And so it's neat to have that. Uh, but the clinicians are affording a lot of that because Scott's a clinician, Miller's clinician, Reese's a clinician doing histopathology and growth.So that's pretty nice. So it makes our system better, but if they don't have somebody like me in the postmortem room, kinda cock of the walk, cause you didn't come in here and walk over me. And if you try to, I will walk over to the clinics and find you and tell you about it. And if you send over a rotten dog that you've done $400 worth of clinical biochemistry and you send it over, uh, on Friday night and we get the re request for necropsy on Monday. What a waste. And I don't allow that to happen without a little bit of kit. Can I write it in a report? The clinicians lose their cool, but we don't send the reports to the owners. They go to the vet clinician or something, cause we're not. And if they want, if they come back with a little bit of an apology, I might change the report and, you know, wipe out all the little notes I put in the bottom. It's just a shame that the owner did not want to share this dog with everybody after doing all this work on it. Somebody gets the hint, right?

Meuten *You think the conditions have a little too much, say a little too much power at the veterinary colleges now?*

King Well, with our new curriculum, they only have a crack at the students for maybe a year, a year and a half. And that's it, all the rest of it is done by big committee, of which many of them are not veterinarians. And that's the shame because you don't have the veterinarians doing that. Now, some of the veterinarian is like that, but, uh, because you know, gave them less work, but I don't think it's good for the students or the profession. We already talked that a little bit. I don't know how that's going to last, but I don't think it'll work.

Meuten *Yeah. Well, in the Cornell system now is just so drastically different from any other curriculum that they're in the country. How about Olsen? Tell us some more things about him and, and in particular, and I assume it's him, but it may, that may be the wrong answer. Who infants, you the most in vet for veterinary pathology?*

King Uh, well, pants here because he was there every day. And, uh, but some of the young people surprisingly yourself and the fact that you picked up on the hypercalcemia of malignancy, That's pretty neat. And some fellows like everybody here knows John Edwards. Yeah. As my, as my protege protege in a way I really don't think you are, you guys made yourself. And I like to think of when I teach, I want to teach somebody for two years, three years, whatever, and make them self perpetuating pathologists. They know lots of the answers, not all of them, but they know how to. Do the post and think more than just a superficially. And I think I'm proud of many of them hashtag, you know, and yourself and Edwards. You guys don't need somebody like me anymore. You can think deeper. Uh, but there's a lot of others who have never done that. I don't think they did enough autopsies. And I think enough autopsies are very important. Uh, and when you share them with 11 other residents, I don't think you're getting enough unless somebody is there and they force a show and tell. And if you're a reticent pathologist, cause we have some at school who have been there eight or nine years, and they're still trying to take their boards. They told me off long ago. So I haven't talked to them since. I mean, I can take a hint. You don't want to talk to me cause you don't like my questions. Sorry. I, I don't know how to do any better. But I have a guilty feeling about that a little bit, because if you upset the people too much, that they don't want to learn from you, you've lost a little bit. And that really bothers me a little bit, not enough to change now, I'll be sorry to, when I go see the big guy up there or something like that or down there, I don't know which, uh, I wished I guess that's a few places where I'm sorry. That I irritated some people so badly by mine, but then I wasn't willing to change and they didn't come and say, Hey, let's, let's bury the hatchet or something and let's all learn together. Something I wasn't willing to change. I do feel sorry for that.

Meuten *Did you start the show Intel's at Cornell or were they not?*

King That's, that's OK. Uh, they learned other ways. But all of a sudden didn't want me to do it first, but Fox and the others spoke to him and asked him to do it because he thought it was a wheelbarrow, all that. And it's all I had at first, but then Roberts, I think it was Roberts bought a big, proper cart that I could wheel around instead of a wheelbarrow. So they did a, he did a good, I think it was Robert.

Meuten *Yeah. And then eventually just kept them in the necropsy lab and they came to you.*

King And at first they all came. Now I Fox came, Hillman's still comes. Mary Smith comes, Fox comes and they see these things and the young clinicians. So you get, say you graduated from Washington state, Missouri or something like that. You're going to come in and let a young. Younger or older Whipper snapper tell you that. They're crazy about what they said about this big lung it's full of air and, and congestion. That was pulmonary congestion and emphysema. And I said, no, the cow or electrolytes were probably a little screwed up as she was dying and she had breathing hard and she gets emphysema. So what next? But they don't like that. Savoir Faire or nonchalance or something, whatever you call it that I, I tend to show things of no significance.

Meuten *I feel it was lucky for me at least to have seen the show and tells an oldest son could attend there. And it got to the point, though, that he, it seemed as if he had to trust your eyes.*

King Oh, absolutely. Cause he couldn't see doodly squat in the last few years, but there was a period of about 10 years before I came back in 68. Um, well, the eight years that nobody asked him back and that really hurt him and he felt bad about that. So when I asked him to come back, you know, we didn't have to waddle in and I'd tell him that. And then he'd give you the stories. Well, I don't have too many stories. Like he had, I guess, Because he got in at the beginning of many very important diseases, the things I show people like this incomplete heart anomaly, I mean, incomplete subglottic, stenotic ring for it's not clinically important. Why worry about it. Except as a general pathologist, you should know what it is. Core temperature gangrene. We've seen core temperature, gangrene. Are you familiar with it?

Meuten *Uh, or at least by that name. I'm not, I mean, either better.*

King You don't know. Uh, it's you know, you have a horse it's Oh, full it's losing its its hoof sloughed. And if they don't check all the other feet, they'll think, well, gee whiz he's left his, Hofi heard it got an infection sloughing, but if they had checked all the temperature, the other four feet. F O U R you would find all of them and he might be sloughing all of them. That one's the first one that fell. And this is due to, in my mind, My core temperature gangrene is you get a high fever for whatever reason and you're cold. Even in the hot summertime, you're cold, you're cold. You shiver. You're cold. You get a high fever. You're Chevy, you're cold. And you'll get peripheral vasoconstriction, so bad that all four feet will slough because you now have gangrene of those feet all because it's like, I know, are you people arguing me on this thing too? On Ringtail? I've seen Ringtail in thousands of rats. When I worked for industry, because we raised all our ATS, I was the only veterinarian, the only pathologist there and stuff like that. And every day in caves that we saw, the cages were all wet and the little rats were cold and they froze and rats controller temperature when the young, by their tail vascular. And they will constrict down ans and pigs in the summertime that lose the tips of the year. Somebody says vegetative and it could either, I said, baloney, that's due to infection, give them a fever. And then they get core temperature gangrene as a result. Now you might throw them from up there. And then somebody says, Oh yeah, thrown in. I said, what do you think they came from? Oh, from the heart? If it's on the right side, but that's baloney. Cause you're then telling me that a little piece broke off the left heart. It started up at broken two exact pieces. Both went up the external carotids or whatever, our internal carotids, and then they divided up and went the irregular branch in both gangrene. That's, that's a story, man. That's not real, but there's no reason you can't get stagnation thrown you when you get core temperature gangrene. So that's something a little bit new and different. I'm willing to argue about. If you say I'm wrong, that's okay too, but I'm probably more right than you think I am.

Meuten *before we get into the new and different lesions? How about some of those that you'd have to take credit for either the discovery of, or a significant part of the identification of,*

King Only because like you did with your, uh, With your hypercalcemia, you saw that kind of stuff, and then you finally put it together. That's, that's what I did. Cause you saw enough, you saw a lot and that's what I have done with a lot of these things that are kind of new and different.I don't think it's, um, all that, that smart, uh, some of them that you, uh, in 19, in 1940, you know, in 19. 19. Oh, 63. I was doing an autopsy on a war veteran, a GI at the VA hospital in Pittsburgh, and I get to his heart and I see these, these areas of damage into myocardium. I said, Hey, good. Look at this man. Uh, what would you think when you get scattered areas of fibrosis in the heart?If I asked you, you would say, well, you had coronaries or something like that. Yeah. And I'm saying, yeah, he's got coronaries. All right. Uh, I mean, he has coronary disease maybe before that, what happened at, at school with all of a sudden, I had this sheet that had these fabulous lesions myocardium, acute lesions, mineralization, uh, fatty change, mineralization, stuff like that. And then, uh, I hauled all, all of a sudden out there and record mechanized. I remember this, it was great. All three of them came out and looked and they said, well, he's probably got white muscle disease, John. I said, well, maybe, but doesn't look at, and he's an older shape. And, uh, he had listeria fibrosis. Well, he hadn't mineral. It only takes 20 hours or less to get mineral one day we, and the old days we like gated the, uh, Uranus on a dog. And, uh, he couldn't get rid of anything. Uh, no. We took out the kidneys actually and they get mineralization in the Oh 20 hours, something like that. Anyhow, uh, that's what I used to be a research type. So on this, uh, the sheep, it's got these multifocal multifocal areas of degeneration of myocardium, all of a sudden said white muscle. No, it's an old shape. And, uh, we didn't know about exertional my opposite at that time, but it didn't matter wasn't that. And then he and Rick had mechanism, they all agreed. It could be white muscle for some reason, lo and behold, it had listeria. So this GI that would died. He had all these multi-focal areas and, you know, I'm, I didn't believe anybody then either. And I don't really know. And lo and behold, I said, but his coronaries are clear. Well, I healed. So, yeah, it'll give me his diet and we'll cure everybody in the world, you know? And uh, I said, no, he has something else wrong with him. Now, remember, I'm doing these, even the people and, uh, at the VA hospital in Pittsburgh without histories, they're there, the MDs there, but he just let me play, you know, stuff like that. So I'm playing,

Meuten *you're a trainee or what.*

King No. I was just a visiting pathologist happened to be veterinary pathologist. And so he's Oh no, that's good. He's got coronary disease. I see. It does not. And he said, you look, I said, well, how could I say he didn't? Cause you know, I give him a little static. How can I say he didn't have it? If I didn't look and then we let it go. Except I say, you know, when I see it, usually they've had trauma to the head. And that guy had a steel plate and old side of his head from shrapnel during the war. And then when he died shrapnel during the war myocardial damage brain, heart syndrome, or neurogenic cardiomyopathy, whopped to the head spinal cord or major nerve plexus. And you'll get these myocardial changes. And if they're big enough, they'll leave scars, you know, 20 years later, I mean a scar, what the heck you can live with a scar. Everybody does. And that was my first case there. So we kept proving that they don't, the humans still don't accept that fully, which is their loss, but we've seen a lot of that. We see it with the kidney gastric stomach, and nobody believed me. So the clinicians twisted the stomach of a dog, and now they built now they're believers.The core temperature is we're talking about the clinician said, well, we think we have it. And they were absolutely on cloud nine. I got car temperature, gangrene. I wanted to say, what the heck are you getting excited about? We've had around for 20 years, you know, but I I'm nice. I just, I wouldn't insult them like that. Take you a long time to sell the brain, heart syndrome to the, Oh yeah. It'll take twice as long cell core temperature, except I have some of it in some of these books. They're not well, uh, Reviewed maybe, but some of us stood the test of time, so I don't worry about it too much. And remember I make the diagnosis usually without the history. And that's what pays off. You guys have some mere cats here. Yeah. You guys have some mere cats. Pictures someplace. Yeah. And I had one in Switzerland. I said, Hey, he's going to have a beautiful, uh, he's got a brain lesion. He had a beautiful brain lesion cause he had that lesion in the heart, stuff like that. So I don't mind fighting the system. And when you go into heart, heart with hardware and a cow, yeah. You know, the piece of wire is going to be that long and about what a cocaine like that, you know, guess what that cow in. They hadn't even opened the heart. They made the diagnosis because it was full of pus and junk and they had an open heart. So I pulled it out of the barrel and I said, and. I told all the students it's going to be this long. Well, thank God because I'm not bologna in them. I'm serious in my pathology. And I happened to be right again. But do as much as I have, you'll be right. You still collect those, put them in your notebook.

Meuten *It's one of the photographs I show the students. When I teach that part. And there's the D one of the major differences between you and me, I didn't take the time to save those over the years. You did. Cause it makes an impact on the students. When I say now this notebook is full of these and they are.*

Well, that's fun. No, that's yeah. That's why I like it. But to have graduate students like you, I wouldn't do it. If I didn't have graduate students. Pick one more in the closing two minutes that, uh, you were a big part of, or one that you want to talk about. Let's do that one for the last bit.

The anesthetic gas machine loan, all these dogs that died pretty quick after anesthesia, for instance, and they lose all the oxygen. they're intubated with, uh, anesthetic gas, which is metabolizable. And if for some reason they don't get air with 80% nitrogen in the lung, Wilton tend to collapse after when it coming out of anesthesia or, well, they're already out of anesthesia, but if the bandages are too tight or something like that, all that metabolizable gas will be absorbed and the lung will collapse more and more. If they don't get bagged with air, not oxygen air here with 80% nitrogen and then they'll die. That's a very interesting, uh, thing. Hmm. Nice new entity. What about the, uh, geez. I feel like you're going to yell at me if this an atypical interstitial pneumonia while it's so typical, it shouldn't have had that name who gave it atypical. I thought that was you Robin Kennedy. Oh yeah, no, I've always called it prolific pneumonia because the only thing in the lung, the alveoli that can respond the epithelial cells. So it's a proliferation of OVO lying cells type two, because, you know, type one is a single nucleus here and cytoplasm going here, maybe another nucleus, a little side of the pipe. You hardly see the lining. And when I first worked on it with Abel, Hey, bill was the first one to prove at Cornell that there was a epithelial lining with the EDM. Cause it was the first DM pictures of it. Hazel took that there is an epithelial lining of each alveolus. You ever convinced the clinicians to use atrophy? Several Bob Kenney at Penn. And that's the only thing that'll save him. Is that your pain? But that was Mack Andy's comment. He said use that because we stopped degranulation of the pituitary. Let's get a little complicated by giving him whopping doses of atrazine. One gram that kicks it, the belly photophobic. Yes, but they stopped degranulation, but it also stopped secretion. It'll save those cows with. No, your dries, your mouth or your trachea or whatever, and they live, huh? Your name. You're going to tell us who you are. Uh, in the, in the very beginning of the tape and the closing moments, we're going to put that stuff in because of the We'll get it in. His name is Don and we'll take a break at this point. Pick up for the third session. Good show.

Meuten *Good. Thanks.*

Meuten *In the, uh, for the last hour, let's make sure that we, uh, talk about some of the, uh, uh, people that either you knew or influence you. And I know we've covered Olson and you've mentioned McEntee and record and so forth, but who are some of the others that, uh, you'd like to share with us?*

King Uh, although they were my teachers, don't forget, we should not forget the pupils, so to speak cause they help make your life.

Or nicer, miserable. And so residents like yourself and all the others that, you know, that I've been associated with me, but some of the others would be like Charlie Barron. He was one of the best men for pathology. Uh, in veterinary pathology. He was a, uh, a clear erudite speaker. He knew what he was saying.

He would question everybody and he and I were, um, What good friends, uh, professionally. And I really respect that, that like he wouldn't, if, if you were giving a talk on primates, you better not say monkey when you're talking about a gorilla and you darn well not talk about monkeys when you're playing with a slow lore, either.

Cause he would, he would speak up in the middle of a thing and give you heck or correct you. I thought that was darn good to put for the profession. I tried it a little bit, but I wasn't quite as smart as he was. So if it dealt with something in the necropsy room, I'd probably even give him even give him a little lip, but he was smart enough not to do that with me, I guess, but he was a wonderful man for the profession.

Then, you know, the what's who, who is doing all well, who was doing this? Or why did it start? Um, uh, cl Davis, Charlie Davis. I met him at Chicago. He, and, uh, at the meetings we used to go to and this whole thing, they, if I, they ACV piece started, uh, at the continuing education center, they're way out in the boonies from downtown Chicago, but it was a wonderful meeting.

Uh, and I met him there and one of the best things I ever learned from the fellow was, uh, if it's green, it's not TB. Cause he, he recalled that he had never seen a positive case of TB that was green pus. And I thought that was, uh, that's, that's helpful, well forth for almost 40 years with me. Uh, there's a little.

Little niche in that right now, our little, little, um, it might not hold all of the time, but pretty close. So I, that would be one of my cliches that I would use in teaching. If it green screen, it's not to be another good cliche. Like that would be a, if it ain't from and ain't pneumonia. And of course I apologize being a Cornell professor from my English, but.

You all got the point. If it ain't from innate pneumonia

Meuten *that was just some John King isms.*

King Uh, and, um, like being full of as a Christmas Turkey or something like that. Full of beans as a Christmas Turkey. Yeah. I don't use them quite as much as I used to. Cause I don't know. Who's going to find fault with them.

Uh, I mean I'm not a beer drinker, so should I take a. So should I take a umbrage at somebody saying, uh, um, beer, beer commercials or something like that, or being a, what is it? The Milwaukee brewers. I mean, why do I care about beer, wine named them brewers? You know, people are getting silly at what they get touchy about.

So I don't want to do that. Um

Meuten *But Charlie Davis and startıng the*

King Charlie Davis. Yeah. Well, he didn't have anything to do with starting it except being the inspiration for it. So the guy that we really should really think who has done more for continuing education in the world now, not at Cornell, not at Ohio, not at North Carolina, but in the world.

And in general in the United States would be Sam Thompson. I remember him. He was a kind of a Martin net because he was in the army and these army guys, they're all like that. You know, they learn how to Sloot and they spend the rest of your life saluting. And I think some of them want you to, even when they're out of the army.

And so Josh with him about that. And I don't think we ever clicked our heels together. That was too Prussian for him, I guess, but I bet he would have appreciated it now. And then, but Sam has done so much for all of us. He made this available to you and I, it's a nice little break from the stinking post-mortem room.

If it's a hot sunny day, wherever we are in the summer.

Meuten *Yes.*

King And therefore he has done more than anybody and, uh, you might not. Like his way all the time. Because when this all started, the cl Davis started, I think for the first several years, I gave seven out of the 12 talks. And at first there was just a few, uh, it free cheer, you know, every month they had a meeting and sunset or what's that place in New Jersey.

I already forgot it. Somerset. Somewhere near there. And I would drive down from Cornell with half a dozen people or four people. And, uh, I'd give the talk for four hours, or I guess it was four hours and I'd just show COTA Combs for hours and say what I thought. Cause these guys had never seen a lot of dogs and cats and cows and horse stuff.

So I would do that and I always enjoyed it. I didn't get paid for it. And, uh, uh, I'm not even sure he paid, uh, he paid the expenses, but it didn't matter in those days we were doing it. And it was a good thing. Cause I was teaching my students cause you know what I showed down there and Somerset, I wouldn't show at Cornell or something like that.

And that worked out very, that was very nice. Uh, then when he started out in Chicago, I went out there and gave maybe three or four year out there and he paid for all this. I mean, uh, for that trip, cause that was Cornell probably wouldn't want to do that. I didn't want to push my luck too hard. And I went out there and, uh, did the same thing.

So I think all of us while everybody, and then when, uh, Charlie Baron died, all of his books were given to, uh, Charlie Davis. I mean, to the foundation and most of them were bound. Charlie, Charlie barons were, and Sam gave them to me to give to either Cornell or somebody else who wanted them. Well, See if he's that nice to give him to Cornell Cornell doesn't need them.

Cause everybody who dies in New York shipping books to Cornell, you know, so they were all sent to Latvia. Now, Cornell paid for the transportation, but there was thousands of dollars involved in just sending the darn things and a sale Davis

Meuten *Where they go?*

King Latvia and Lithuania. Um, can't remember if it's one or the other, cause it wasn't Estonia, but it's Stony.

Meuten *Why was that?*

King They didn't ask, I guess. So I only sent it to the people who asked, but Sam gave me all of the, all of the books and they were bound and uh, just, you know, the, uh, American, I mean the vet path journal and all that, they were all sent over there. So in Sam's glad for that because you know, no sense wasting them at Cornell.

Meuten *Hmm.*

King Uh, let's see. Who else? I don't know.

Meuten *You work with any of those folks or it was mostly at meetings that only overlap.*

King Yeah. I had much to do with them. Yeah. Uh, Leon Saunders, I Oh, He has been, he is a perfectionist, he's a pain in the butt at times for that, but he's wonderful. And because he's so competent, I liked him at times.

I argue with them. I mean, not too much professionally, but he's a purist. And these, uh, he actually gave me heck within a month or two ago because it took me 15 years to read the history of Russian. The veteran medicine of Russia? Well, I had a copy of the book. I don't know where it went, but I got another copy and I read it and reading a lot of dry 42 letter names of, uh, you know, whatever it was kind of dry.

So I forgot them, but it was a very interesting book cause he's a fabulous writer, uh, Leon and he's, you know what the heck he was? He's almost 80 or something now. And he's no kid. So, uh,

Meuten *It's actually a fireball.*

King Yeah. And he's a wonderful man. So you could learn from him and he started the journal, you know, the ACV P journal.

Meuten *What does he think of your photos? He like your coat of crumbs.*

King I never heard him complain. Hmm. I don't know if everybody likes the blue background. I do, because there's nothing biologically blue except. Your eyes, aren't their green jealous, but there's not much too much as blue. So that's why I chose that background and I didn't choose it arbitrarily.

Uh, I took lots of pictures, were black, red, green, whatever. And I asked many people what was the best background. And I got out of most of them that blue was the best for the things others say, Oh no black while I don't know, I liked blue. And I said, well, why not use it?

Meuten *I asked that question mostly because of his, a perfectionist aside.*

And hero's big and just put this back, specimen down, take a picture.

King Yeah. Cause that's how we saw it. And I didn't mind highlights. I still don't mind highlights cause that's how you see them. Um, but I remember arguing with him, Oh, this is a great thing. Out of Chicago, we had the, uh, he was always keen on eyes, Leon Saunders and he was keen on eyes and he said, Uh, Oh, you have to do all this special fixation and all this stuff like that.

And I said to her, cause I did eyeballs and sure you have an artifact here and there, but I didn't worry about them too much. I mean, if it had an inclusion bodies and some of those cells, it was distemper is nobody's, that's not hard to do so what, anyhow, we also have eyeballs and he told everybody how to cut the culottes and do it all properly.

So I went down in Hudson. We had 12 pigs to autopsy. That means 24 eyeballs. You're all killed quick. And I put them in S acid, um, our boons and alcoholic, uh Zenker's and formalin and none. Uh, didn't put any calcium chips, neutral formula and stuff like that. I put them in this whole battery of, of uh fixatives and then we cut them all in and we had the, almost everybody was around.

Including the eyeball people evaluate them, which was best, which was best. They couldn't decide. So what's that mean to me? Little smell. That's all you need. And I think I might've set Leon Saunders world back a little bit, but I was willing to argue with him and, uh, John stopped fidgeting and, uh, So that ended up like that.

And I told him that, but he's never really complained to me. All of a sudden we have an older son, short course every year at Cornell this year will probably be the last year. Cause I'm leaving it unless somebody picks it up at Cornell. I doubt if they will. Um, they didn't like the way I did it, but now I wrote him a note and said, well, I'll let you guys do it now.

And I don't think anybody's going to pick it up. Well, that tells you one thing. And, uh, and I tell them all off, I say, they're lazy, but it's, um,

Meuten *Getting helps.*

King Yeah, it does. Yeah. And they're very cooperative after that. And, uh, but, uh, Leon was in on the, uh, establishing the Oleson metal in general diagnostic pathology, research and teaching, or general diagnostic pathology, teaching and research.

And he came up to Cornell. One day when we're establishing it with the one of the past deans, we had my, one of my chairman's were there and, uh, no sense of naming people, but

Meuten *Yeah.*

King And, uh, dr. Crook was there and several others and somebody said, well, they expect to get the oldest in metal someday. And he wasn't a basic diagnostic pathologist.

He wasn't, uh, Research a yes, but molecular biology stuff.

Meuten *Yeah.*

King And Sandra says, well, I've been the head of research at a big commercial or industrial company industry, and a Smith claimed French, I guess. And he says, and I have yet to see anything. Those guys have turned out that was worth something. And he really put him down.

Meuten *Huh?*

King The research is his laboratory. He didn't tell my guy off, but he was telling him, you know, around the side that it was, you know, they haven't done much for veterinary pathology, these basic researches for human stuff, getting grant money. But even it hasn't been that great. And every time you get too many PhDs in a system like Cornell or any others on the faculty, what do they teach?

Or what if times get rough right now, money is being pinched. If those guys don't have money, what can they do in research? Because they're not getting money, what can they do in teaching veterinary students or, or service? You know, necropsies not a darn thing worthwhile, or they can give a lecture. Cause we do have one guy who gave PCRs a what's that PCR.

Meuten *Are you asking me quiz questions? quiz questions,*

King PCR, you know? Yeah. What the, what reaction? Yeah.

Preliminary has I forget, but I listened and I actually got something out of it. So he was, I didn't get the name. Uh, but I was impressed.

Meuten *Write it down.*

King Yeah. I better do that PCR. Yeah. And I thought that was very nice.

But after five minutes, what else would he have to give to us? As veterinarians as veterinary pathologists, nothing. And, um, and, but that's what the bucks are. Cause I think our Dean, for instance, he gets, if we get a million dollars from the, the army, if they were crazy enough to give us a million dollars for research, the Dean gets 600,000 of it.

Meuten *Hmm*

King Cause that's their overhead or whatever they have to pay for their share of toilet paper and paper clips and pencils and water, whatever. And I understand that a little bit, but fender medicine couldn't do it itself. Cause we got lots of stuff. The MD types don't have a clue about

Meuten *A FIP is hosting us, but this clearly is not very linear.*

King I don't understand.

Meuten *Well just as we work our way through other topics. Yeah. It started off with the people. And then that was with the toilet paper scenario.*

King I don't know.

Meuten *We tend to wander*

King yeah.

Meuten *Conversation.*

King Okay. Yeah. Well get me back in line

Meuten *And I wanted to stay on the people part of it and finish up with Saunders and see who Sunderland dimension.*

King Saundra's great. Uh, and all of you, you can't forget your wives. My wife, she's 50 years next year. And, uh, it's been wonderful. It couldn't be better and you need somebody, you know, it's supposed to be 50 50. She might say it's 90 10 in my favor, but I don't think it's that bad, but I admit it. Uh, there's a joke goes around sometime.

They call her Saint Saint Marie for some reason. And I don't have a reason. I don't have a guest.

Meuten *We all know*

King St. Marie

Meuten *Did you ever, uh, do you participate in her birdwatching and that's hers?*

King I take her there and every now and then if there's the rare bird alert and she's got to travel 300 miles North.

Uh, ever see a great gray I'll sit in the pool and just turn his head around like that. What a stupid thing to do. And his 400,000 people all watching this stupid bird turning his head around because he was blown 4,000 miles off his track, you know, but I had a driver up there, but on the way up, some kid gave a fabulous talk on the Monarch, butterflies and their migration route to Mexico and stuff.

So I learned something. So I didn't mind doing that, but that's about the only way. She went to the Antarctic. And who do you think paid the renters rent downstairs that she collects. And, uh, and then she went to the Danube and she saw all the birds there and she's been every place in the world. She's one of them.

She's the keenest birder going.

Meuten *She says she is the Saint to tolerate you. And she's a very lovely person.*

King Thanks. Okay. Now what

Meuten *I haven't been able, I feel to get you to say enough about some of the, uh, early recognition of the diseases are those that you really had a part of. And, uh, nobody would believe you're humble, but I've got to get you to bring out some of that, uh, information*

King If it was, uh, if I had studied it and tried to make the answer, I would think I was smart, but I didn't study these things.

So. Give me a hint as to which ones you want. I don't care.

Meuten *Well, the world to judge whether or not you were smart as somebody outside of this room, but, um, uh, we covered the brain heart. What about the vitamin K induced renal toxicosis or red maple or a Brown dog? Gutter. Uh,*

King Oh, myo met a pleasure. That was Sam Thompsons.

Uh, the Brown granules in the dogs that you see in the gut it'll make a. Uh, it used to be called maple sugar intestine and knock nibble did this back in 1918, I believe, or 1923. He a biliary officially the dogs and all her guts became Brown, but us Brown, good Brown to be as Brown as this, uh, this chair.

Um, and then it gets lighter like the rug and, uh, then you can barely see it. Well, I graded them one to six. This would be a six. The rug would be about a four. And I could see a two, I couldn't see a one, one was always histological, but Sam called him leiomyoma metaplastic and he wrote it up originally like that.

And I had a hundred cases, but then Don Cortez came along from, uh, New Zealand and he went, he was at, he was a Connecticut of all places. You were there for a while, weren't you?

Meuten *Yeah. Then current again.*

King Yeah. And he did his PhD on it to show that it was a vitamin E deficiency. A thing. So, but I had already had a hundred cases and I reported on it somewhere, but, uh, mine was just cause I saw it like that.

It was a fantastic disease. And then I didn't see it from 1960 until about 1968. It disappeared. I don't know where, and then you just see a few cases every now and then as a vitamin E thing. Okay. What's what's the other one you asked?

Meuten *Uh, vitamin K toxicosis and vitamin K. Is that a real, is that a real thing?*

King Yes, that's a real thing. Some veterinarian back in 19 early seventies, he had, uh, treated a horse and the horse got sicker than heck, and he didn't know why. And it had blood in the urine and all this stuff. And, uh, he didn't tell me why, but I autopsied the horse four years later because it went downhill.

And my autopsy, they had the funniest kidney disease. I didn't know what it was. And it was segmental. It was a segmental, pigmentation and fibrosis. And that was the first clue that I ever had of single dose renal disease. And I usually. For anybody in the audience for, or liver, what causes PostNet chronic scarring.

If I pushed you and asked you while I'm not quizzing you here, but I would ask my kids, my kids remember some of my kids are 40, 45 years old. You know, when they come to be a resident or something

Meuten *You referred to as a kid now.*

King And I would ask them, well, how do you explain if you're looking at the whole kidney?

This area is damaged. This area damage in this area is partly damaged while you must explain it in my humble opinion, because it is humble.

Meuten *Of course.*

King Yeah. Unless you want to fight it. And, uh, and that is that you have, you know, five vessels going to any part of your liver, 5,000,005, 5,500, whatever number you want.

But let's for easy numbers. In my mind, you could five vessels. How many of them are working any one time

Meuten *Three*

King Three. So if the poison is only exposed to the kidney or the liver for, you know, 20 seconds after you have ingested it or inject, injected it, whatever it'll affect this area, that area in that area.

And won't hurt these areas. And if it's enough and severely toxic enough, it only went there, there, and there, and really damaged it. And you'll get these areas of necrosis or pigmentation, like in the kidney. If it's absorbed, goes to the kidney quickly and then. It's diluted and unheard anymore. Then you'll see this single dose effect.

And that's what makes this post, the chronic, uh, liver and post degenerate kidney. And the same goes for vitamin K. Cause that's what happened in these vitamin K horse. He was getting foundered and the veterinarian loaded them in years after I send it out as chronic renal disease, multifocals, something like that.

Pigment attorney . He told me he did it. Well, subsequent to that rebuke and Everett, everybody else has proven it. You need a degree of dehydration to get it. Uh, probably the horse was dehydrated. I don't know, but I imagine so we see it and it's, it explains a single dose effect. Very well. Here's you're working at what you want to ask about, right?

Meuten *Here's your common. New and different ideas and lesions and domestic animals. And gosh, I don't know how many pages it is*

King But it's far too many to discuss, but maybe you see one you like to know about

Meuten *There's some, there are some in here that I know that you've highlighted. What about the shipping fever of horses?*

King The Australians just work that out. I would usually ask my, my students and never, well, what's the most common cause of pneumonia in New York state. And I could ask you that cause you were up there for awhile and it would be shipping fever, pneumonia of horses, where they tie the horses head in such a way that he cannot throw his head and snort and clean his nose like you and I.

I guess, you know, if you're real farmer, you can do it with your thumb or however you do it and then snort and you'll, you'll, uh, clean your darn sinuses or whatever. Think you do well. That's what happens to the horse. Any Australians actually did that and proved that if you hold a head in a position, they can't do it.

The postnasal drip will drip into the lungs. If there's not a lot of dust on the ride, then you'll get a little bit of inhalation cranial eventually. And it's a fabulous entity. Uh,

Meuten *Now when you cover this, when you go through your Kodachromes*

King Yes. Because it's something new and different, and it is the single most common cause of pneumonia and horses in New York state that doesn't hurt them very much unless it's lots of material they bring down and then you'll get a good inhalation pneumonia, and always secondary to that.

Uh, I love the fight. This one for anybody is the most common cause of inhalation of empyemia, which is pissing. The chest anywhere is a ruptured lung abscess. Now I say that without reading the history. I say that without knowing ahead of time, if I see the lesion, it's going to end payment. That's a difficult one too, to teach all the interns and residents.

The problem there is we have new residents and interns every year and they come from every Podunk university, Ohio, North Carolina. I haven't got one of my proteges, one of my spies in there teaching them this stuff you got to, the clinicians will come and say, Oh, that sounds like bull who's ever heard of that.

And then you have to start at square one again, for them.

Meuten *We had a calf with a big pulmonary abscess and I had left it at that and he said, well, what'd you find? And I said about pulmonary abset yes. And you made me and you participate in it, uh, pass all the puss and so forth through a sieve.*

King You remember that?

Meuten *Sure. Yeah. And an old hall.*

King Old hall. Fantastic. You got a good memory for it.

Meuten *Well, there was a lot of stress at that time and I think that's the other reason people remember that.*

King That's great. Well, I made some impression on you.

Meuten *Oh, it makes people a believer too.*

King Yeah

Meuten *It doesn't take too many.*

King We did that sewer colander.

Yeah.

Meuten *Yeah.*

King Found the old house

Meuten *Seems like with red maple when they was first. Observing it in New York, I seem to recall, bud tended about, had it down to that. It was a mix up in the some fertilizer. He got mixed into some feed and they hadn't maps up and we're tracing it through new England and New York.*

And we're just about ready to incriminate the company.

King That turned out as we all know it was red maple, but it always followed storms. Real good storms. The leaves wilted to make this lesion. And when I looked at it, I said, it's a pigmentary nephrosis and something damaged the blood. I didn't know what it was.

Cause all I got was a biopsy in those first few cases. And then we said, no, it's a poisoning. And uh, one of the, and finally somebody believed it because when the farmer brought in the tree, he said, well, the horse was eating this and he gave it to them and they fit it. Darn. If they didn't get the lesion, I wasn't in on that part of it.

So it's not me, uh, uh, which is okay. And I don't mind not being in on it, except that I said it was a poisoning because that's what make this pigmentary nephrosis. And that, that turned out pretty good. We're lucky on that one.

Meuten *I guess our vet students getting enough exposure to vet path today, especially in terms of using it as you just did as a investigative tool.*

King I don't think so because , they're taught case-based things and so much detail that I don't think they're getting enough, uh, because they can't ask the tutor. Who's teaching that cause he's probably not a veterinarian. And so therefore they're probably getting cheated a little bit. Maybe, maybe not. And maybe it does make them read more material.

But Donald,

Meuten *Yeah*

King This is a book and I don't care what book it is. And you've got the price on it.

Meuten *That's against your signature inside of it.*

King They're all very good.

Meuten *Yes.*

King Okay. Uh, now I hand that to you and you're a sophomore student or junior, senior, whatever. And I say, well, you'll get the information in here.

And what do you think of all that info?

King There's it all gospel you bet. Cause I,

Meuten *however, I'm glad you beat me to the answer.*

King Very good. Because you know, darn well, some of this stuff is absolutely wrong. And is one, if you look in there and on, the nose of the cow has got little cysts, I said, I saw it in Mulligan Terrell fever, where you can see it in any cow. You look at it. If you look enough cows, I mean, not any cow, but you can see it incidentally. And I have no idea what caused it, but had nothing to do with me willingly Tarrel fever, except the first case, uh, first few cases or something. Cause when you want to see it, million Terrell fever, you'll look at all the rest of them, Charles fever or something for the same thing, low and Bo, but you won't look at the other ones in between, and then you'll see it in the next one. Hey, Terrell fever lesion. And it wasn't. So that's what I mean. That's what happens in a. And some of these pictures, but you as an undergraduate, you don't know which ones, if I gave you the study, you would have to learn every one of these as gospel. Cause you don't know it isn't gospel and you didn't bring it to a guy like meals. Well, that's junk. That's baloney. This is absolutely crazy. And that's what they're missing.

Meuten *It's, it's perfect that you just went through that in that way for the camera, because that's how you taught us pathology as sophomores, we all had to by Jones and hunt, I think it was a requirement.*

King Smithton right.

Miss Ms. Jones. And we'd bring it to class and he'd say, okay, open up a certain chapter, and then she'd start telling us what the X out, what to believe, what was BS, what was bunk?

King Yeah

I can remember my classmate Marina and I were sitting there saying, I don't believe this guy is better than the book he's going through here and tell us what to believe and what not to believe. But part of it also was that he added the perspective to what was so rare. Call me collect if you ever see it and what real common things that you are going to see, where were

Meuten *we're going through here? We just went through another*

King right. Dorsal colitis. That'll worth the comments about stretch, stretch ulcers.Yeah. This isn't a sexism thing on women, is it? Oh, I wasn't even on stage when he said that. Cause I know I'll get blamed for it.

Meuten *That's the nice thing about being here with you. That's right. That's who they'll remember?*

King Ah, yeah, the right dorsal colitis was, uh, dr. Tom Vaughan. He was at Cornell for those few years, uh, making a self more, wanted as a Dean down in Auburn. And that's why he went to Cornell. I think. Cause then when they lost him, they knew what they lost. Cause I thought he was a gentlemen. Good Southern gentleman. Did you ever shake hands when it's done? He was out, he had it muscle and stronger than Rick Rickman's. Yep. That's the other fellow to consider him and Rick, anyhow, he sent me a horse over and I say, well, he, we did the autopsy. I run a, I'm a little hard on the postpartum room because if you don't, the clinicians will start telling you when to do the post and stuff like that. And then it all goes to heck in a handbasket. Yeah. So, uh, he sent the horse over and did it and beautiful small colon. And I say, well, somebody sculpted it. And, but nobody could explain how they could get the, the hot water scald all the way down to the small intestine to the right doors for the colon. And then it turns out though, and I didn't know this, that prostate glands involved and prostate gland in his high concentration in that area. I don't know why. I don't know the basics for some of these things as it isn't a duodenoscope. So in both the fools, you get enfolds, you get the burn in the epithelial portion of the stomach and in the duodenum. Whereas in horses, you get it in the right dorsal, colon, anytime you lose mucosa, as you know, you can take that gut and do that, and you'll stretch connective tissue. Cause there's no mucosa and it'll tear because it's just a Dematis. And you'll get these stretch ulcers. There are any mortem because you can see the edges are trying to heal and all that, but it's a new and different lesion. And that's why I have it. And what's new here. The band, I mean, a band, I mean, are Buddhists, all it is a nonsteroidal. I don't know which they are when I went to Australia and showed these, Oh, those guys all get down on me in a hurry. And one vet in Western New York said he cussed a little bit. My wife said don't cuss today's so I'm being very careful. And he gave me Holy heck in front of the whole audience because I say this band, I mean, did it. And, uh, and I had the gross lesion there to show him. And, uh, he says, Oh, cussed a little bit. I use that stuff like, like water. Well, you don't use that stuff like water in dehydrated animals. Cause now. I think who's, uh, who's the girl veterinarian at the lady veterinarian, excuse me. No, the other one. Uh, who's not there at Creech gun. Yeah, Diane. Yeah, she was the one who published it. Uh, but we had seen it for a long time before, but we just didn't publish it on the band. I mean the right dorsal colon, she did good work on that. And we, they reproduced it at school too. So it's a nice lesion.

Meuten *Hey, while we're talking about diseases, what's right. What's wrong with the Bible. What's it say about trophic rhinitis.*

King We see it and trophic in Taiwan or at, even at, uh, in Ethica, Cru changed the diet on the pigs and we don't see it anymore. So that's pretty good. I think it is nutritional. If you look at it, trophic rhinitis is bilaterally symmetrical. And how many infections have you ever had mumps as an adult? You probably got one big, uh, one big, uh, male go net. And one little one. Why not both. It's not bilaterally symmetrical many in most infections. Aren't bilaterally symmetrical. So why does say everybody say trophic rhinitis? Is, and for that reason, in many times you see trophic rhinitis, you section the consci or whatever the turbinates, and you don't see any inflammation. Now somebody says, Oh, it's Pasteurella toxin or something like that. I don't happen to believe it, but every time I present it, I tell people the two things and I know everybody. I know everybody wants to make its board to teller or Pasteurella or something like that. I just can't accept it. And I don't yet, but I'm almost open-minded Leonard had some controversial opinion, always has, and probably always will. But the crook Lennon, Cru. Yeah, he's a, he's still there and he comes in every day. Although he's retired, he, uh, is pretty, I, I need, I need him. I like him. Because I send all the kids, the residents over with any bone problems.

Meuten *So he still looks at the bone lesions.*

King Yup. If you ask them again, when you get older, you get a little more crotchety.

Meuten *Yeah.*

King People are a little afraid of you, just like I'm worried about becoming, you know because I get a little more set in my ways. I don't believe them. That's not quite fair to them, but I don't know what to do about it. That's age.

Meuten *If you looked at Leonard and certainly think of the bones, and you said the other specialists are the different systems that she could.*

King I include him in that specialty.

Yes.

King The fact is I still include them as a Cornell attribute.

Meuten *What would you like to be remembered for, uh, in the field of veterinary pathology?*

King I cared enough to be mean to you, so you should learn. I don't give a dang if you believe me or not, as long as you've learned it, because then you will be you'll remember it. And I think it's good information. I don't know what else to say to a question like that, but I didn't mind being mean, I dread it a little bit for the people I've turned off, but if I really turned them off because that's real life, you know, someone's going to tell you to go fly a kite. I mean, in the real world, that's, you're full of beans yourself. Dr. Mutan.

Meuten *Um, have they come back to say thanks to you some years later,*

King every now and then somebody does point out and makes your day, week and months easy after months. I forget it

Meuten *but perhaps justifies the next encounter. Torture.*

King Yes.

Meuten *So teaching certainly is one of your greatest influences on the profession.*

King I would hope so. I've worked at it. But I've also been very selfish because I know my way has been the best and you know, that's full of beans, but I pushed it because I really thought it was the best if I didn't. Why would I be stupid and do that? Yeah. But I would have won more friends if I had been a little bit nicer, but I had no, I mean, I don't. Yeah. I don't know how to handle that either.

Meuten *Did you have, uh, goals along the way to be something other than what you are? chairperson?*

King Oh, no, I didn't want to be a chairperson. I know I'm too hard nose for that. Cause if you didn't work as hard as I did, I'd probably be upset. I'd try to make your work as hard as I did. Yeah. Cause there's no excuse. Like I washed up the Postmortal many other days after show and tell six 30 at night show and tell, I come back at eight 30 and nobody had cleaned it up. So I saw I'm not against work, but I was a little ticked off at everybody, but one of them was a Spanish fellow and I think I'd already told him, well, the guy's coming back in to clean it. And he didn't. So I did because I'm proud of the postmortem room, even as old as it's getting. But I'm still proud of their darn place. It's usually pretty darn nice. Anyhow, I have, I need specimens for show and tells to for the oldest son, of course, coming up in August and other places. Yeah. Well,

Meuten *we haven't mentioned the, uh, show and tell that goes on the road. I actually take the van, load it up with. How many buckets, five-gallon buckets,*

King probably 1500 pounds of guts. And I go, we always hope never to have an accident, at least a really bad one. Cause they're going to try and put this big heart in me. Cause I'm the oldest son, the little cat heart and the little girl and went with us here, you know, cause her ear is over there. What if we have that kind of accident? Gosh, forbid. But anyhow, that's something that has gone over very well. And I do all the driving because I like driving. But we sing. And one year we had Germans, French, Spanish people. We sang every song from Jack in the original language, you know, stuff like that. And it's a good trip on the East coast drive. We stopped at the animal medical center on Sunday afternoon, put it all in there, icebox, 20, 20 big buckets like that. And then, uh, the next morning at, uh, eight o'clock, we have a show and tell until noontime, the kids who go with me six, seven, or eight of them. For whatever. Uh, they go and visit the animal medical center or in town, but they better be back at 12 cause I'm leaving at 12 and we pack it all back. It goes in clots and uh, in the paper, plastic bags and inside these big plastic containers. And then we haul that and then we go to the new Bolton center and from the new Bolton center to Blacksburg, to Raleigh your place. And then. Athens Georgia, and then Tifton, Georgia, and Florida. And we have a show and tell every day and you guys always carry the, get the ice forests. We put them in a plastic bag on top because we should have a refrigerated van say,

Meuten *what's it smell like by Florida?*

King Uh, but every night we put it in the refrigerator and it comes out cold in the morning for show and tells. And in a lot of time, it stays cool. But it's not as good as the old fashioned clots with chloral hydrate, which is difficult to get. And this last year we went to a and they, and you guys always take care of all my expenses except for the van. And I get a week off and, uh, Cornell pays for the van. I don't know if they know that. Uh, well, my chairman will never see this probably so. I'm not sure he'll somebody will tell them, they'll show it to them. They'll lie. It's way over there.

Meuten *When you get to Florida, is that where you don't leave it? Yeah.*

King But on the way you guys, sometimes you save stuff. Let me take your stuff on, take ours on down and that's good. Or I'll photograph it. Cause I'll bring it even back and photograph it. If I didn't believe you, what you told me and I can't prove it at the time I show and tell it, I'll cut it in and prove you're right or wrong. Anyhow. Yeah. This time we went to Columbus, Ohio. Uh,

Meuten *how'd? They like it.*

King Oh, they all like it. Oh, everybody. I haven't, it, they all said to come back. So I've been back several times to all, and then Knoxville was Slawson and Oh yeah, we go two months in Starkville. I would be in Smith and still in Starksville. Yeah. His home is down there, but he comes here every summer. But he's retired from teaching Clinton path. Oops, sorry, touching that machine. And then we go to Baton Rouge. They always have a crayfish boil, broil boil. I don't know. And, uh, for, for all of us in beer. And, uh, then we go down by the Gulf of Mexico. Remember this last time we had three Spaniards with us. They had never seen the Gulf of Mexico. So we all walk out. And the Gulf of Mexico and then get back in the car and run like heck to Tuskegee. I stayed with a guy in Alabama who was in the army with me in 1946. Oh my goodness. Hadn't seen him in 50 years.He's got a veterinarian for daughter and he's a friend of Tom Vaughn's. So we stayed two nights with him and then we went to Tifton cause at the Southeastern path meeting, we go to, and

Meuten *so you do a show and tell at Tifton?*

King Yes. And we do that at their diagnostic laboratory in Tifton, after the steak dinner on Saturday night. And they always welcomed me. So I'm not too obnoxious, I don't think, but everybody's scared of me in our post-mortem room when they get through. I don't think I've ever had a group say that or. I think most of them would say, it's the best rotation they've had in the vet school for two weeks of learning hard work. Cause I don't let the seniors out. I mean, we have, we have a 24-hour service every night and weekends. I mean, when they're on duty, they're stuck two weeks and the post, one of them, they hate it when they get there. Cause they've heard all these bad things, but I'm such an angel. Why don't they all love me, you know? And uh, but they don't when they start, most of them do when they finish. Because sure. I joke with him, I kid him, and stuff like that.

Meuten *But you go to the necropsy lab every day still.*

King Oh, almost every day. Sure.

Meuten *But would they still have someone else quote on duty?*

King Oh yeah. Cause I'm not on duty all the time. Like almost like I used to be, cause I kind of refuse. Uh, I go out there and I look and if they don't, if any of them get, you know, and the faculty gets tough about it. I just back off and look at it and won't say anything to anybody, but the students will come and bug me. And it's the wage or the residents.

Sure.

King Yeah. And that's okay. I don't really, I'm not there to hurt anybody. I'm just there to say. Why, why don't you think of that? You know, like in Pima we had him pay me, dad. They said, no, it's, it didn't have a lung abscess. They didn't feel the whole thing alone. And I, I don't give the faculty, heck I'll give that resident heck and they know I will, but they like it. Most of them like it because they know I'm trying to teach them. I think. I don't do it as nice as they think I should maybe, but you have to should be truck drivers. I have an application, a whole blank of them that you can tear off and write in and get an application. Are we getting the message?

Meuten *Yeah. That it's starting to come to an end. You've indicated if I asked you how you wanted to be remembered professionally. It was for the teaching.*

King I think of necropsy.

Meuten *And how about pathology personally? I hope the person,*

King I hope my son loves me when I'm dead and my wife too.

Meuten *you had a chance to go through this dance again. What would you do differently and what would you keep?*

King Just being nice. I'd be a little bit nicer to the family. I'd do the same thing again. I don't think as much. I probably keep my mouth shut a little more. Cause it's. I can't make a big dent when the rest of the faculty all wants I'm in a research instrument or something. And I don't think it's worthwhile or a new faculty member. I think they're dodos we shouldn't get them. Somebody came up for tenure not long ago. I said, but he's not a veterinarian. He doesn't teach veterinary students. And he was supposed to have done this and that. And I say, no, well, my mine's only one vote. He didn't get it. But there are 14 others who gave it to him. Well, I'm known for being, for saying that and cause it's how I feel, but they're nice people. I mean, if he was in some other department, I'd vote for him, certainly, but not in veterinary pathology where it doesn't work. That's really being hard. Cause it's not his fault. It's whoever hired him in the first place, his fault,

Meuten *uh, dr. Coggins often said that we seem to end up with it. Two different groups or two different populations when we have the non-DVMs and DVMs at the veterinary college. Is that how you say, how did you feel?*

King Hey, how are we Evans at school? Do you know? Yeah. Oh yeah, man. Yeah. If you want to know about why what, here's a fish, it's dead and you want to know, he wouldn't know why it was dead. He wouldn't know. But he knows that's a bottom feeder and that's how that's where his lips are going down on the bottom. And the others got like this. He knows that kind of stuff, which makes your work as a pathologist better, but why do we need 36 of them on the faculty? I mean, one of those guys and he knows snakes, he knows birds, and that's what we should have. And if you want more of them prevent, prevent pre. But our people don't realize that cause they think, Oh, all these molecular biologists and get all the research funds. Slossen with a 13 faculty member, one Ph.D. faculty member, uh, he's got as much reefers research funds as our department has and he's doing wonderful. So there is money for veterinarians, a few. Now it's not $742 million for five years or something. But nobody's starving to death there.

Meuten *I wonder if dr. Evans could start his class off today, the way he, uh, Uh, started it off. How was that? In 1970, when I have eight, he passed a bone around, through the class, and then we had to identify it. And of course, it was that immediate. And I think that was part of Cornell's education for so many of the people that were there were this question and answer. Uh, and then no one knew, and it was the us penis of a walrus. And I don't know if he could start it off that way today.*

King No, you couldn't. That's sexist and somebody would say something about it. And that's, that's a reminds me of the S penis and the, uh, secretaries. Did you want to capture that one? As we conclude it would be, it would be a nice, humorous way to end it, but if you don't want it.

King I know, I understand whether or not, because this is national television.

Meuten *We're at the end. You go ahead and say something that you wanted to, uh, conclude with. Cause I've certainly enjoyed this and you know, how much I respect you. And, uh, without a doubt, your teaching method, as unique as it might be, it's right.*

King I'm honored that you had me for such an occasion, but I'm also giving somebody credit. I'm not quite sure who that they picked a wonderful young man too. Grill the old man, so to speak. And I thank you very much for it. And I think the whole organization, all of our fellows on the machines and the bright lights and all that. Thank you very much.

Meuten *Good. Thank you.*

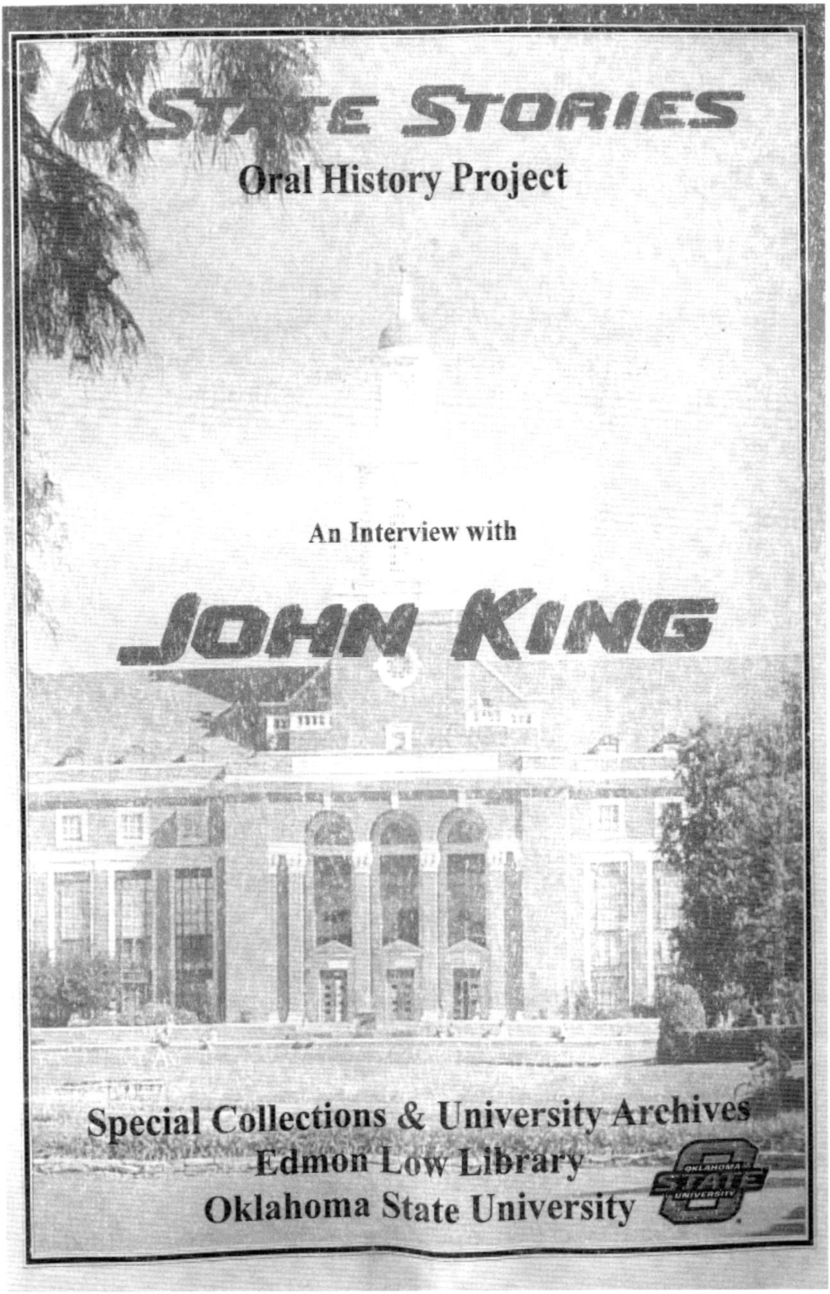
O-STATE STORIES

Oral History Project

An Interview with

JOHN KING

Special Collections & University Archives

Edmon Low Library

Oklahoma State University

Oral History Interview

with

John King

Interview Conducted by
Jennifer Paustenbaugh
October 31, 2008

O-STATE Stories
Oral History Project

Special Collections & University Archives
Edmon Low Library • Oklahoma State University

Interview History

Interviewer: Jennifer Paustenbaugh
Transcriber: Samantha Siebert
Editors: Latasha Wilson, Tanya Finchum

The recording and transcript of this interview were processed at the Oklahoma State University Library in Stillwater, Oklahoma.

Project Detail

The purpose of O-STATE Stories Oral History Project is to gather and preserve memories revolving around Oklahoma Agricultural and Mechanical College (OAMC) and Oklahoma State University (OSU).

This project was approved by the Oklahoma State University Institutional Review Board on October 5, 2006.

Legal Status

Scholarly use of the recordings and transcripts of the interview with John King is unrestricted. The interview agreement was signed on October 31, 2008.

O-STATE STORIES

AN ORAL HISTORY PROJECT OF THE OSU LIBRARY

About John King...

John M. King, a 1955 graduate of Oklahoma A&M College (OAMC) of Veterinary Medicine, is a veterinary pathologist. He was reared in Massachusetts and served a four year stint in the Army where he was paratrooper. He married in 1947 and with the support of his wife he earned an undergraduate degree from the University of Delaware. He then used the G.I. Bill to attend veterinary school at OAMC. He went on to earn a PhD from Cornell University and served faculties at Washington State University and Cornell.

Dr. King has lectured extensively around the world and across the United States in his specialty of veterinary pathology. He has published several editions of *The Necropsy Book* and the two volume set, *An Atlas of General Pathology*. A collection of his worldwide experiences is published in a volume *Have Knife, Will Travel, 1975-1998*, available at libraries at Cornell University and Oklahoma State University.

Over the course of his career of over 50 years he has taken over 50,000 photo images of pathologic specimens; many of these can be found on the "Dr. John M. King's Necropsy Show and Tell" website at http://w3.vet.cornell.edu/nst/ .

Dr. King has received numerous awards including a 2008 Distinguished Alumnus Award from the Oklahoma State University College of Veterinary Medicine.

John King

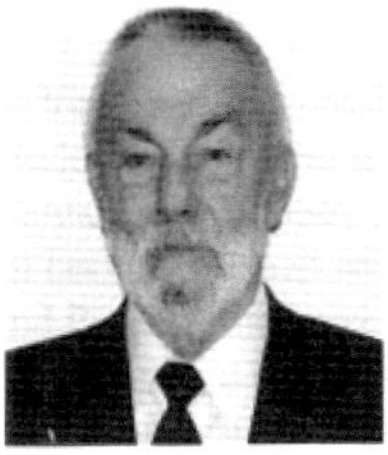

Oral History Interview

Interviewed by Jennifer Paustenbaugh
October 31, 2008
Stillwater, Oklahoma

Paustenbaugh *This is Jennifer Paustenbaugh and it is Friday, October 31, 2008. We are here in the Dean's Conference Room in the OSU Library. I am with Dr. John King, who is a distinguished alumnus of the College of Veterinary Medicine. I am also joined today by Dr. Sidney Ewing, an emeritus faculty member in the College of Veterinary Medicine, and Heather Moberly, the Veterinary Medicine librarian, who are here to assist me with this interview.*

Dr. King, thank you very much for taking time out of your busy schedule at this conference to join us today for this interview. I know that you were a graduate in 1955, and while most of our interview is going to focus on your time as a student here at OAMC and then your subsequent career, could you tell us a little bit about your family background, where you grew up, and any other information you'd like to share about your pre-OAMC days?

King I am honored that you are taking this information and that you think I'm worthy of it. Thank you very much. I was raised in Massachusetts and I don't remember much of my really young life. But when I was seven, I was sent to a boy's school because my folks had split up and I had no place to go. I had three older sisters, they went with the three aunts that we had, but I had to go someplace. So I went to this school for ten years. I saw my mother twice a year. And to this day, I thought it was wonderful and I had a good time there. I've had a good time most everywhere in my life. At that boys school, it was a farm school, you did all the jobs that you'd do at a farm, all the crops, all the harvesting, everything like this. And it was very worthwhile.

Then I had four years of the Army and those four years were a blessing because I got in the paratroopers. I made 50 bucks extra a month, that was fine. But the 48 months that I had in the Army, in the Service, the four years gave me 48 months of education under the G.I. Bill. And that's what I used primarily for the vet school. The pre-vet work I did in Delaware a little bit and I worked, and my wife was working. I got married in 1947 while I was still in the Service, and she kind of put me through the University of Delaware because I didn't want to use the G.I. Bill until I got into vet school.

Your kind Dean McElroy out here at the Veterinary School, he was a classmate of the Dean of Professional Students, those who wanted to go on to professional schools, he was a classmate of that Dean. And so I wrote to Oklahoma to get into vet school because Cornell wouldn't take me. They had just one from Delaware and Pennsylvania a year to go to Cornell. So he wrote to the Dean and to me, and said that, "If you want to come to Oklahoma, why don't you keep up your good grades, even come to Oklahoma, and possibly apply from Oklahoma?" I did that. I had a wonderful time doing it. I met the best man at my wedding, his family lived here in Broken Arrow, Oklahoma and it made a very good place for me to go on weekends to their little ranch. I incidentally picked up lots of Indian arrowheads on their property. That was nice.

When I got out here and met Dr. McElroy I had an interview here at the veterinary school and I made it. I think I made it mostly because I was a paratrooper in the Army and one of the faculty here was a paratrooper in the war. I was in the Army before the atom bomb went off, but I didn't get into any fighting. I had a good time in the Army too because I knew they couldn't shoot me, I was too fast, I was too young. So you can't shoot young men. Maybe the guy next to me, but not me. But anyhow I didn't have any problem with that, getting into vet school. Well I had a little problem—physics was a son of a gun. We had to take physics to get in in those days, and that was—I was not that smart. I had a good memory, but I was not that smart as a student. I had to work—every grade I got, I had to work for. I didn't get anything easily.

When I finished after five years here at Oklahoma A&M College, I think it's nice that it's changed in a way, but either way I was very proud. Our son was born here at the hospital, the older hospital in Stillwater. All in all a wonderful time in the vet school. Of course there was a little animosity somewhere along the line because every damn Yankee they accepted into the veterinary school kept out an Okie. And that wasn't looked at too nicely. But it happened and I was just so proud to get in.

Paustenbaugh *So were there any specific incidences along those lines that you recall?*

King Yeah. I wasn't the best cowboy in the class, but close to it because I would run horses around in the paddock that were all the ponies that the university bought for use, and I would get out there with the ponies and ride them bareback. But the only way I could get on was to get them running, then I could swing up on them, hang in their mane. But doing that, and there's eight, ten, fifteen ponies, I would swing sometimes too far and fall over on the other side between all these horse's legs. But it's interesting, the horses will not step on you if you're soft because they think it's a hole and they might break their leg. At least that's what I was told, and it worked out that way. So that was one of my better thoughts. The football games were wonderful. I was disappointed that Oklahoma A&M didn't beat OU, but that was part of life.

Paustenbaugh *When you lived here, did you live in Vet Village?*

King Oh, yes. I think they had a Vet Village, or they just, no it had to be there, because there were Army barracks. But the one we lived in was the south one, at least the one that was between the veterinary school and the main campus. Not the one up at the end of Knoblock. I didn't get to live up there. We were in the Army barracks between the vet school and the regular campus.

Paustenbaugh *So I take it your quarters at that time were pretty spartan?*

King They were wonderful. They were Army barracks, but they were wonderful. I have no complaint on that kind of stuff. Actually it was better because the buildings were being demolished slowly and I think after we left they didn't last very long, at least the ones down here, not up on vet village. We were able to do what we wanted in those buildings pretty much. I had a dog and I had a hole in the wall. I could let the dog out without going downstairs to let her out. She went out on her own and came back. So things like that. We had a good time.

Paustenbaugh *So you came to Oklahoma from Massachusetts via Delaware. What was your impression when you first got to Stillwater?*

King Oh my goodness, we're a long way from civilization! When we got out here, driving from wherever we drove, we went to Broken Arrow quite a few weekends, because that family had a lot of eggs and vegetables and things like that that they gave us. And the G.I. Bill of $105, I think it might have been $10 more than that when I was married, but we welcomed that kind of aid.

Paustenbaugh *Sure.*

King And also I was welcomed by the fellow who was in charge of the large animal clinic, [Dr. Woolf]. He gave me a job in the library in the veterinary school. It didn't pay very much, but every nickel counted in those days. He did it I think to help me, I'm not sure he needed it. But I thought it was wonderful of them to do that.

Paustenbaugh *What did this student job entail?*

King One or two hours a day I would go down to the library and either put the books away or work with papers or file them. It wasn't very much work. Of course, as a veterinary student, we worked in cleaning the stables and things like that [as part of the education]. But I was an eager little beaver and I think I learned a lot in veterinary medicine, but also in getting along with people, I learned a lot.

Paustenbaugh *Do you recall how many people were in your entering class?*

King Thirty-two.

Paustenbaugh *Thirty-two. And that was about typical for that time, wasn't it?*

King Yes, but we lost a lot of the students. I think we lost eight from our class; maybe there were 40 that started. But we lost eight, now that was an awful lot. But it made us prouder that we stayed in, the fewer that stayed and...

Ewing *These eight who were lost were academic casualties?*

King Yes. Some of it was intimidation in the sense that when you get in vet school, "Oh boy, I finally made it into vet school!" But you can't be too proud or you can't be too happy with that because you haven't passed any exams. When you pass the first exam, well you can't be too cocky because you have to get through another course. And then you still can't feel free, that you have made it. And I think it's four years of that that many of us worried about. And we actually thought about it. But some of the young people who are there, it scared them that they knew they were going to have to work. It was very hard. And a couple of them I actually know, they said, "We can't keep doing this anymore, it's just too much" and they left the school. And they hadn't even taken exams, well maybe one or two, but it was just too much studying. But most of us liked it. So it was just a few people.

Paustenbaugh *You mentioned that to get into the vet school you had to take physics and how difficult that was for you. Your first year, what was your most difficult class?*

King It was well organized. We knew what we had to do. I don't remember anything really that bugged me. When I went on for an advanced degree, you had to pass German and it took me four or so years to study that just a little bit each year until I finally passed. That was even worse. It was worse than anything, worse than in Oklahoma.

Paustenbaugh *Now I understand that June Iben was the first female veterinary medicine student here and that she was a member of your class. Do you recall her?*

King I recall her very well. Especially one day when we, this is a little bit risqué, but you have to do rectals on cows to see if they're pregnant, otherwise a cow without a calf, a dairy cow, you lose a couple months money in milk production. So we would be doing a rectal on a cow or something and one of the wise guys, maybe me, I don't know, would say, "Hey Iben, I got you by the ovaries!" when we're in there seeing if they're pregnant. She finally got tired of that and she lowered the boom on the whole class. And most of us kind of smiled, but we respected her for that. That was great. We've been friends ever since because she's in western Pennsylvania and I'm not too far above the border in New York. We've helped her out a couple of times when she needed help. She had a fabulous practice until she had a wreck on her motorcycle. But she's still practicing and working with big cats. That's what she most has worked with, big cats, lions, tigers, bobcats, you name it.

Paustenbaugh *Interesting. Were there some professors that you especially remember having very positive interactions with or who really influenced your career?*

King Dr. Peterson was remarkable, even on the way out here for this trip, as I drove across the fields, I remember the whole class going out on some days with Peterson looking at and identifying poisonous plants. He was wonderful like that. Dr. Friend helped him, but Dr. Friend was always low-key. He helped Peterson, but he was low-key. Guys like—oh! I had a big run in with Dr. [Newton] Tennille, because I was always doing something a little bit different than most of my classmates—I don't know why. When I did that one time I took some radiopaque material and I injected it into the aorta of a dog who had lost its leg. I wanted to see where the vessel, the main vessel that I might have to work on when I took the leg off surgically, I guess it was hurt somehow, and I wanted to see where the vessel stopped so that I knew that if I could give it this radiopaque material, take a radiograph every second or two, I could see that. It worked fine, I was able to see it, it all worked fine.

But Dr. Tennille was out of town at the time, so I asked one of his assistants if I could do all that. Yes, but Dr. Tennille gave me holy heck [on his return]. And then at the end of the semester he gave me the lowest grade you could give anybody without flunking them, because if you flunked in those days, one class, you're out. So he didn't flunk me, but I went in to ask him, I asked, "Why did you do that?" and he says, "Because your attitude needed a little bit of come-uppance." Something like that. I hated that at the moment! But ever since I wished I had listened to him a little bit more and paid attention. And even on the way out here, of all the people, he made almost the biggest impression on me for my life. Not for the education—well for the education. He was smart, he was capable, he was a great big heavy man, but the best hands you can imagine. If my bone was broken, I'd like him to fix it. But as it turned out, even on this trip, 2008, I thought how wonderful he was to try and help me. I wish I had kept my mouth shut.

Paustenbaugh *The folly of youth, huh?*

King Yeah.

Paustenbaugh *Early on in the college's history, there weren't really a lot of opportunities for research, and yet there were some faculty who had an appreciation for research. Can you talk about any of those people?*

King I had no interest, I've had no interest, except on the practical application doing a necropsy—that's an autopsy on an animal. I would rather do that than worry about little nitty gritty things in research. Dr. Panciera, he said he worked for 50 years doing what I've done all my life, and I still like it, but he's now into research himself with hepatozoa, a parasite in dogs, and he's absolutely on cloud nine doing that research, finding out that it's coyote fleas that are involved or it's the egrets—I'm impressed with his interest. I didn't have that interest, I never had it. I liked to do another autopsy and see why, or go to the farm. And that was the best opportunity was to go to the farm at the end of the week or something, whenever I had opportunity, to find out why that farmer had those diseases that we autopsied during the week. I did the same in Australia, I did the same in South Africa. They gave me the car, they gave me the permission, they gave me the gas. It was wonderful to do these things. But that's an applied basis. I didn't want to do research. And I didn't know anybody who really did anything in those days, they probably were, but that's my ignorance, not their fault.

Ewing *You did know about Dr. Krull working at Cornell in the summer time...*

King Well he was probably the most renowned individual I knew at the veterinary school, but I didn't know what he did. He came back one year after he had discovered the dicocoeleum, the liver fluke, and he talked about it but—you know I already said that Peterson was one of the best practical teachers, but I think Krull would be the best scientific teacher that I had. He was fantastic. He was nice about it. He was the one who gave us most pop quizzes. At the top of the paper it might say "Pop!" It's a pop quiz. I misspelled 'scissors' on one of those darn things! He was wonderful. I knew him a little, I knew where he worked at Cornell and in the creek behind my house when working on that. I went to a farm subsequent to that where he did his original research with the liver flukes. Very good. Probably I wouldn't know of a better researcher in veterinary medicine than Krull and I'm glad I knew him when he was here.

Paustenbaugh *So given the fact that you said you weren't really all that interested in research, what was it that lead you to Cornell to pursue a Ph.D.?*

King In order to get a Ph.D. you have to have [a research project] at Cornell you don't have to have residence credits for classes you take, you have to have a finished thesis signed by your major and minor professors. When I got to Cornell there was a whole bunch of dogs that were dying with Hepatitis X. Nobody knew what it was, but it turned out to be aflotoxin in peanut meal, spoiled peanut meal. I had six bags of ground raw ingredients that I could use with dogs and it was a nice research project, I learned more in that research project than—I learned one heck of a lot. But it wasn't something I was going to do the rest of my life, just work on research projects.

I would go to farms where they lost an animal or had a foal that's got a broken leg. They said the mare kicked the foal—well sure, mares might kick the foal, but most of the cases over 50 years I've found that the animals had soft bones. That's why they broke, the mare might have kicked it, and then I'd do the autopsy, I'd find a rachitic rosary, that's the enlarged ribs junction, and I would say, well I made the diagnosis. This is rickets, but it's not due to a vitamin D deficiency, it's the vitamin A that's really at fault, because vitamin A is anti-vitamin D. I don't know if the rest of the world knows that now, but it honestly is to my mind, and I did it on each [different] case as it came into the post-mortem room.

That's a kind of applied research. I'd try to reproduce it by giving them this diet. I did a little bit in pigs—oh! Incidentally I forgot, I worked with rats for six years at Carnegie Mellon University and I did have time to do some of these research projects and I enjoyed that too. But I've enjoyed everything I've done. I would rather do autopsies and not basic research.

Paustenbaugh *And I understand that you have a website that is utilized very heavily by veterinary medicine...*

King Thank you for your librarian here.

Paustenbaugh *Yeah she's great.*

King Over the years I probably would spend two hours a day taking, sometimes longer, but average, no at least an hour a day taking Kodachromes of every [good] specimen that I autopsied. I would do it on the whole carcass or I would do it when it was partially opened or the individual lesion. And the slides were all marked in a very specific fashion so I could find almost any slide, or Kodachrome 2x2, in ten, fifteen seconds from the whole collection. And there's 50,000 of them in the collection. Now they're not 50,000 diseases that I've worked on, but one time I would do this heart lesion and "gee it's a great lesion," I'd take a picture of it, but it's only on the inside of the heart. Then the next time, the next case, well most of it would be on the outside of the heart, I could see the muscle lesion so I'd take a picture of that. Many of the students wanted pictures for their senior seminars that every one of them had to give. So I took a lot of pictures.

When I went to the farms for any problem, pigs, horses, or cows, I'd usually take a picture to show all these calves, they're not gaining any weight, we don't know why, what's the problem. You go there and in New York, it's cold and the barn walls are wet. They're lying on wet bedding. And if you want to get cold, just get wet and let it evaporate and you'll get cold. These calves didn't get enough to eat and they'd all be starving. But the farmer didn't want to believe it. The clinicians didn't know about it really. That was my job as a little applied research to this necropsy case. So I would do those things.

Paustenbaugh *You almost sound like a veterinary CSI type of person.*

King Well I did enough of them that it was very interesting. And it helped the veterinarian, it helped the owner and I would take pictures of all these, so here they are.

Paustenbaugh *And what is the website called?*

King Well, it's necropsy, it's got a big long thing, http://W3.vet.cornell.edu/hst. I don't use it very often, [like my own phone number!] (Laughs)

Paustenbaugh *I heard it was called Dr. King's Necropsy Show and Tell.*

King Yeah, at Cornell when I got there, at the end of every week we would have show and tell. Sometimes we'd have it twice a week we'd have so many specimens. And I would just stand there and discuss what I found [for only an hour]. Another good thing about that, from Cornell I would carry once a year for a week, I would take four, five, or six graduate students, foreigners or vet students, usually graduate students in pathology, and we'd go down to all the veterinary schools on the East coast. And not only vet schools, the Animal Medical Center in New

York where Dr. Krull was for awhile, and then Pennsylvania, then Virgina, North Carolina, Georgia, Georgia Veterinary School in Tifton[,Georgia] and Gainesville, Florida. We'd take a week to do that. And I would take hundreds of specimens in Klotz solutions that kept the color, kept them soft, and I would show them at each one of these places for two or three hours in the morning and then drive like heck to the next place. It worked out pretty good. All these lesions I would discuss, but every now and then they would save specimens for me, trying to test me because I would bring out my specimens and I would have a couple hundred of them, and they would bring out 25 or 30 to show me, to quiz me. And that worked, it was very nice for both of us.

Actually I'm going to do that in Baton Rouge in December this year, the same thing. They say, "Well you know we're saving a lot of specimens for you." And they're going to see if I know them, because I don't use histories usually. If I get a carcass I open it up, make the diagnosis if possible, and everything I find should fit the history because that's where it came from. But I don't want to know the history first because I'd be prejudiced. And sometimes you might take a shortcut knowing what they found, I don't want to know that. I've done that all my life, I've enjoyed that. Roger Panciera does that a little bit here also. I don't know how much he does, but I'm sure he does it too.

Anyhow, we started at Cornell with a wheelbarrow. I'd go to Fox's and Roberts' and Kirk's class with a wheelbarrow of stuff. Then after awhile I got to a stainless steel push cart, and then after awhile we get to this Necropsy Show and Tell on Friday afternoons at 4:30 every day, well sometimes every day, but almost always on a Friday, save all the stuff.

Paustenbaugh *So it seems like doing an autopsy or a necropsy, I mean there's a lot of art involved in that. How did you learn that art?*

King Well, Dr. Peter Olafson was a grand old man in pathology and he used to do something like that. And then Roger [Panciera] did it because he got his Ph.D. there. When I got there a couple years later, I learned from Roger and Olafson and then I developed my own way in some of the techniques. Because you don't have time to waste in trying to open something. So you open a gall bladder. It doesn't take me long to do the gall bladder. But I open it onto the white surface and if there's any, flukes floating in the bile, I'm going to see the flukes in that bile with a white background. And so you do that just automatically in every autopsy. In every animal [with a gall bladder] you break the rib against the curvature, that's easy. When it's once broken, you can cut the costochondral junction to hunt for a very specific lesion that's not well described anywhere because people don't do it.

So I try to teach a single technique, it [sometimes] takes me four hours to do a—no, I can do a horse in an hour. That means taking out the brain also, if there's nothing wrong with it. Or a cow. And a dog about 20 minutes. I can finish that dog and I'll tell ya, if there's a lesion, I bet you I won't miss a lesion very often. Or I shouldn't. But I do the whole thing and at the end of it you can ask me, "Well, what did you think of the adrenals?" Hardly anybody looks at adrenals. That even came up here in the last couple of days—pigs have a nice disease called PSS. The cause of that disease, everybody says they get muscle lesions. Well, some do, they all don't. But what they all have, almost 99% of them have small adrenals. But if you don't look at adrenals in *every* animal you won't know that. So I push that kind of stuff. And I've got a lot of pictures for it. That's part of show and tell [and takes a lot of time].

Paustenbaugh *So was that Dr. Olafson's approach? That you didn't read the case first, that you went ahead and did the necropsy?*

King No, I don't think so, because a lot of people fault me for this. They fault me in the sense that "Well, why didn't you read the history?" But I should tell you, I never throw the carcass out unless I've read the history, even afterwards. But I would have seen if there was a brain tumor, I would have seen a prolapse of the hindbrain, if there was whatever, I would have seen that. And it will fit the history that I get with the animal. I have a cocky attitude—if it doesn't then they're wrong, not me. And that has caused some problems personally or whatever. I'm not that easy of a guy to get along with. It's like I don't ask students their names very often because I expect the student to know their name, whereas I will ask them, "Well, how did this tumor get from here to there? Through what vessel circulation-wise?" So I'll ask them things they have to think [to answer].

Paustenbaugh *So after you got your Ph.D. at Cornell, what did you do from there?*

King I went to Washington State to teach for a couple of years. I had a little bit of a hard time there because the expression is "You can always tell a Cornellian, but you cannot tell him much." I heard it several times out there, because I was a typical Cornellian. And then I went to work for industry doing rats and mice and monkeys and stuff like that. But that all got to be very routine, because you keep the rat for two years and you do the autopsy, and it doesn't take long to do them, with a sharp knife. I should say something nice about knives: if you don't have a sharp knife, don't do the autopsy. It's work, you can't push the dull knife through the meat. You can't open up the ureter on every horse and every cow, every dog with one knife. I don't use scissors. I can open up a cat's ureter with my knife because it's sharp. So there's different ways of doing these things. Some people would just be appalled that I didn't read that history first. But I'm not gonna miss nothing. And that's important to me.

Paustenbaugh *You mentioned that you had been in Australia and South Africa. Tell me a little bit about that. What led you there?*

King I did the same thing in those locations. I went to South Africa. If you have to study something for the whole country, you're going to be a pathologist. Well in America, if you want to study pigs, you don't go to Cornell. If you want to study beef cattle, you don't really go to Cornell. You're not going to see many as a pathologist. So in order to see these animals in the United States, you kind of have to go where the pigs are, where the cows are. But in Australia and South Africa, everything comes in to a central lab. Certainly in South Africa. But I just came back from Peru a few weeks ago, and the same thing, they bring the animals in and I don't really want to know the history first. When it gets to be a nervous case I have to know the history but I've already got the brain, I've already looked at it. If it's not obvious. Now saving some specimens, if there's any hint that you want urine, well you'd take it as you do the autopsy, it only takes ten seconds.

So when I'm down in South Africa, the animals would come in and I'd do a complete autopsy. In Australia, a complete autopsy of an aborted calf. You do all of it because you will find that you will find everything that's wrong, darn near everything. But I've been everywhere doing this. I had a year in Argentina doing it, a year in Brazil. I was in Korea in April this year for the month, so that's what I do. I do autopsies without a history. And most of the time, by doing these autopsies, necropsies, even while I was in Korea, I find things they've never recognized before, only because I'm looking at them, at the little things. You do a complete autopsy, you'll find them all.

Paustenbaugh *So are you working with students, teaching them your techniques? Or are you working with professionals or both when you do this?*

King Surprisingly, when I go to these places—if I'm there for a year, I'm usually on the faculty or the staff of the veterinary school and I serve my time like they serve their time. But then I show my Kodachromes to the students and to the residents, all are different, nice Kodachromes and then there are students there. But I don't interfere with their method of doing things, because it upsets some people. It shouldn't, but it does and it would upset me, because they just do it a little bit different. But they do a good job. Let's see, what was more to that question, there was something else?

Paustenbaugh *I was just interested in if you were going there in the role of a faculty member or working with professionals in industry…*

King I usually worked with the pathologists and the resident students. I didn't work with the undergraduate students unless I was going to be part of their faculty for a year, and then I'd have to show each student that. But I would show the techniques to all the residents, and some of them did exceptionally well with it. Many of them came to the United States—actually that's one of the reasons I got to go to these places, because many of the students had come to Cornell, and then they'd go home and they invite me there. So I go, I usually don't get paid, because Cornell [sabbatical] pays you half salary for a whole year or full salary for six months if you go. I usually tried to go for a year because it's easier for my wife and my son and all. I'd do the autopsies with the residents and graduate students and I'd have show and tells at most places for them also. They all liked that because I had enough experience to ad lib that this is something a little bit different how often you see it, and it's just a different way of doing things.

But I did it as unknown and when I went down—I was in Georgia and I did the autopsy, and it should have had a certain lesion in the reticulum, it should've had a piece of wire going through the reticulum to kill the cow with what's called hardware disease. I did the autopsy, I couldn't find anything. I found a hole. But what did it? And they had already found it. It's usually a piece of wire about four or five inches long with a curve in the middle of it and that's what allows it to go through the wall easy. But they had already taken it out and they wanted me to find out that I couldn't find it so, "Hey King, you goofed up." Well, I didn't. But it was a fun thing and I accept that. I want them—because if I put you on the spot to ask you questions, everybody else around that table, the only reason I'm asking you is because all the others don't know the answer either. Then I pick on you. And other people find that, "Well, we're worried about King." But as soon as they learn this is the technique that I'm using, it works.

Paustenbaugh *It sounds like you travel very extensively and in doing so, do you see unusual things that you haven't seen here in the states?*

King Well right now I have a publication being printed. It's true stories of a different kind. It's 104 stories there, and I'll bet you, 90% of the pathologists in the United States haven't seen those lesions or understand the pathogenesis, the mechanism for its development, because they're different. If you open up a cow and you see its abdomen has got peritonitis and fibrin and some ingested, it's leaked out, then you know it's got a ruptured intestine. But why do cows get ruptured intestines? Especially five hours after calving. Well then you do the autopsy and you find out that you don't have to ask the farmer, you don't have to have the history—or I don't have to. I'd look at it and say, "Hey, you put a couple chains on that calf to help the cow deliver and in doing that you had a loop of intestine in the pelvis and the calf coming out, it compressed the intestine, and the loop that's in the pelvic canal ruptured." Hardly anybody to my knowledge has ever seen that and put the two of them together, that it was due to owner-assisted parturition problems. It happens, nobody sees that, I don't know why not. And yesterday Roger says, "That was the best thing you could have said," when I gave a talk here, he says, "That's the best thing to teach these guys, they've gotta look at everything when you do an autopsy or necropsy." Thanks, Roger.

Paustenbaugh *The title of the book that you just mentioned is...*

King Well actually it's *King's Necropsy Book*. I could've said *Olafson's Necropsy Book*, but he didn't teach it all this way. He had his own way of doing things. Every animal I do has to lie on its left side, right side up. And then as soon as I get to something—and if you don't, if you do it another way, then you don't recognize what's instantly not right, whereas I do everyone the same way. Now there are other ways of doing it than King's, than my way, and that's in my necropsy book. I've written all of this down in a necropsy book. And I've got the smells of pathology. You can make different diagnoses just by the smell. If you open the abdomen up of a horse and he's got kidney disease but you smell a strong urine odor and then you look at the colon and it's purple, then you say, "Well he's got uremic colitis." Not many people have ever seen or really heard of that. It's one of my true stories, because I've got dozens of these cases, I'm not talking about one.

Ewing *Would you like to say anything about the conversion of your Kodachromes to an electronic medium?*

King Very good. Over the years, the last five or ten years, I had a gal who I paid part-time and the school paid a little bit. She took all my Kodachromes and she digitalized them and she did a good job. I had two secretaries I paid on the side, one was free but another secretary in Wisconsin, she was a veterinarian, actually a nurse and a veterinarian. I wrote up the 23,000 Kodachromes that I put down. I went through the whole file and I chose 23,000 and they were all good cases. I wrote a history for each one of them. The animal, the tissue, the description, a brief description: white spots, connective tissue, whatever. Then I gave an etiological diagnosis, the cause if I knew it, I gave a morphological diagnosis just to fit the description, and named the cause if I knew it.

Then I gave, what I like on the whole thing, my personal "comment, note." What it amounts to, it's what I think about that case, no matter what you think, this is what I'm thinking. Then I can pull up any one of those by any of those titles, I can push "cow, liver, parasites bile ducts" because somebody looked there and found them, little red ones or something like this, Dicrocoelium, or lung worms. I can pull that up within 20 seconds or so out of my Kodachromes.

Now, when I retire, what am I going to do with all my Kodachromes? I got 27,000 that aren't on the webpage. What am I going to do? I'm at Cornell, Cornell didn't want them. They already had a copy of every one of them that I took, or almost every one, and nobody was going to work on it. So I said well, if they don't want to, I will. But now you also said—when my wife and I got married, we've been married 63 years or something, and we just moved to a smaller house. Now what do you do with a married collection of stuff of 62 years when you go from nine rooms down to three? That's been the hardest work we've done in ten years! Because which picture do we want, which whatever do we want? But how do you get rid of all 50,000 Kodachromes?

So I called up many people everywhere. I said, "Do you have any interest in any of these?" I got about 20, yeah we'll take them. But they didn't want all of them and they wanted a history for every one of them and whatever, but they were very nice. And I got rid of—oh, of course I have extras. You know, I've got Dr. Bob Garman's rat tumors. I mean and that's eight carousels of 80, that's what, 640 Kodachromes of just rat tumors. So I've got to give these to somebody. I finally worked it out when I went down to the AFIP, the Armed Forces Institute of Pathology, and those people have access to the library—Library of Congress, I don't know, but the National Library of Pathology, and they took it. They said they'd gladly have it, they're going to digitalize the other 27,000 and I didn't have to throw them out. Because a lot of people have thrown out their collections because they're—and it's not easy to make a good collection. That's why they ignore them, throw them out. I couldn't do that to mine, at least I hoped I didn't have to. And thank goodness they helped [as each picture was labeled with case ID, animal, tissue and diagnosis].

Ewing *You recently gave Oklahoma State University your parasitology notes and included your own personal notes as well as those that Dr. Krull handed out, and even included some of the old examinations. And this, I was interested to see, was professionally bound. Did you have anything to say about how you came to do that and how you chose to pass it on to Oklahoma State?*

King I have been proud since I left Oklahoma State that, maybe excepting some well-trained veterinary parasitolgists, I am as good with parasitology in the autopsy room as anybody. Maybe not Roger Panciera and maybe some other people, but I don't take second seat for anybody in *parasitology* in the necropsy room doing autopsies. And most of that I learned from Krull. He gave us these handout notes and my own comments to help, and I put it all together. But it was the most valuable, single collection of any information I've ever had, from anybody. You know, not a published book like Jubb & Kennedy or things like that, but Krull's was all practical, more in my line of thinking. It wasn't all the stuff that came from the literature where somebody who's not a pathologist, for instance, who did the autopsy and he thought this bloody gut was a lesion; he didn't recognize it because he's not a pathologist, he didn't recognize that it wasn't a lesion. So that's written down for the disease he was talking about, or he thought he was talking about, he made that diagnostic a lesion. That's bologna! Krull didn't do that, it was all his own work and his notes that *we* added to the side. My notes, the test that Wally Carter took from Krull, a couple that I took that I didn't get good grades on. But I didn't sit back for anybody on that.

Let's see, yeah that's where those notes came from. And it's like when you read Olafson's textbook of pathology, he didn't write it, but he had a textbook of pathology that he used for teaching and he wrote his little notes on the side. That book is more valuable to me than almost anything else. Rickard's notes that he put on the side of the books that I got from him, they're wonderful and there are comments on the side. I didn't know you were going to treat my book as well as you are, or my collection. I think it's wonderful that you did and I think it's worthwhile. It's still got the most veterinary parasitology information than any book I know. Much of the stuff that's written today is by Ph.D.'s. They're okay, it's fine, but if they're just a Ph.D. and not a veterinarian, they can't speak the veterinary language. They can't serve as role model for a veterinarian. So I don't put the guys down, because I don't do their research, I don't even know what they're talking about anymore. But in the post-mortem room they wouldn't dare walk in and say, "Well I don't believe you, John." I'd tell them, "Well okay, yeah." You know.

Paustenbaugh *I understand that you are being honored this evening as a distinguished graduate of the College of Veterinary Medicine. Can you talk a little bit about that?*

King I'm humbled by it and there's nothing I can say except that there are more people I think who deserve it than I do. Because I've done what I wanted for 50 years, the way I wanted, and they allowed me to do that. I'm just so pleased at that. And should I be proud of it, being such a whatever? I don't know.

Paustenbaugh *Well it is a very nice honor.*

King It absolutely is. And I'm not sure I deserve it. But thank-you very much.

Ewing *I know that many veterinarians who already had Ph.D.'s, who wanted to become members of the American College of Veterinary Pathologists, came to you when they were preparing to take the examination for the ACVP. Can you talk about your role in helping young pathologists get ready for that hurdle?*

King Only through Cornell and the graduate students who came there. Now there's an organization called C.L. Davis Foundation. Sam Thompson started that because C.L. Davis was a government pathologist in meat inspection, one of the best. He did a fabulous job. Well, there's a lot of old-time veterinarians like Olafson, or Rickard and McEntee, who are fantastic people, smart, capable and everything. Sam Thompson, he was in the Army for a number of years, he and Charlie C.L. Davis, were good friends. I had started the Olafson short course at Cornell. And that meant that every year we had a week's meeting of Kodachrome presentation. Olafson was still alive actually. But then Sam Thompson said, "John, why don't you come down to New Jersey and give the Kodachrome presentations?"

I went down there and gave four hours of Kodachromes on a Saturday morning. I'd take half a dozen Cornell residents or whatever in pathology down with me and we'd come back that evening. I did that every month for the first year or two, but then Sam Thompson started getting new people other than John King because I was just running out of good Kodachromes. So he started getting other people and from that, I did mine for 30 years [at Cornell] until I was getting ready to retire at Cornell. But he had done the same thing with Kodachromes and he had started doing it a little more often, he started doing it at the Armed Forces Institute of Pathology whereas I just went down from different schools. He had big classes.

My Olafson short course, the people would come from all over the world for a week and they got, what, 40-some hours of Kodachromes. But then I had to stop because my information was only on necropsies. But then we had DeLahunta for the brain, he's probably the world's best veterinary neuropathologist. And then we had Danny Scott on the skin. And they started giving their specialties. So I got out of it a little—I still give general stuff in the post-mortem room. But they started doing their specialties.

If anybody asked me what they should do, should they be a generalist like John King or Roger Panciera, I'd probably say no. And the reason is I don't know, and probably Roger doesn't know, all the basics that we should know about any one disease. Sure, you know the Rabies virus, but you don't know how to culture it, you don't know what's new and different. I think everybody almost—I think I'm going to get arrested for heresy or shot, but I think being a specialist you can give more. But you need a generalist like King, you need a generalist like Panciera. So there's room for all of us, but I would think I might go into specialty. Eyeballs. I mean, how many veterinarians know anything about eyeballs? Well, a lot of them go to ophthalmology. But when you've got six species to look at their eyeballs, it's like the human, the MD guys, they only work 24 hours a day. And the veterinary pathologist, if he does it all, and he only works 24 hours a day. I hope I got the numbers right. And therefore I think you can learn more—if I have a brain lesion I don't understand, I go to DeLahunta, if I have a skin lesion, I go to Miller or Scott, if I have eyeballs, I go to Reese. Because I am a general pathologist, and I work at it. But I have to go to those experts [for the final in-depth info on these subjects].

Parasitologists. Now there's a problem. Many parasitologists don't have a clue about the average veterinary problems with parasites. One best example I had there was one of the young parasitologists came into the post-mortem room and said, "Can I borrow some knives and instruments to do some autopsies in the field?" and I said, "Sure. Why some?" "Well I'm going to take some students with me to do the autopsies on the sheep to show them the parasites that are killing them." He did take them, he took the company car or the van, he took out everything, and they killed five of the guy's sheep. And that was okay, but didn't make a diagnosis. And when he didn't make a diagnosis that was embarrassing to him enough so that he came back and he said, "John you're right, I should've been a veterinarian."

I had another clinician in a seminar, they did a lot of work on the woodchuck. I used to do a lot of woodchucks and they still do them at Cornell, they got a five million dollar grant to work on the woodchucks and stuff like that associated with hepatitis and hepatitis in humans. I just did the autopsies and the histo—you know, an autopsy means histo gross and histo pathology, you just don't do the carcass and then quit. Then the senior student who was giving a seminar finished his seminar and I asked, "Well, was the dog autopsied?" Many times they're not. But he spoke up and said, "Yes, it was autopsied." But it didn't sound right, the autopsy results, to me. So I asked, in the seminar, all the veterinary students are there, a few faculty and whatever, and I says, "Was the animal autopsied?" "Yes." And I asked, "Well was it done by the Pathology Department? By a pathologist?" He didn't know how to answer that. But all of a sudden some guy in the back, who was in charge [of the woodchucks], he says, "Yes it was autopsied, and I did the autopsy." Oops. That's good. I didn't say that. Now I'm thinking, "Uh-oh." But anyhow I spoke up, I said, "I beg your pardon? You cannot do an autopsy." He said, "What do you mean I can't?" I says, "An autopsy can only be performed by a trained observer of pathological detail and you don't have that training. Otherwise you're like a slaughterhouse guy who does 400 cows a day, he's not a pathologist either. But, will you call me a surgeon because I've done six spays on dogs?" And it was quiet.

Moberly *I was wondering, with your website, is it to be a virtual show and tell or as a review tool? Because we use that feature a lot.*

King People do that. So we wanted to make it as well-rounded a webpage. I didn't know how to do any of this. I didn't know how to put it on there. So a guy named—whoops! Gee I forgot his name. The guru in the computer, he did all that. There's also a big webpage from Georgia. They have a quiz section in there and I don't use that, I haven't used that very much, but I think they copied the technique. They didn't copy it, they just used it. And if you find it valuable, that's wonderful. But I really didn't have much to do with that part of it.

Moberly *When you were designing the page, did you ask the programmers to do the quiz part? Or did they ask you if they could do the quiz part?*

King I think I'm surprised it's on there. Because I don't think I said, "Hey, let's do that too." I just didn't think that far along. I don't think I had anything to do with it really.

Moberly *Before we began the taping, you were telling me about how you organized your Kodachromes. Would you tell us that for the camera, because I thought it sounded like one of the best visual classifications I've ever heard of.*

King The first thing you must understand when you're making a collection of Kodachromes is that the Kodachromes have to be marked in a certain standard way. So my Kodachromes, they have the post-mortem number or the accession number from outside, nothing to do with the webpage, but some identification number, autopsy number or necropsy number. And over in the top right it's the species: cow, dog, horse, and if you want to make it a little bit better you would make it bovine or canine or cat. But I wasn't that fussy at the moment, so I accepted, when I say, "Oh it's a cow," well it's a cow. It doesn't mean it's a milking cow, it just means it's a cow—bovine.

Underneath that it has the tissue: liver, kidney, lung, adrenal, whatever. That's in the top right and on the bottom you have the diagnosis. If you have any room for anything else, you can put something else. But those things are on every slide and every time you look at Kodachromes you pick it up and you turn it right-side up and you face it down, that's where you put the number: top left. If you don't, you get a lot of exercise moving the pages around, hunting for which is the right end up. Don't do that, it's too much time and effort. Then we, from there, my 15th big collection on the wall about three-quarters of this wall of notebooks, you know, standard three-ring binders, [color coded pages,] and I would have liver, liver, eight books of liver. One of them on a horse, maybe two of them on a cow, one of them on a dog, one on a cat, pig, sheep, goat. Now I can also go to the wall and pick out adrenals. And I'd just pull out the book on adrenals and that'll be probably one book. I pick that out and it's got all the species in there because I didn't have more than that number of pictures to put in the file.

As I pull it out, the notebook, it's in front of me, I look at the top of the page holding 20 Kodachromes: if that's color coded orange I know it's a horse; if it's yellow I know it's a cat; if it's white I know it's a sheep—because sheep are so anemic, so white tissues, just for that reason. So that's color-coded. Now I'm down, aren't I? I'm down from the kidney, I'm down to the species. Then I've got the color, when I go inside the adrenals I can just flip the page and up at the top of the page of Kodachromes I have nutrition, viral disease, bacterial diseases, trauma, whatever the classification of the lesions are. And then I can pull out all the trauma cases that affected the adrenal glands—there aren't that many, but I can do that in just what, 20 seconds, 30 seconds. It's a good way of doing it. [Also I have a miscellaneous group which has many that are not easily categorized.]

Paustenbaugh *That's a system that sounds like a librarian would have been proud of to have devised.*

King Well there's a woman at Cornell who's done a lot for me, Susan Whitaker, she's a librarian *par excellence* and she helps everybody. She helped me a lot because I needed a lot of help. But she's fantastic help, to have these kinds of people. But it's good to have good technicians because every case that you've heard me talk about, if it needed histo-pathology, I had to give it to the technician. And then I got the slide and every glass slide has been saved at Cornell. Now they're throwing some of the stuff out, but that's their business not mine. I had my 50 years to do what I could.

Paustenbaugh *Is there anything that we didn't ask you that you wish we had?*

King How did my wife help me? How did my wife help me and how did all the other pathologists [and students help me]? We couldn't have done it without their forbearance in all the time we spent in the necropsy room. Cornell was lucky. We were able to do the autopsies 24/7. And we did them 24/7. Some schools aren't that lucky. We were lucky because I didn't mind coming in any time. My wife allowed that. Some schools, if you don't have the pathologists who are around who aren't that interested because they have research projects they're busting their hump trying to do, I didn't have research projects. All I had to do was another autopsy. That was wonderful for me, and my wife allowed it. She didn't appreciate the smell when I came home. Even though I had taken a shower and changed clothes. I might not have showered. Then I'd have this odor, this aura, around me and it just drove her up a wall. But my coveralls and all that I could just leave at school and that was nice. So I do appreciate that. And my son. They had to put up with it. I'd take him to a football game maybe, but if I had three horses to do in that afternoon I'd take him to the football game with a buddy and then I'd go back and do the horses. Not that I was dedicated because there were other pathologists around, but some of them were researchers and they didn't have their heart into it even though they might have done the work. Their heart wasn't into it. And if they didn't save the specimens, I wouldn't have any for show and tell. And therefore, if I did the autopsy, I had the specimens for show and tell every week. But there's a lot of people I owe everything to, but I have to mention my wife, Marie. She made it all possible.

Paustenbaugh *We appreciate you taking the time, again, to meet with us today. That was very generous of you.*

King Thank you very much, ma'am. I hope I didn't talk too much.

Paustenbaugh *Oh no.*

King Everybody says I do.

Ewing *You can't get an oral history if they won't speak up and we appreciate it.*

King Thank you very much.

Paustenbaugh *Thank you and again congratulations on your award tonight.*

------- ***End of interview*** -------

Interview with Nam-Yong Park at Kendal Ithaca

Nov. 9. 2014

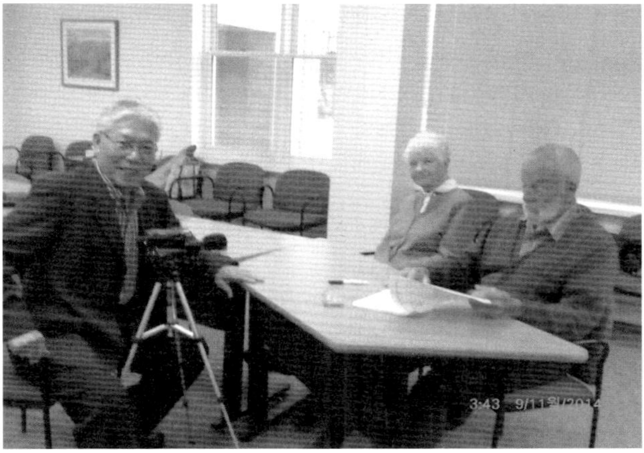

Here is your town, Kendal Ithaca Community. Is this seminar room reserved for a couple of hours? For today's interview, I came from far away Korea with preparation of a lot of complicated things. Mrs. Marie thankfully attended the event. I had been thinking about the following questions in advance.

Park *What particular incidence or reason you can remember that inspired you to choose the field of veterinary medicine?*

King I was raised at a farm home school for boys and somehow was the one of eighty boys who took care of the sick animals, domestic or wild, and who helped the visiting veterinarian when he was called.

Park *Of all the field of specializations why did you choose veterinary pathology?*

King I believe I thought I'd get the best answer as to why the animal was sick especially if it died and I necropsied it. Even as I started in my very short time in clinical practice, I was immediately very disappointed with the few answers from a necropsy

Park *Was there anybody who influenced your decisions in life?*

King There were several people that had a big influence on my life decisions, Pop Sanford, the head of the boys school and Dr. Dinsmore, Wellesley, Mass, the author of the first veterinary book I read, "The Horse Doctor" and Dr. John Bentinck-Smith at Cornell and Dean George Poppensieck also of Cornell standout as fantastic individuals to emulate for me personally.

Park *What is your favourite animal? Any reason why you choose this particular animal?*

King I guess my favorite animal would the cow because they can have so many things hurting them and they often suffer through them alone and they need our help.

Park *During your childhood days was there any particular anecdote or incidence that you consider very memorable? Why did you consider this as a very memorable anecdote?*

King A cow at the boys school did not come back for milking one evening, but finally wandered back completely blind with bilateral ophthalmitis. I pitied her so as I cared for her and she never complained. I also set a leg trap near a fox den and forgot it only to find a skeleton in it months later. I vowed to make up for that stupidity somehow.

Park *When you joined the military service why did you choose the army? Was there a particular reason you volunteered to join the airborne divison?*

King It was wartime and, like all boys, I thought it was the thing to do and the airborne was a special challenge.

Park *While in the military service, was there somebody you can consider as your "buddy" or "best friend"?*

King Being a Yankee and going to Camp Croft, Spartanburg, South Carolina for basic training, I learned early of Johnny Rebels and immediately had to defend myself. A good buddy told me how to let them hit first, but never last.

Park *What is your favourite sports? Do you play this particular sports, or are you just an avid fan? In professional basketball, baseball and football which is your favourite team?*

King I guess I liked football best, but never had time at a boys farm school to engage in organized games especially, I guess, because my farm knee boots were lousy to run in. I also had no money to be an avid fan and attend real games. I can't stand watching basketball as we never played it. The Yankees are great, but not this year.

Park *What is your favourite hobby? Aside from being a professional veterinary pathologist do you have a particular skill which you practice regularly?*

King I collect old veterinary instruments, clean them up, wax, identify and label them with a veterinarian's name, school and location and donate them to local museums including the one started at Cornell. I also make sets of Shaker (Religious culture) Oval boxes as a hobby.

Park *As a young soldier in the army assigned in France did you have any pleasant or unpleasant memory encounter with beautiful French ladies? Where you able to communicate using the French language? How about French cuisine, any particular comments about the French food?*

King As a young soldier in France and in the US Army I might as well have been on the moon in regards to outside of army life. Germany was more interesting as I tried to find relatives when I was on leave there, but I had no luck at all. The whole area was bombed but good.

Park *While in the military service was there a very memorable* *incident or anecdote that you cannot forget?*

King I trained in what I believe was the only paratrooper school in Germany, with the 508th Parachute Infantry Regiment in getting ready for Japan when the atom bomb went off. We all thought that was neat.

Park *How did you meet your wife? Please tell us your "courting days" which finally led to your marriage? Why did you have only one child, was it a choice or a natural phenomenon beyond your biological control?*

King I was in the service and just returned from Europe and I would take all the education and training classes I could qualify for, if nothing else, to get me out of guard duty and K.P. (Kitchen Patrol). I signed up to take a track and wheeled vehicle course at Aberdeen Proving Grounds in Maryland. I was at Fort Bragg, North Carolina with the 82nd Airborne Division after returning from Europe and this gave me a chance to see another part of the country. While studying to be an electrician, I attended the USO dances at the Proving Grounds base and met this beautiful girl at one Friday night dance and asked her, "Dance, Ma'am?" Guess that started it off and it has lasted sixty-five years so far. She came down from Wilmington, Delaware with the USO bus and had to return after the live band dance every week. Classes lasted for three months, but then we kept in contact for nine months til we were married in Wilmington. I once took a big chance to thumb a ride from Fort Bragg, Fayetteville, North Carolina to Wilmington, Delaware on a four day long weekend pass to be with her, but the MPs caught me one day late and I got a one day AWOL write up on my permanent army record. It was worth it.

We even got a short furlough to Daytona Beach after we were married and as she came down to Fayetteville, NC to meet me she was on the train that she got on in Wilmington. In Washington, DC at the train station the conductor asked her if she wanted to change her seat and she said no. That was a slight faux pas as segregation was still in effect and she was supposed to move to another car for white people only. On arrival at Fayetteville she was on the last car at the far end of the station and I almost went back to camp thinking she was jilting me. She had a long walk as I stood at the white people area far ahead and worried.

Now, of course, after losing our son at the age of forty-seven, we are sorry for not having another child.

Park *Was there an incident during your married life that you consider very important and memorable?*

King Our son's death, of course, was the most horrible event. One of the nicest was going to school in Oklahoma and getting my DVM in 1955 at Oklahoma A &M and then my PhD from Cornell in 1963.

We lost a dear friend who was at our wedding by his death within a year, but it led to meeting his mother and father from Tulsa, Oklahoma and being invited to go to Oklahoma and get into veterinary medicine there. A wonderful experience.

In 2002 we lost our son unexpectedly from cardiomyopathy, an unexplained enlargement of the heart common in red cows, cats, pigs, dogs (Dobermans mainly) and others. We had been in Florida only five days and to get a phone call from someone saying they were sorry for his death so unexpectedly was a shock.

Park *What is your favourite food? How about your favourite menu cooked by your wife?*

King My favorite food is bread pudding. At Hillside , the boys school, we had cereal, meat, potatoes and green beans and tomatoes that were canned by all the boys picking,ending, boiling and canning them ourselves with Pop the overseer.

Especially the tomatoes, which I loved then and still do. I was a honcho for canning them into two quart jars. Quite an operation really.

My wife is a great cook, but I've made it easy for her as I'll eat just about anything that won't eat me first. Except jello, I hate it. I do like coffee jello, however, made with leftover coffee with milk and sugar. I've rarely met anyone who has known it existed. My favorite menu includes spaghetti and meatballs.

Park *Please tell us about your life as an academician in the university. How about the reason why you thought of the idea of making the world famous "Necropsy show and tell"?*

King I don't think an academian's life is all that different than many jobs. A lot more responsibility in being there for classes and knowing your subject very well. I guess there is something to knowing how to get the students interested day after day, but most professional students come to class for the information they expect you to have. My rather main theme was to show them lesions, changes in body tissues and organs and ask them questions about why, how, what, etc, making them think for each question. I would hardly ever ask them their names as, of course, I expect all to know their names, but as pathology is a "moving thing" always changing as lesions do then I'd want them to think of what happened to change what normally should be there.

Sure what is in front of them is the lung, but how is it changed from normal, what probably caused the change, etc? I would then expect a pathologist in training to give the reason for their answer.

The happiness for an experienced general pathologist is that with many necropsies already under his belt he can immediately relate one lesion to the next and then to another ad infinitum to understand the whole story and explain it to the younger pathologists. With a relatively few necroposies this would be hard to do otherwise just from looking at selected specimens from someones collection.

The Show and Tells actually began as a simple wheelbarrow full of yesterday's great lesions that were pushed to Dr. Fox's and Dr. Robert's classrooms for their early morning classes of juniors and seniors to demonstrate the lesions. It expanded to Fridays as the last class of each week, saved in Klotz solution for good preservation, color and pliability.

These specimens were even kept for several weeks in the Springtime when Show and Tell became the Cornell Road Trip to the south in a covered van with five or six graduate students, residents or seniors who wanted to visit the seven schools along the way. We presented at each school who hosted us from eight to noon from the seven or eight containers of Klotz and specimens also carried in the van, before scurrying to the next school or facility south.

These Show and Tells were even enlarged to become the Olafson Short Course given yearly at Cornell for young pathologists from all over the world actually attending the one week intensive Show and Tell by all the specialists such as Dr. Sandy de la Hunta in Neuropathology, Drs. Danny Scott and Bill Miller in Dermatopathology, Dr. McEntee in Reproductive pathology and Dr. Ron Miner in Electronmicroscopy and others in their specialties.

A Show and Tell session was usually given at the end of the day's necropsies in the countries visited over the years whenever lesions were found for demonstration. Klotz, however, was not usually available for long term preservation in these countries.

Park *During your long years service in the university as a veterinary pathologist was there a particular necropsy case you cannot forget which you consider as a very memorable incident? Why do you consider this case as very memorable?*

King One of my most interesting cases has been the finding of young cows lungs being enlarged ,usually wet, heavy, slightly firm diffusely in relatively suddenly dead animals. Certainly a toxic agent can be suspect. A farm visit or direct questions are called for. You necropsy the animals and find the above lung lesions which histologically show a marked proliferation of the alveoli and finally someone has discovered that some chemicals cause this result with the higher oxides of nitrogen being one of them. One researcher says it was probably the brown gas found at the bottom outside of newly filled silos. Many cases are presented with the affected cattle indeed stanchioned near the bottom of the silo. However others may be at the other end of the barn with no easy access to the brown gas. In other cases a farm visit shows that the only silage source is a trench silo many yards away. So we changed our great answer to the idea that cows eruct lots of gas during the rumen fermentation function, but how to prove it. Its been known for sometime that by catherization of various gastroenteral vessels that a certain amount of volatile fatty acids are produced in the rumen, eructated and subsequently inhaled to be absorbed from the lung. Now one has to prove this and by asking the students to think of a way, the idea proposed and used was to use a tracheal canula in one sheep so that it breathes only air from under its neck at the canula's opening. Then another sheep does not get a canula so must breathe eructated rumen gas. Now fill the rumen of both sheep with anesthetic ether. Which one goes to sleep and why? The sheep without the canula does as it is the only one able to breathe eructated rumen gas.

Park *You are considered as a very important figure and icon in veterinary pathology not only in the USA but known throughout the world and you had enjoyed a long life span. Can your share with us your "secret" for a long life?*

King I believe my long life span in veterinary pathology has been because of an enormous collection of very good kodachromes made available gratis to the world on my website http://w3.vet.cornell.edu/nst and my availability allowed by Cornell with sabbatical leaves and other leaves for a total of about eight years to all parts of the world many times without pay except for my wife and my expenses. Having the many graduate students from overseas certainly allowed my contact with their institutions and my willingness to travel using my collection. There are many young pathologists now with their own digital images of very great quality doing much the same as I did for so long. Dr. John Edwards at Texas A&M is a great example. The unheralded person who has done more for teaching veterinary pathology throughout the world is Dr. Samuel Thompson of the C.L. Davis Foundation. Sam actually started the foundation by having individuals, including me, give Saturday afternoon classes in his home in the late 1950s and he has continued, to this day, to support and manage this fantastic veterinary pathology education worldwide.

Park *Was there a case when your diagnosis was questioned and challenged? If there is such an incident how did you resolve the conflict?*

King Concerning questioned and challenged diagnoses I've made over the years have, to my mind and for the most part, taken care of themselves by people knowing of them and then recognizing their own cases with at least some explanation. I have had a good one by one of my former residents that I may have goofed dealing with a lung lesion in horses caused by a virus that I did not see the viral inclusions in the lung, but Dr. K. Williams did, but alas I have no access to my original nor to his at this time. I'd rather believe his as I had no explanation of my own, but am surprised by the discrete lesions of fibrosis multifocally scattered in the lungs. I welcome the discussions involved if we can communicate on any case. You show me yours, I'll show you mine.

Park *You had been to many countries as a veterinary pathologist* *or visiting professor or consultant. Which particular country do you consider very memorable? Why?*

In your long years of teaching in the university producing lots of veterinarians is there a favourite student or group of students you will always remember? Why?

King This is a very difficult question as each country has its high points and low points. I can honestly say I'd love to go back to any or all of them because they all have great cases and even better they have interested students and many student groups would wish I'd come back sometime as they welcomed my openness with their questions and my answers. The faculty at almost every institution would even stress that the reason I was invited was because of this openness. All are to be honestly congratulated for being open themselves.

Some faculty, not pathologists, were a bit cold because they may have listened to any of my talks, explanations or comments, but not being pathologists would not really understand my point being made. Again remember my talks and interpreter for me was for English and misunderstandings could easily occur. Overall, however, I do not recall very many disagreements. Politeness I guess.

Memorable country: this is a great question as all are different in their own way. I think Israel was the friendliest in that the people went out of their way to be friendly knowing we were guests. I felt Brazil and Argentina were like the USA of fifty years ago with fantastic potential in animals and natural resources.

India was a large country with lots of smiling faces.

Taiwan was the busiest with everyone doing their thing and even the most inaccessible plot of ground would be cultivated. Their women did much of the general labor, but were always polite and smiling.

Greece had the best dressed people in the world I saw, even the everyday worker was nicely dressed.

South Africa was still working with apartheid, but was more like the USA than any other country overall. I was so impressed that apartheid was abolished without a blood bath.

The French were surprising in that they were amazingly friendly as we were told to expect otherwise.

Italian students have a handicap in their teaching as they have accepted a sometimes arbitrary handling by their professor that no American student body would accept. The students were among some of the most interested I taught and would come to class early just in case I was early.

I felt really sorry for the Mexican students as there are so many of them trying to learn, but not with much hope of employment after graduation. All seemed happy though.

All the countries have beautiful countryside and cities as we do, but ours are somewhat more spread out.

Maybe a major downside is that in most countries the students do not tend to ask too many questions. Afraid of being put down, afraid of getting on the professors bad side, afraid of classmates jealousy. I guess all could be considered more so than I recognize here very often. In general there are differences, but no better or worse than ours.

Park *As a final gesture, do you have a particular motto in life which you follow? Do you have a message, especially for the young generation of veterinary pathologists?*

King Be glad when you can ask questions at almost any time and place without penalty or worry. I learned pathology at an active facility with many different species. Maybe in this day and age you can be more valuable as a specialist in organ, species of animal or maybe even technique. It is not likely you can be an expert in all, there is too much to cover all the bases, but don't worry, you'll find your niche if you study at a good institution.

Park *Did you have a natural affinity for pathology when you were starting out or was it more of a conscious decision to pursue?*

King I think I have always had an inordinate interest in finding out what is wrong with the body or what went wrong to cause death. I think if we do a complete necropsy (animal autopsy) we will find the answer. As a thirteen year old boy I killed my first cow for meat, not thinking it was good or bad for the cow, just that it had to be done by someone and if I could do it and get it done, and get it done well, that was a good enough reason to do it.

Park *Your contribution in pathology has had strong impact on veterinary education. Which of your best characteristics have led you to your success as a person and educator?*

King I believe that doing complete necropsies, and doing them well, will give us the answers especially if we do enough of them and not just one or two. As always, asking "Why" is the key question and asking it of the students, and then giving them your ideas, will help them arrive at the correct answer.

Park *If you could go back at any point of time in your life, and tell yourself something from the future, what would you say to yourself?*

King Because my future is already here, and maybe a little "gone," I would tell myself that when you see a great question, but no answer, you should somehow make a note of it to make you think of it again. Lately I've asked several people what two or three things they now wish they had followed up on. I think the two things I am most sorry I d id not learn to do is to type and especially to learn to draw what I have seen.

Park *You have travelled the world and seen veterinary education in less fortunate conditions. What are/ were the limitations in veterinary education in those countries and how do you think will they be surpassed?*

King I think that the biggest problem is that students are afraid to ask questions. Some limitations I've noted is that teachers do not ask questions enough to make the student think. You must make the student answer the questions within the group as we know the whole group might not answer the question correctly and they will be glad it was not asked of him or her. Make them all think. Of course with four hundred students in a class you cannot ask all of them a question, but "pick on" a good student you know will not be afraid to answer rightly or wrongly. That will get them to think.

Another thing of importance is to have the best and easiest to use equipment, for instance, sharp knives. It is demoralizing for a weak student to be exhausted and dread cutting up another carcass.

And while doing a necropsy, maybe the teacher can ask questions of the "what if" type to take the place, in part, if there is nothing there. Make them think.

Park *Now you have lived a full life. Is there anything else that you still wish to see or happen?*

King I would still like to do necropsies or see new and different lesions and diseases. Have the slaughterhouse people save out the good lesions in Klotz, a good holding solution, and take them out one at a time and discuss them without history known to all. Then get the proper answer at this type of Show and Tell. I would love to do it today, but most faculty would consider it too aggressive.

Park *If you could give three pieces of advice to young generations of aspiring pathologists, what would it be?*

King Students in pathology, do as many necropsies as you can of fresh carcasses with a good pathologist who will answer all your questions within reason and will ask you questions continually. I would think mechanistic questions as to why and how.

Do complete necropsies, but in as easy and fast fashion with a good, sharp knife as the first tool. I do not mean mass produced lesions, but mixed lesions as seen in any active diagnostic facility.

Young or old pathologists, do not forget to always end up getting full histories and even better VISIT THE FARM or the facility. You should not just look at the carcass. I will bet that over the years I've increased my percentage of known diagnosis to fifty percent or more with farm visits.

Park *What new fields of pathology do you think will be most useful and promising in the future?*

King Specialization. I believe it would be better for the pathologist to know as much as possible about any one organ, tissue or disease instead of a limited knowledge of a great number of entities. I have necropsied many animals in depth, but I cannot answer in depth questions for most of the specialities like neropathology or dermapathology and I have to go to the specialist myself to get the answer.

Park Thank you for taking time off for interview. As a commemoration, a video was shoot at the same time. The video camera was for 220 Volt, so I had to purchase a battery for a long time shoot on Amazon. For a change of scenery for Marie King, I play "Power of Love" by Helene Fisher, your favorite song, as a closing mark. Thanks a lot.

John King's Black Box Lecture : Refer to Davis-Thompson Homepage's Portal

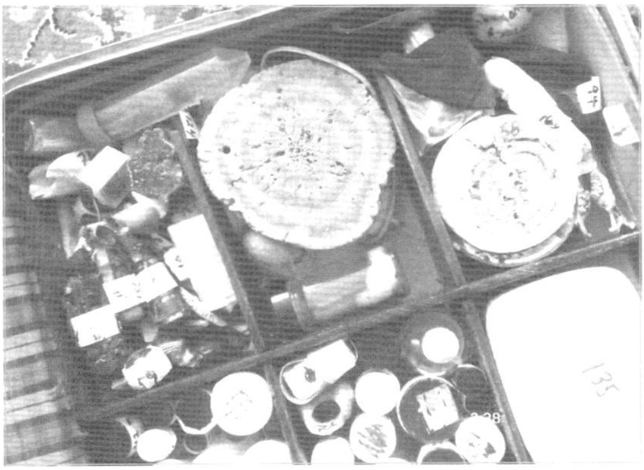

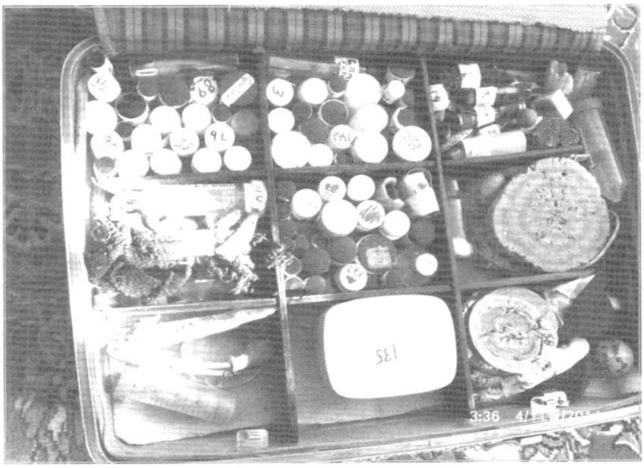

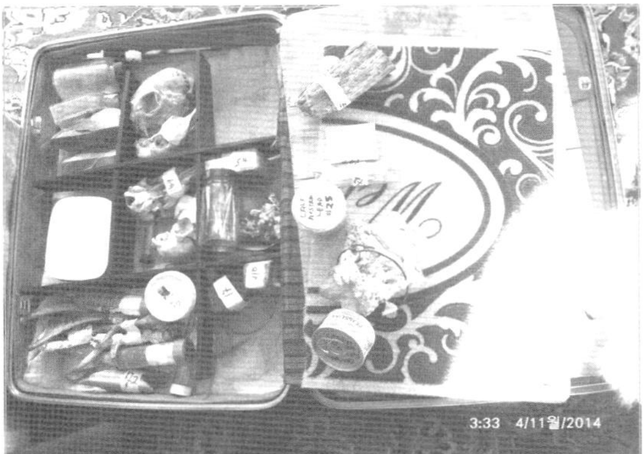

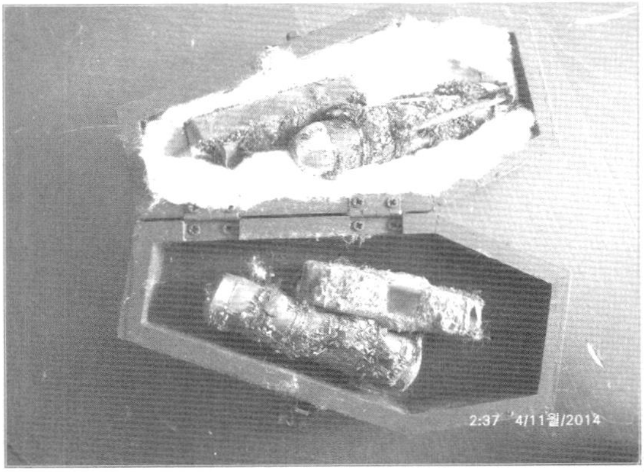

Supporting Letters for Harold W. Casey Teaching Award 1997

C. L. DAVIS
FOUNDATION
HAROLD W. CASEY
TEACHING AWARD

JOHN M. KING

ALBUQUERQUE, NM
NOVEMBER 18, 1997

CHARLES LOUIS DAVIS D.V.M. FOUNDATION
AWARDS RECEPTION
Albuquerque, New Mexico
November 18, 1997 5 - 7 PM

Introductions

Presentation of Donation to the Registry of Veterinary Pathology

Student Scholarship Awards

Armed Forces Institute of Pathology	Dr. Dana P. Scott
Cornell University	Dr. Kristin Freels
Colorado State University	Dr. Mary Jo Burkhard
Louisiana State University	Dr. Uriel Blas-Machado
Kansas State University	Dr. Cynthia Bacmeister
Michigan State University	Dr. Phillip Clark
North Carolina State University	Dr. Paula Blackshear
Ohio State University	Dr. Eric Blomme
Purdue University	Dr. Nicholas Macri
Texas A&M University	Dr. Cheryl Guyer
University of California-Davis	Dr. Melissa A. Chechowitz
University of Florida	Dr. Kristin L. Henson
University of Georgia	Dr. Mark Abdy
University of Illinois	Dr. Laura Anne Gumprecht
University of Missouri	Dr. Roger A. Van Andel
University of Pennsylvania	Dr. Amy Usborne
University of Wisconsin	Dr. Elizabeth Mauldin
Virginia Tech and	
Univ. Of Maryland	Dr. Jeff Wolf
Washington State University	Dr. Dorothy M. French

Journal Scholarship Award
"Spontaneous Cardiomyopathy and Exopthalmos in Cotton Rats" (Sigmodon hispidus)
Veterinary Pathology Vol. 33:375-82, 1996
S.D. Sorden and T.C. Watts

Barbara Jean Thompson Service Award
H.J. Holshuh

Harold Casey Teaching Award
John M. King

Closing Remarks

UNIVERSITY OF FLORIDA

Department of Pathobiolgy
College of Veterinary Medicine

PO Box 100145
Gainesville, FL 32610-0145
(904) 392-4700 ext. 5800
Fax (904) 392-5426

November 11, 1997

Dr. Annette Gendron-Fitzpatrick
University of Wisconsin
Madison WI 53706

Fax: 608 - 265- 2698

Dear Dr. Gendron-Fitzpatrick:

I am pleased to acknowledge Dr. John M King as nominee for and the recipient of this year's Herald W. Casey award. The committee has selected a very worthy nominee in that Dr. King certainly fits the spirit and thrust of the award.

John King has been my teacher, mentor, trainer and friend for many years. He has inspired me as he has others to pursue a career in Diagnostic Veterinary Pathology. I am grateful to John for what I am and for providing me with the knowledge base from which I started my professional career. John King convinced me to see things his way, the King's way, and trained me to keep my feet on the ground and my head on my shoulders. I am very thankful to spend several years in the "Kingdom" at Cornell's College of Veterinary Medicine.

There are three major events during my years at Cornell that I would like to share with the rest of the world and to add to the King memoirs. First, I belong to the class of 1972-1976, the years where John King was at his best. This turned out to be good luck for me and my co-resident, Jim Inhelder, in that we did and saw many cases on the necropsy floor (about 1500 each per year). Second, I did not like the man initially and during my first encounters with him at the Animal Medical Center at New York City. As a matter of fact, I avoided John by finding all kinds of excuses not to be around him. It is for this reason that I obtained a reasonable training in human pathology by disappearing to the Bronx VA when John was in town. Only through scheduling mistakes did I get caught by him on occasions and to be invited to war movies (he enjoyed the Germans loosing) and to apple pie after the movies. I confess that made all the difference and I turned around to change from a Saulus to Paulus. Thirdly, I became tremendously impressed by John King's diagnostic skills of smelling the correct diagnosis of an animal disease. Case and point: John rushed one day with his typical squeaky shoes through the necropsy room to reach his car in the back by the loading ramp. As he passed the necropsy table where I was about tho start the necropsy of a cat he made the

Equal Opportunity / Affirmative Action Institution

diagnosis of FIP on an unopened cat. He was right of course as this was the final diagnosis of the cat necropsy. How did he know? John has the sixth sense for pathologic lesions.

With fondness will I always remember the formative years at Cornell while being a resident and graduate student. John, I owe you a lot. I respect your keen eyes and skills for a quick and (mostly) correct diagnosis. I admire your stamina.I enjoyed your Friday Show and (story) Tells. God bless you and your family and please stay around for many more years. Stay healthy and happy.

Best wishes and good luck,

Claus Buergelt
King's class of 1976

UNIVERSITY OF
WISCONSIN
MADISON

November 10, 1997

Dr. Annette Gendron
380 Enzyme Institute
1710 University Avenue
Madison, Wisconsin 53705-4098

Dear Dr. Gendron and members of the selection committee:

This letter is to express my overwhelming support of Dr. John M. King as recipient of the Harold Casey Teaching Award. I am one of the newer and perhaps one of the last trainees (a.k.a. "King clones", "grunts" or innumerable expletives) to have been graced and tormented by the most caring and demanding teacher I have known.

I met Dr. King during my residency interview and I will never forget: "Why the hell would they want to hire you anyway?" The next year was rocky as it took me a while to grow accustomed to his antics. When I stopped fighting and started listening, I developed a passion for veterinary pathology and genuine admiration for this enigmatic man.

King is a bulldog with one hell of a bite. He demands quality work and attention from his residents. He incessantly quizzed us on the spot regardless of whose company we kept (dean, student or diener) and promptly carried out the proverbial chewing of one's gluteus maximus when the response was incorrect. After rounds, I would spend countless mornings with my head inside a barrel labeled "not for human consumption". And memos continuously circulated--such that we all bear witness and learn from our mistakes and the mistakes of others. It might sound unconventional by today's politically correct standards, but John King taught me to be a competent and efficient diagnostician with a broad knowledge base who doesn't bow to textbook dogma.

Some of his theories are imprinted in my memory: the coconut theory, the well known prisoner of war story, meteorites to explain our most preposterous conclusions, the flush of ruminal drinkers, cirrhosis-the King way, parasites, toxins and lungs galore. I rarely finish a conversation with former residents without one saying "King was right about so many things." I recall one day, a visiting Brazilian resident consented to lie prostrate on the rounds table while King pretended to stomp on her liver--none of us in that group will ever forget the liver's response to traumatic injury.

School of Veterinary Medicine
Department of Pathobiological Sciences

2015 Linden Drive West   Madison, WI 53706-1102   (608) 263-9888 FAX: (608) 263-6573

He often took residents on farm calls to investigate herd problems. One such incident involved the mysterious death of two donkeys with no gross or histologic lesions. At the farm, King observed a row of shrubs that had been mowed down a week earlier and abandoned on the side of the pasture. He carefully nibbled the bark of those fallen shrubs and finally said "cherry trees--cyanide." When the distraught owner, a burly middle-aged woman wearing a black leather duster, asked him if he thought her donkeys suffered, King replied, "Ma'am, if I choked you with my bare hands would you suffer?" She looked at him strangely and said, "I guess not for long." And King replied, "You bet your sweet ass."

King never stopped pushing me and never gave me a break. Underneath his gruff and sometimes tactless disposition, he treated me fairly, with respect, and always gave credit and praise when it was due. I think Dr. King is an outstanding educator-demanding, inspiring and above all--caring. On my last day in Ithaca, King and I went out for coffee at the Manos diner. As usual we chatted about everything... neat places he has lived, the infamous boys school, strange clothes women are wearing today and finally he said endearingly, "you know... shit-for-brains, you're all right."

Sincerely,

Elizabeth A. Mauldin
Clinical Instructor in Anatomic Pathology
University of Wisconsin-Madison

UNIVERSITY OF
WISCONSIN
MADISON

10 November 1997

To-Whom-It-May-Concern:

I am writing in absolute support, without reservation, of the nomination of Dr. John M. King for the 1997 Charles Louis Davis Foundation for the Advancement of Veterinary and Comparative Pathology Harold W. Casey Teaching Award for Veterinary Pathology.

There are very few individuals that have had as much influence in the training of people in Diagnostic Anatomic Veterinary Pathology as John King. And I suspect that there will be very few individuals to come that will have as great an impact on the discipline.

His notoriety, as well as his stature in the field of anatomic pathology preceded him and influenced my course of study early in my veterinary medical studies. I suspected that to be trained by John King would mean that I would be trained by the best. And to that end, I tailored my curriculum in veterinary school with the sole goal of a Residency in Veterinary Pathology at Cornell University. When that offer came on a cold snowy evening when I was up to my elbows in horses with Salmonella at New Bolton Center the winter of my fourth year, the diarrhea didn't seem so terrible.

The first six months of my training were a bit rocky. I had come to Cornell to pick John King's brain for all it was worth. But I guess he read my insistent questioning as an arrogant attempt to "prove King wrong." And we all know where that will get us (unless we have proof to back up our claims) - written off as a useless piece of garbage and not worthy of his attention. I couldn't understand why I was being ignored, but worse yet as if I was invisible. In retrospect, I suspect that I appeared to be doubting what he was saying. I have been known to come across as insolent; with an attitude. But John King was always available for the young people with an interest. And after I insisted on an audience to explain myself, and apologize for my overbearing demeanor, he came to see me for who I was - someone who had an insatiable hunger to suck his brain of any and all information and to benefit from his expansive experience. From that time forward, I became a constant target for his prodding and questioning and pressure to respond to his inquiries - a result that was not always comfortable, but was always meant to push me to think and evaluate and learn. Many people don't like the way he teaches; some don't even understand his methods, but for me, the two-by-four to the back of my head was the best technique for my learning. Socrates would be proud. I know I am. His unusual, to understate immensely, scenarios of lung disease (If I **** in your left lung), kidney response (tie off your pe***), and lesion distribution (Coconut theory), to mention a few, may have alienated or outraged some (many things that John King does has that effect) but I know one thing for sure, you never forgot the answer, or the principle that he was illustrating.

School of Veterinary Medicine
Department of Pathobiological Sciences

2015 Linden Drive West Madison, WI 53706-1102 (608) 263-9888 FAX: (608) 263-0438

UNIVERSITY OF
WISCONSIN
MADISON

I know many trainees may have taken some of the things he said personally, or were taken aback by his gruffness, and at times vulgarity, but this is John King and was never meant to be an attack on the individual but instead was supposed to get you fired up, and filled with "piss and vinegar" so you would "show John King" your interest and progress, and that you wanted and could learn. I for one knew I was on his shit list if he didn't mutter an expletive deleted or two during the course of the day. And with their utterances I was secure in the knowledge that I had had a good day. His constant pushing enabled me to develop the discipline and work ethic that has got me to where I wanted to be - a diagnostic anatomic pathologist doing clinical work and teaching at a veterinary school. I know that as a result of John King's teaching I have achieved this end.

I have been called on more than one occasion a "King clone." I wear that label proudly, and I am secure in the knowledge that his continuous tirades, harangues, and ravings have provided me the best possible training in anatomic pathology and will continue to influence my efforts to improve my skills and lifelong learning. I have always said with greatest conviction that if I could only know what John King has forgotten I would know something about pathology. He deserves this award as much as any past recipient, and his influence on me will be a part of me until the day that I die. Thank you Professor King.

Howard Steinberg

Howard Steinberg VMD, PhD, Dipl. ACVP
Clinical Associate Professor Veterinary Pathology

School of Veterinary Medicine
Department of Pathobiological Sciences

2015 Linden Drive West Madison, WI 53706-1102 (608) 263-9888 FAX: (608) 263-0438

James A. Baker Institute for Animal Health
College of Veterinary Medicine
Cornell University Ithaca, New York 14853
(607) 256-5600 FAX (607) 256-5608

Nov 11, 1997

Dr. Annette Gendron
Research Animal Resources Center- Univ. of Wisconsin
380 Enzyme Institute
1710 University Ave.
Madison, WI 53705-4098

I am writing in enthusiastic support of Dr. John King's nomination for a Harold W. Casey Teaching Award.

I completed a residency in Veterinary Pathology at Cornell University from 1992-1995. Dr. King is a consistently enthusiastic teacher; he is always present on the necropsy floor to answer questions and ensure that every required joint is opened. His comprehensive gross pathology slide seminars ensured that I barely had to study that section for the boards. He can provide an accurate gross diagnosis for practically any shapeless hunk of tissue, and anyone who has attended the weekly "Show and Tell" knows that he does so with style. The many heated discussions I have had with him over the microscope served to deepen my understanding of pathologic processes (his tolerance for the opinions of others is legendary!) and how histologic appearance of a lesion translates into its gross appearance.

For both the duration and enthusiasm of his teaching activity, I cannot think of anyone more deserving of this award.

Sincerely yours

Caroline J. Zeiss BVSc., Dip ACVP

UNIVERSITY OF ILLINOIS AT URBANA-CHAMPAIGN
COLLEGE OF VETERINARY MEDICINE
at Urbana-Champaign

3231 Veterinary Medicine
Basic Sciences Building
2001 South Lincoln Avenue
Urbana, IL 61801

217 333-4291
217 333-4628 *fax*

November 10, 1997

Dr. John M. King
Department of Pathology
College of Veterinary Medicine
Cornell University
Ithaca, New York 14853

Dear John,

I am pleased to provide a few comments and reminiscences on the occasion of your receiving the well-deserved Harold Casey Teaching Award. Our common history began nearly 30 years ago in 1969 when you were teaching Special Pathology and I was a sophomore veterinary student at Cornell. You introduced us to your unique teaching style by stating that we should bring Jones and Hunt (Fourth Edition) to class and you would tell us what was incorrect in the textbook - everything else we were responsible for. I have that old book on my shelf and in my own teaching of Special Pathology I still refer to the line drawings in the margins of the book that I copied from the chalkboard to better understand the importance of lesion distribution.

After nearly 6 years of practice, I longed to continue my training in veterinary medicine. When confronted with the choice of any veterinary specialty, I chose pathology because John King seemed to be having more fun than any veterinarian I had ever met. So I returned to Cornell as an intern, resident and graduate student in the Department of Pathology and began to take full advantage of sitting at the master's feet and absorbing as much knowledge and enthusiasm as possible - I also learned a thing or two from you!

My teaching vocabulary is full of "Kingisms" such as "coconuts from spaceships" which humorously and effectively drives home the concept of the fertile soil theory or endothelial selection, depending on the decade in which one is teaching. I will forever be in your debt for instilling in me the enthusiasm I still have for the teaching and practice of pathology.

What I owe most to John King is that he taught me, by example, the value of logical thinking and deductive reasoning in problem solving which I use daily in my activities as a diagnostician, teacher, research scientist and administrator. I will always be in your debt and will always be proud that I was one of your trainees in the Olafson-King tradition. I am also proud to call you "friend."

Congratulations of receiving this well-deserved and long-overdue recognition for all you have contributed to generations of veterinarians and veterinary pathologists.

Fondly,

Howard

Howard Gelberg, DVM (71), PhD (80)
Diplomate ACVP
Professor of Pathology

I would certainly like to add my support to John's nomination for this award. I have many fond memories of my time at Cornell and especially the famous show and tell sessions in the PM room. John is a gifted teacher and has unique and effective way of getting his message across.

New Zealand veterinary pathologists still have fond memories of the sabbatic he spent down under.

Donald Arthur
Cornell Pathology Resident 1988-1990

FROM: François Dargent, DVM
Former Cornell Pathology Resident
2, rue de Hesse
75003 Paris - France

TO: Dr King Compilation Book, Attention Dr. Annette GENDRON
C.L. Davis 1996 Harold W. Casey Teaching Award for Pathology

October 23, 1995

It is with very sincere pleasure I write to support Dr King's nomination for the C.L. Davis 1996 Harold W. Casey Teaching Award for Pathology.

The description of this Award fits so well Dr King that, as we say on this side of the Atlantic ***"If it did not exist, then one should have invented it for him"***.

I first met King as a new arrived Cornell Pathology Intern in october 1986 and still remember his warm welcoming smile and friendly handshake. I also still remember his high level of energy, his "working" clothes and his seemingly permanent presence in the necropsy room. After meeting all the other Faculty members, I knew right away Dr King was different - althought not yet sure in what way.

After a few weeks, I realized how much Dr King enjoyed his job: he just loved pathology and, most importantly, teaching all what he knew. Of course, he was very impressive, but not intimidating. ***He pushed you to look, to see, to find and to know.*** He knew so much that sometimes I felt he knew more than all others together. He knew how to replace the findings "in their places" and in the clinical or breeding context. He was great at teaching how to sort out normal variations from true pathological findings and his large experience had taught him what was really significant in really explaining the death or the disease. Also, when he did not find anything, I was confident nobody else would have done better.

I also remember very human attention from my times with Dr King: on saturdays, he would take the interns and residents on duty for coffee-donuts breaks: one cannot forget them in the cold Ithaca winters! Dr King had traveled overseas - including in France, not for vacations if I remember well - and knew how foreigners feel. He was at all times very thoughtful with me and my wife, inviting us many times at his house for parties and Thanksgiving dinners.

Dr King, thank you. *Merci* for having been such a great teacher, making the necropsy rotations enjoyable moments, *Merci* for your contagious love for Pathology and *Merci* for being such a warm and honest person.

From the desk of **Xiantang Li**
BVM, MS, PhD, Diplomate, *ACVP*
Phone: 773-834-0676
Fax: 773-702-9152
Animal Resources Center & Committee on Comparative Medicine and Pathology
The University of Chicago, MC 1030
5841 South Maryland Ave., Chicago, IL 60637
li@arc-1.bsd.uchicago.edu

July 18, 1996

Dr. A. Gendron-F.
C.L Davis Foundation:

Dear Dr. Gendron and C.L Davis Foundation:

I am very pleased to write a letter to strongly support the nomination of Dr. John M. King for the Harold W. Casey Teaching Award. I can see nobody in the field of veterinary pathology who deserves the Award more than Dr. King.

Dr. King has been a figure of veterinary pathology. When people talk about veterinary pathology, Dr. King's name will invariably comes up. When people talk about Dr. King, they really talk about veterinary pathology. With a knife, Dr. King has traveled around the world. He brings pathology specimens from all over the world to train his students, residents, and other trainees. He takes pathology specimens to all over the world to train veterinarians and pathologists at all levels. For any animal diseases that we could think about ***Under The Sun*** or on the earth, Dr. King would have a gross and/or histologic specimen(s) for us. Dr. King has seen so many gross and histologic lesions that he has put forth many theories about the mechanism of many diseases. Many of his theories have been approved scientifically, and some are being approved sooner or later. Thus, he has contributed to the education of virtually everyone who performs necropsy on animals and who looks at animal tissues through a microscope.

There could not have been a more dedicated teacher of veterinary pathology than Dr. King. Dr. King has trained so many students, residents, and other trainees. He always goes to such extraordinary lengths to make sure that his students, residents or other trainees do not miss any educational opportunities. Dr. King saves, transports and shows pathology specimens up and down the east coast, up to Florida, almost every year. Voluminous collections of gross and histologic lesions prepared by Dr. King have greatly enhanced the learning opportunities at Cornell University and around the world. Because of Dr. King, most of our students, residents, and other trainees at Cornell University are well prepared for the gross and histologic parts of the ACVP certifying examination. Because of Dr. King and other pathologists at Cornell, many of us passed all parts of the examination at once.

People often say *if you live long enough, something good will eventually come to you.* For me and for the veterinary students and pathology residents who have fortunately gone through the training program at Cornell University, we are truly lucky. A good thing comes to us before we wait too long, i.e., we meeting Dr. King in our early professional life.

Thank you very much for considering this letter seriously.

Sincerely,

Xiantang Li

CORNELL
UNIVERSITY

Department of Pathology
New York State College of Veterinary Medicine

Ithaca, New York 14853-6401

November 7, 1997

Dr. John M. King
Department of Pathology
College of Veterinary Medicine
Cornell University
Ithaca, New York 14853

Dear John:

Heartiest congratulations on receiving the Harold Casey Teaching Award for 1997! This recognition by your peers is certainly well deserved. Both as a former student of yours in the late 1950's (while you were a graduate student) and, more recently, as a colleague in our different roles as professor and dean, I have always admired your zeal for pathology as the means for solving so many of the riddles of life and death. Your infectious enthusiasm for teaching and command of your specialty have earned you the respect and affection of nearly four decades worth of veterinary students, residents and graduate students. In an age that looks increasingly to molecules for answers, you have demonstrated on a daily basis the larger truths that can be revealed by careful observation at the necropsy table.

John, you are one of Cornell's modern-day legends! I am proud of our association and appreciative of all you have done to advance the discipline of veterinary pathology here and around the world.

With all good wishes,

Sincerely,

Robert D. Phemister
Professor

THE OHIO STATE UNIVERSITY
HEALTH SCIENCES CENTER

College of Veterinary Medicine
Department of Veterinary Biosciences

1925 Coffey Road
Columbus, OH 43210-1093
Phone: (614) 292-5661
FAX: (614) 292-6473

Columbus, November 4th, 1997

It is a great pleasure and honor for me to support by this letter the nomination of Dr. John M. King for the C.L. Davis 1997 Harold W. Casey Teaching Award for Pathology.

Dr. King, also known amongst his residents as "the boss", has, as most people of the veterinary community know, an incredible knowledge in diagnostic pathology and amazing teaching abilities. During my two years of residency under his direction, he has impressed me with his knowledge, ideas, and enthusiasm. Most people, however, do not know the human qualities of Dr. King. Dr. King is always (any day of the week, any hour of the day) present to motivate, support, or help.

My best moments with Dr. King were probably on the roads throughout the U.S. He would talk for hours, sharing his impressive knowledge of American history, of veterinary history, or of the world, but sooner or later the discussion would finish on Pathology. The boss and his pathology trainees were having quite a lot of fun in the van. I remember, however, that we, the trainees, were suffering a little bit when Dr. King was singing "O Sole Mio". I guess Fabio did not know what he was doing when he taught us this song. I remember how quiet, slow, and sad was Schurman Hall when he was out of town; there was just somebody missing!

I came to Pathology because I had a strong interest in that field. Dr. King taught me Pathology with excellence, patience, enthusiasm, and intelligence, but most importantly, he made me enjoy Pathology. Without any doubt, he is a unique teacher and deserves this award. Thank again for teaching me, Boss!!!

Eric Blomme, Dr. Met. Vet., Dipl. A.C.V.P.

The most comprehensive health sciences center in America

College of Dentistry / College of Medicine / College of Nursing / College of Optometry / College of Pharmacy / College of Veterinary Medicine / School of Allied Medical Professions / The Ohio State University Hospitals / The Arthur G. James Cancer Hospital and Research Institute

C'est du Pays de Voltaire et de Victor Hugo, au pied du château royal d'Amboise d'où nous parvient (parfois) l' inspiration géniale de Léonard de Vinci, que je viens modestement supporter la nomination de John M. King pour le "Charles Davis' 1996 Harold W. Casey Teaching Award for Pathology".

Dr. King est à la Pathologie ce que Edson Arantes do Nascimento dit le Roi Pelé est au football (pour la traduction, lire ce que Magic Johnson est au Basket Ball). Démonstration:

Tout comme Pelé, Dr. King est le Roi du contre-pied. Tout le monde pense que Haemomeslama ilei résulte de migrations parasitaires, que la sténose rectale du porc est une séquelle de Salmonellose, que la tubulonéphrose rénale est obligatoirement diffuse....etc (j'en passe et des meilleurs). Eh bien tout le monde à tort, tout le monde sauf Dr. King ("Prove me wrong !").

Dans la salle de nécropsie, Dr. King est comme Pelé sur un terrain de football, un Seigneur. Comme tout un chacun, il voit, il touche, il sent, il goûte même parfois. Mais comme seulement de rares personnes qui excellent dans leur domaine, il dirige, il anticipe, il intègre toutes les données avec une rare virtuosité.

Avec le Dr. King ou avec Pelé, le jeu est simple ("Keep it simple"). Quand tout apparaît compliqué, Dr. King nous dresse un schéma pathogénique que certains qualifieront de simpliste, qu'il faut simplement qualifier de génial.

Dr. King et Pelé sont des Passionnés. Ils sont à l'origine de nombreuses Passions, ils sont à l'origine de mes 2 Passions.

Summary for the few people who may have missed a few French words. I spend 3 years at Cornell University and Dr. J.M. King was my mentor. I learned from him that Pathology, like Soccer, is an Art. Many of the players are good, only a few are more: they are Artists. The "King" Pelé was an Artist, Dr. J. M. King is an Artist.

Dr. Jean-Loïc Le Net

Centre de Recherche
B.P. 159 - 37401 Amboise Cedex - France
Téléphone: (33) 47 23 77 78 - Télex: 750 907 F
Télécopie (fax): (33) 47 23 79 95

Pfizer

Télécopie/Facsimile

Pathology Associates International
A Company of Science Applications International Corporation

SAIC An Employee-Owned Company

1/3/95

Dr. Annette Gendron
380 Enzyme Institute
1710 University Ave.
University of Wisconsin
Madison, Wisconsin 53705-4098

Dear Dr. Gendron:

For myself and the great majority of veterinary students and pathology residents whom have had the good fortune to pass through the necropsy room at Cornell University, there could not have been a more dedicated teacher of pathology than Dr. King. There is a recipe for success with Dr. King. A student must listen, show interest and think. Dr. King supplied the rest. I know of no other teacher that would go to such extraordinary lengths to make sure that interested students did not miss a worthwhile educational specimen. He even transports specimens up and down the east coast almost every year. The educational pyramid (with King at the top) that develops from this type of commitment is mind boggling. It is difficult to engage into a meaningful conversation about veterinary pathology without Dr. King's name coming up. He has trained so many pathology residents, shown so many gross lesions, put forth so many new and different lesions and ideas that he has, in one way or another, contributed to the education of virtually everyone who looks through a microscope at animal tissues. I can remember at Cornell, when they were first putting together some computer assisted pathology training programs, Dr. King was asked to contribute a picture of cranial ventral pneumonia in cattle. He contributed 25 pictures because he said that they were all different and anyone interested in pathology needed to see all 25 to really understand cranial ventral pneumonias in cattle. Anything less fell into the category of "No Interest".

I can think of no one in veterinary pathology who deserves the Harold W. Casey Teaching Award more. There is certainly no one in veterinary pathology since Dr. Olafson who has had more influence on his students. When I finished the ACVP certification exam, I had a new 2-week old baby (plus 2 other children), no firm plans for long term employment, and my family and I were about at the end of our financial rope. However, the only thing I could think about as I exited the Gross exam was "How am I going to face King if I fail this part?" That feeling was typical of the effect of Dr. King. Thank you for taking the time to consider this letter.

Sincerely,

Mark T. Butt

Mark T. Butt, DVM, Diplomate, ACVP

15 Worman's Mill Court, Suite I • Frederick, Maryland 21701 • (301) 663-1644 • (301) 663-8994 FAX

The American College of Veterinary Pathologists
875 Kings Highway
Suite 200
West Deptford, New Jersey 08096-3168

(609) 848-7784 FAX # (609) 853-0411

Office of the President

November 6, 1997

Dr. Annette Gendron
Research Animal Resources Center - University of Wisconsin
380 Enzyme Institute
1710 University Ave.
Madison, WI 53705-4098

Dear Annette,

It is my distinct pleasure to submit this letter in support of Dr. John M. King for the Harold W. Casey Teaching Award for Veterinary Pathology from the Davis Foundation.

I was honored to have served on the same faculty with John in the Department of Pathology, New York State College of Veterinary Medicine, at Cornell University, from 1976 to 1985. This was my first faculty position following completion of my post-DVM graduate program. The responsibilities of this position were fairly typical of those associated with most entry level assistant professors of pathology, i.e., one is expected to be a somewhat competent morphologic pathologist. Yet, it was in this position and a direct result of John King's expertise, that I learned most of whatever competence I have in diagnostic pathology.

John was not as his best in the classroom, but put a knife in his hand, a bucket of assorted body lesions in buckets of Klotz solution, and an audience of budding young veterinary students and blossoming pathology residents in front of him, and he was THE BEST. Who else besides John King could pack the bleachers adjacent to an ash-spewing incinerator in back of the necropsy room for Gross Rounds at 5 o'clock on Friday afternoons?

There's no question, that John has his own opinions about pathogenetic mechanisms -- and that he does not hesitate to tell anyone who is willing to listen! The trick with John is to determine where the fact stops and the speculation starts; but then again, he with the most forceful and cogent argument becomes the most believable. It's tough to argue against John's catalogue of pieces of wire "just so long with shaped just so," recovered from reticulopericardial tracts of cows with hardware disease.

My personal note to John would be: Thank you, John, for your friendship and mentorship. Because of you, I hope to have rendered a few correct diagnoses...and for the incorrect ones, I can always use the phrase, "Well, King says...!"

Sincerely,

Gary L. Cockerell, DVM, PhD
Diplomate and President, ACVP

TUFTS UNIVERSITY

School of Veterinary Medicine

Department of Pathology

November 7, 1997

To Whom It May Concern:

I have known Dr. John King since 1978 and I appreciate his great contribution in morphologic pathology, and I appreciate also his high quality of teaching. I would highly recommend John for the Harold Casey Teaching Award.

Sincerely,

Joseph Alroy, DVM

200 Westboro Road
North Grafton, Massachusetts 01536
508 839-5395 ext. 4800
Fax: 508-839-7936

FACILITY FOR COMPARATIVE STUDIES
THE HOSPITAL FOR SPECIAL SURGERY
535 east 70 street; New York City 10021
phone: (212) 606-1437 ① fax: (212) 717-1192
E-Mail: BraytonC@HSS.EDU

Cory Brayton D.V.M., Director

Dr. Annette Gendron
RARC 127 BIOTRON
2115 Observatory Drive
University of Wisconsin
Madison Wisconsin 53706
Tel: (608) 262-1239
Fax: (608) 265-2698

August 30, 1995

Dear Dr. Gendron,

We the undersigned, former students of Dr. John M. King, wish to nominate Dr. King for C.L. Davis' 1996 Harold W. Casey Teaching Award.

Dr. King is unique in his approach to, and his reverence for Pathology and students, and he has made an impact on the lives and careers of us and of many others. All who encounter King remember something of the encounter: a joke, an insult, a story – and usually some pathology. His worst insult to anyone is "You have no interest". He teaches that anyone who has enough interest can learn Pathology. All great teachers teach differently, yet all have something in common: their love for their subject and for teaching their students.

We and many other of his students and former students, and colleagues look forward to seeing Dr. King receive this award in recognition of our appreciation for his 'interest' in Pathology and in us.

Cory Brayton, DVM

Tracey McNamara, DVM, ACVP
Head, Pathology
The Animal Health Center
The Wildlife Conservation Society
The Bronx, New York

5 November, 1997

C.L.Davis Foundation
c/o Dr. Annette Gendron
FAX: 608-265-2698

To Whom It May Concern;

I am writing to express my support for Dr. John King as a recipient of the C.L.Davis teaching award. Dr. King was in residence and in action during my four years of graduate study at Cornell, 1980-84. In my experience, above all other things, John King was a teacher. His dedication to this task was total and profound. To his students he could be kind or harsh, forgiving or demanding, a delight or an dreaded experience, a friend or not, but he never was disinterested. He lived and breathed his discipline from dawn to dusk; he was always there to review a case and give an opinion. He spent hours and hours assembling and distributing teaching materials to current students and to former students. He cared immensely that his students should learn anatomical pathology, that its place as a discipline should not be lost in academic veterinary medicine, displaced by concepts of life as molecules and genes. He demanded that pathology as a discipline maintain its place in the service of society through veterinary practice. The taught his students to do this with total dedication. All honour to him for this.

Frederick A. Leighton DVM, PhD
Professor and Head

Department of Veterinary Pathology, Western College of Veterinary Medicine, University of Saskatchewan
52 Campus Drive, Saskatoon SK S7N 5B4 Canada Telephone: (306) 966-7280 Facsimile: (306) 966-7439

Angell.

ANGELL MEMORIAL ANIMAL HOSPITAL

350 South Huntington Avenue • Boston, MA 02130 • 617 522 7282 • FAX: 617 522 7356

DEPARTMENT OF PATHOLOGY

October 4, 1995

Dr. Annette Gendron
RARC 127 Biotron
2115 Observatory Drive
University of Wisconsin
Madison, WI 53706

Dear Dr. Gendron:

I am pleased to write a letter supporting Dr. John M. King's nomination for the Harold W. Casey Teaching Award, for there are few Veterinary Pathologists who have dedicated themselves to students of the discipline as much as he. Dr. King's skills as Diagnostic Veterinary Pathologist are among the finest, but more importantly, his ability to spread enthusiasm for Diagnostic Pathology and teaching are second to none.

Daily Pathology Rounds (Show and Tell) led by Dr. King are instructive for undergraduate veterinary students, pathology residents, pathologists, and clinicians. His entertaining style brings many whom do not have a "burning" interest in pathology to these sessions, and, in spite of themselves, they leave with increased understanding of a particular lesion or case and a better appreciation for pathology. I attended my first "Show and Tell" when I was interviewing for veterinary school. At that session (which was over 20 years ago) I still remember learning, "If it's green, it's not TB," and he frequently used a word I had not heard before, "infarct." Since everyone else seemed to know what he meant, I was too embarrassed to ask, so I looked it up when I got home. That's the type of interest a good teacher should inspire in his students.

As a veterinary student, my interest in pathology grew. Part of that was due to Dr. King's encouragement. He was there to teach anyone and everyone who was willing to put in the effort to learn. Dr. King's "tell it like it is" style is, admittedly, not for everyone, but almost everyone who listens to what he has to say goes away with a better understanding of some aspect of veterinary pathology. Dr. King encouraged me to pursue Pathology as a specialty and I am glad I did. His dedication to resident education outshines all others in his Department. Residents, past and present, acknowledge that no other faculty member is as interested in their education as much as Dr. King. Even if he wasn't on duty, residents could always call on Dr. King for help with cases, in the post mortem room, or across the double-headed microscope. He always had the time to share his knowledge and experience with us.

In 1985, I moved south and started to attend the Southeast Veterinary Pathology Conferences in Tifton, GA. As I got involved in the Conference, I had the opportunity to invite Dr. King to attend as the invited Conference Speaker, a dubious honor since it is without financial assistance. Not only did Dr. King come to that conference, but he has attended the Tifton Conference every year since. He has made the trip south an annual event, bringing along buckets of lesions and a group of residents. Dr. King and his troupe stop at veterinary schools along the way, giving a "Show and Tell" road show at several institutions. Dr. King's desire to share good cases inspired him to initiate the Diagnostic Pathology Specialty Group Sessions at the annual meeting of the American College of Veterinary Pathologists, which began in 1987. More recently he has initiated a diagnostic pathology meeting, similar to that held in Tifton, in the northeast. The first meeting of the group is to be held later this month. The pathologists in this area are looking forward to this meeting with genuine excitement.

Dr. John M. King truly fits the criteria set by the C. L. Davis, D.V.M. Foundation for the Harold W. Casey Teaching Award. His influence is passed down among his students. I am proud to consider myself one of them.

Sincerely,

Lois Roth, D.V.M., Ph.D.
Director, Clinical Laboratory
Angell Memorial Animal Hospital

October 13, 1995

Dr. Annette Gendron
RARC 127 BIOTRON
2115 Observatory Drive
University of Wisconsin
Madison, Wisconsin 53706

Dear Dr. Gendron:

This letter is written in support of Dr. John King's nomination for the 1996 Harold W. Casey Teaching Award for Pathology.

As a fourth year veterinary student at Washington State University I first "encountered" (that is precisely the correct terminology) John on my rotation through the Necropsy Service. His irascible, outrageous personality, coupled with his talented and enthusiastic conduct of Necropsy pathology endeared him to most students. Irreverence for the system and total disregard for convention typified his approach to academic life.

That was in 1961. Upon accepting the position of chairman, Department of Pahtology, Cornell University in 1975, I found myself being his boss. The above outlined traits that I had observed as a student had not changed one iota during the intervening years. Initially, life was not easy for the new chairman, nor was it for John -- now under the thumb of a former student. However, his internationally recognized disciplinary skills, his love for student interaction at the necropsy table, and his insatiable appetite to perform before any audience (be it large or small) enabled him to exercise his craft. He became a legend in his own time, affecting more than three generations of future veterinarians.

John King is first a pathologist, second a fiercely loyal Cornellian, and thirdly, a cream puff -- despite all the noise, buckus, tantrums, bullshit and irreverence.

He is one other thing -- without a doubt the best hands down gross veterinary necropsy pathologist in the world. As such, he is a most fitting recipient of the Casey Award.

Sincerely yours,

Robert M. Lewis, DVM
Professor of Pathology

RML/cyh

CORNELL
UNIVERSITY

College of Veterinary Medicine
Department of Anatomy

Ithaca, New York 14853-6401

Dr. John F. Cummings
Phone: 607-253-3559
Fax: 607-253-3541

October 5, 1995

Dr. Annette Gendron
RARC 127 BIOTRON
2115 Observatory Dr.
University of Wisconsin
Madison, WI 53706
FAX: (608) 265-2698

Dear Dr. Gendron:

This letter is written in support of John M. King's nominations for CL Davis' 1996 Harold W. Casey Teaching Award for Pathology. It has been my pleasure to know Professor King for the past 32 years, first as teacher and later as colleague. I know no Pathologist with experience in postmortem diagnostics that can rival that attained by Professor King. It is based on this experience that he can speak and teach with true authority.

The breath of his knowledge is truly astounding. As a student many years ago I can still recall then Ph.D. candidate King filling in a Parasitology Class on stomach worms in ruminants. His presentation on this subject was far better in clarity and clinical application than any the class had or would receive from the Professor in charge. His enthusiasm and lively exchanges with students have made their learning experience highly enjoyable. While Professor King is very effective in the standard lecture format, his instruction on the necropsy room floor in a hands-on mode cannot be surpassed. This "show and tell" as he calls it has been a truly memorable experience as all the alumni and alumnae of the College will attest.

I can identify a great number of outstanding pathologists, but none have the unique gifts that John M. King brings to teaching. He is truly one of a kind. I recommend him most highly for this award.

Sincerely yours,

John F. Cummings, DVM PhD
James Law Professor of Anatomy

JFC/chw

Genetics Institute, Inc.

One Burtt Road
Andover, Massachusetts 01810
Telephone (508) 475-9214
Telefax (508) 475-0085

GENETICS INSTITUTE

A Subsidiary of American Home Products Corporation

Page Bouchard, DVM
Head of Preclinical Safety
April 8, 1997

Dr. Annette Gendron-Fitzpatrick
Room 380 Enzyme Institute
Research Animal Resources Center
University of Wisconsin
1710 University Ave.
Madison, WI 53705-4098

Dear Dr. Gendron-Fitzpatrick,

I am writing this letter in support of Dr. John King's nomination for the Harold Casey Award for Sustained Excellence in Teaching of Veterinary Pathology for 1997. I was notified by Charlene Fernandez of Cornell University about Dr. King's nomination. I was trained in the Anatomic Pathology Residency Program at Cornell University from 1990-1993 and worked very closely with Dr. King during that time. During my time at Cornell I came to appreciate Dr. King as a unique and treasured gift to our profession. Dr. King has been the most inspiring and influential person in my professional life and I am honored to support his receipt of this award.

Dr. King is widely known for his passionate and entertaining style as teacher of pathology residents, DVM students and undergraduates. His primary teaching responsibilities over the years have been focussed upon gross pathology and the necropsy room is his stage. His presence in the necropsy room has long been synonymous with diagnostic excellence at Cornell. He has always shown an infectious enthusiasm for gross pathology and this is best appreciated by attending his weekly "show and tell" gross pathology rounds. His greatest strength as a teacher is with small groups in the necropsy room, at weekly diagnostic pathology slide reviews, or in kodachrome reviews. He is widely known for his style of challenging residents in public forums and pushing them to perform to his high standards. While this style does not suit everyone whom he has taught over the years, it does leave a lasting impression and forces people to learn the material he believes to be important. While his public challenges and critiques of people are sometimes taken as personal criticism, most people soon recognize that he holds the best interest of his students and residents foremost in his concerns.

Dr. King is one of the most caring and committed teachers that I have ever known. He is committed to excellence in teaching and service and would make any sacrifices to help students, residents of clients of the Pathology Service at Cornell. He has generously donated his time to planning, promoting and hosting the Olafson Short Course on Diagnostic Pathology for many years. While he has always maintained that the Short Course is not an ACVP Board preparation course, it has long served as such. He has also generously donated his time throughout the United States and the world to visit, teach and learn from all who have invited him.

As a pathologist, Dr. King is without question the worlds authority on gross diagnostic pathology of domestic animals. This is the legacy for which is known worldwide and is the area of expertise that he has conveyed to the many student and residents whom have passed through Cornell over the past 30+ years. He has always emphasized the importance of practicing practical pathology with a focus on important findings and de-emphasizing the common artifacts and non-lesions encountered on the necropsy floor. Dr. King has been responsible for describing and characterizing more "non-lesions" of diagnostic importance to the training pathologist than anyone in the world. He encourages a balance between quality and quantity in diagnostic work in the true sense of teaching and service in a busy teaching and diagnostic service.

Dr. King is a true "one of a kind" and his contributions to the profession have been unparalleled. His appreciation for gross pathology are unique and, unfortunately, under appreciated in today's pathology training programs. His presence and legendary reputation in veterinary pathology were the primary reason that I chose to train at Cornell and I can say without hesitation that I learned more useful and professionally applicable skills from Dr. King than any other individual. He has positively impacted many people in veterinary pathology and has been the most important person in my professional career. I love him as a teacher and a friend and take great joy in his receipt of this award. The Harold Casey Award will be honored by it's association with Dr. King.

Gratefully submitted,

Page Bouchard, DVM, DACVP

UNIVERSITY OF FLORIDA

Department of Pathobiology
College of Veterinary Medicine

PO Box 110880
Gainesville, FL 32611-0880
(352) 392-4700 ext. 5800
Fax (352) 392-9704
Castlema@ufl.edu

November 7, 1997

Dr. Annette Gendron
C.L. Davis Foundation
380 Enzyme Institute
1710 University Ave.
Madison WI 53705-4098

Re: Nomination of John M. King for Harold W. Casey Teaching Award

Dear Annette:

I am delighted to have the opportunity to add my letter to the substantial body of support for John King's nomination.

I had the good fortune to be on the pathology faculty at Cornell with John between 1979 and 1986. John is clearly the most enthusiastic and colorful teacher of pathology whom I have ever encountered. His "show and tell" presentations in gross pathology at the New York State College of Veterinary Medicine were legendary and well attended by students, faculty, and pathology trainees. His ability to hold an audience spell-bound with his picturesque stories of diagnostic pathology and anecdotes were most impressive.

From my own personal perspective, I believe that I learned more practical diagnostic veterinary pathology working with John than from anyone else I was exposed to during my training period prior to ACVP boards. A key that I perceive in John's success is the sheer strength of his personality. It can be simultaneously seemingly overbearing, and potentially intimidating, but also warm and caring. This basic strength of personality and communication coupled with diagnostic pathology experience that is matched by few made him a must-see fountain of knowledge if you were somewhere near Cayuga's waters.

John King is a pathologist with many creative and original ideas that he intersperses with fantastic demonstration skills of gross lesions in specimens and kodachromes. Many of his ideas, to say the least, are controversial. To the hungry mind trying to learn pathology, it is only a matter of time until one begins to doubt that 100% of what he says is true (although it certainly is the gospel). To the young pathologist who thinks for himself or herself, this is a tremendous stimulus for self-study and learning.

John King is one of the true greats in the art of teaching and diagnostics in veterinary pathology. His spirit and enthusiasm for the subject has few peers. It is with appreciation and gratitude that I count myself among the hundreds of pathologists who had the good fortune to study pathology under his considerable influence.

Sincerely,

William L. Castleman

William L. Castleman, D.V.M., Ph.D.
Professor and Chairman

MICHIGAN STATE
UNIVERSITY

May 28, 1997

Dr. Annette Gendron-Fitzpatrick
Research Animal Resources Center
Univ. Of Wisconsin
127 Biotron
215 Observatory Drive
Madison, WI 53706-1087

Dear Dr. Gendron- Fitzpatrick,

I am pleased and honored to add my letter of support for the nomination of Dr. John M. King for the Harold Casey Award for Sustained Excellence in the Teaching of Veterinary Pathology.

As is the case for many of us I believe, my awareness and appreciation of Dr. King's unique abilities as a teacher evolved slowly over the three years I spent at Cornell. In truth, it is only since I left that I have begun to understand Dr. King's influence on his trainees.

Although no days are boring or uneventful when training with John King, two days stand out in my mind. The first begins on a midsummer morning. Dr. King, myself, another resident and several senior students are discussing the previous days cases. This is my first week of duty and I cannot do anything right. Every answer, every explanation I give is turned inside-out, unfolded or taken apart. What sort of teacher is this I wonder. He argues with me, pokes holes in all my attempted answers and scorns quotes from textbooks. This professor does not want to hear the facts I have memorized and is not impressed by what I have learned in the past. Frustration wells up and I think to myself, "How will I ever learn from this man?"

For many months to follow, every decision and diagnosis I made was questioned. This was often a painful process and to be honest, tears of frustration, self doubt and anger were shed. Gradually I began to find my equilibrium and I also found that Dr. King not only questioned his trainees, but his peers, and himself as well, always pushing to be a better pathologist. I saw how passionately he molded and cajoled us into believing what we saw, not simply seeing what we had been taught to believe.

A month before I left Cornell, Dr. King and his wife, Marie, took several of us sailing on the lake one summer evening. As Dr. King effortlessly sailed his boat, he was the funny, charming, fascinating man he reveals to us over time. And as I watched him, I realized, "How did I ever learn before this man?"

COLLEGE OF
VETERINARY MEDICINE
Department of Pathology
Veterinary Medical Center
East Lansing, Michigan
48824-1314
517/353-4697 or
517/353-5275 or
517/353-9160 (East Fee)
FAX: 517/432-4008

Just recently, I have come to know that great teachers are defined by the legacy of men and women they train and not by the techniques they use daily to teach us. Because of his legacy, John King has become a dominant figure in veterinary medicine. He is a link to our past because he sees through the eyes of great men, like Dr. Olafson, and he has defined the future by influencing nearly every veterinary pathologist of today. I know that all of us who have been so fortunate to see pathology through Dr. King's eyes will carry on his legacy.

Kelly M. Credille, D.V.M.
Diplomate, A.C.V.P.
Department of Pathology
Michigan State University

Dr. Kurt J. Williams
Dept. VM: APC
School of Veterinary Medicine
University of California
Davis, CA 95616

Dr. Annette Gendron-Fitzpatrick
380 Enzyme Insitute
1710 University Avenue
Madison, WI 53705-4098

11/6/97

Dear Dr. Gendron-Fitzpatrick,

I'm writing this letter to you today to fully endorse the nomination of Dr. John M. King as this years recipient of the Harold Casey Award for excellence in teaching.

My association with Dr. King goes back to my days as a resident at Cornell. To be truthful I had never heard of Dr. King as I applied to Cornell for the residency and his presence there had no bearing on my desire to go there for my training.

First mention of him came as I was discussing my impending move to Ithaca with the pathologists at my alma mater. When they found out that I would be heading to Cornell the first thing out of their mouths was not a "congratulations" or a "good for you" but rather, a "look out for Dr King". They filled my mind with stories of a hard-bitten pathologist that was prone to fanciful theories on the origin of disease in animals.

This experience didn't stay with me when we finally moved to upstate N.Y.. It all came flooding back to me though when I went in for my first day of "orientation". I'll never forget being introduced to Dr. King. No sooner had the handshakes ended that he dragged myself and the two other new residents out onto the necropsy floor to see a "good case".

That first case that he shared with us was so illustrative of the essence of Dr. King, and the reason that I hold him in such high regard both as a pathologist and as a teacher. He always put our education at the top of his agenda and it always was presented in an inimitable style.

Now, back to that case. We walked out on the floor to find a heavy load of necropsy cases. At any institution the first year residents always feel a little overwhelmed just in learning their way around the facility, and we had the added pleasure of being grilled on this case. On the far table of the room there lay a young foal that was nearly completely necropsied with a bucket of Klotz sitting next to it. Dr. King retrieved the complete pluck out of the bucket and asked us our opinions. We all sat there stone silent for a time until he finally pulled out our meager answers. We were all able to identify the abscesses in the lungs, but there was obviously more that he wanted us to note. We never did find the other more subtle lesion in the caudal and dorsal fields. It was our first exposure to Rhodococcus associated with Pneumocystis carinii .

The fact that Dr. King made the association between Rhodococcus and Pneumocystis in foals is remarkable enough, but what is even more remarkable is his intense desire to share it with his residents.

When I say his residents I really mean HIS residents. Although, we were all in the employ of Cornell University we were, and still are to a certain extent, his foot soldiers for veterinary pathology. Never have I ever met a person with such an intense interest in their field, nor do I expect to ever find another like him. His zeal for veterinary pathology was infectious for many of us that had the good fortune to work with him.

I'll never forget the many times that the residents room door was flung open, and those of us that weren't on service at the time were jarred back to reality from reading our slides, etc.... by the sound of his voice asking the very simple question-"anybody in here interested in pathology ?" By the time we all had our headphones off of our ears and our heads turned toward the door the specter was gone, already 2/3 the way to the necropsy floor. He of course knew that we would all be there in short order to hear his interpretation of the latest material to come to the floor.

His presentations of case material, both the spontaneous, and weekly "Show and Tells" that we all attended were a blend of the most unusual nature. He could take a case of Fusobacterium in the liver of a cow and blend it with anecdotes from his days growing up in a boys school, time in France during World War II, and his days working with Peter Olafson. There just aren't people around like him in our profession now and I doubt there will be any to follow. In this day of computer-based learning he is one of the last of a disappearing breed that likely will never be replaced after he retires.

Because of all of these reasons and many more I feel lucky to have had the opportunity to have worked with him for the years that I did and even more fortunate to have him as a friend. He is the quintessential teacher, and a most unique individual.

Sincerely,

Kurt J. Williams, DVM ,Diplomate ACVP

EPL®

EXPERIMENTAL PATHOLOGY LABORATORIES, INC.
P.O. BOX 12766, RESEARCH TRIANGLE PARK, NC 27709 (919)544—8061 Fax: (919)544—7289

September 29, 1995

Dr. Annette Gendron
RARC 127 BIOTRON
2115 Observatory Drive
University of Wisconsin
Madison, WI 53706

Dear Dr. Gendron:

I am writing to applaud the nomination of Dr. John M. King for the **C.L. Davis' 1996 Harold W. Casey Teaching Award for Pathology.** Dr. King is a colorful, memorable teacher who inspires learning. He taught me the very basis of pathology upon which the rest of my knowledge rests. Perhaps the most important of all his teachings was "A necropsy is a once in a lifetime event! Any tissues not collected, any data not recorded, any observation not made will be gone tomorrow with the barrels into the incinerator like new snow on a sunny day." He encouraged the art of keen observation and mulling over often small, seemingly unimportant observations to make a case come together into the correct diagnosis.

To a fault, Dr. King demanded unconventional approaches to diagnoses with rejection of authorities or conventional dogma. Many of his students have gone on to make really important discoveries because of their change of perspective about the pathogenesis of a particular disease.

Dr. King is demanding and gruff but he is willing to teach those who are interested in learning and freely shares his tremendous experience and knowledge with the most ignorant, naive fledgling pathologist. His caring heart and support of students over the roughest times often was the difference in success and failure.

He is a great man.

Sincerely,

Suzanne Botts

SUZANNE BOTTS, D.V.M., Ph.D.
Pathologist

SB:asc
Encl.

EPL®

EXPERIMENTAL PATHOLOGY LABORATORIES, INC.
P.O. BOX 474 HERNDON, VIRGINIA 22070 (703) 471-7060 Fax: (703)471-8447

October 6, 1995

Dr. Annette Gendron
RARC 127 Biotron
2115 Observatory Drive
University of Wisconsin
Madison, WI 53706

Dear Dr. Gendron:

It is my understanding that Dr. John M. King of the College of Veterinary Medicine of Cornell University has been nominated for the Harold W. Casey Teaching Award. I am so pleased that Dr. King has been nominated for this award and I support the nomination sincerely and enthusiastically.

John King is unsurpassed in his ability to teach gross diagnostic pathology and histopathology in all animal species. When, as a senior veterinary student, I was selecting a training program in veterinary pathology I was advised by Dr. Charles Capen of The Ohio State University to study under Dr. King since my interest then was diagnostic pathology. I have been grateful to Dr. Capen all these years for his advice and his part in securing me a position in the pathology training program at Cornell University. John King's first and foremost dedication is to teaching his pathology students. His great experience and knowledge, combined with his great humanitarianism, make him first rate as an educator and a human being. It is a privilege indeed to be able to say that I was one of John King's students and that I am also his friend.

Dr. King is highly deserving of the Harold W. Casey Teaching Award. The impact that this man has had on the careers of numerous pathologists is tremendous. His emphasis on keen observation at the time of gross necropsy is, I believe, the key teaching that enables his students to succeed in veterinary pathology. John King loves to teach and his enthusiasm for veterinary pathology is contagious. What a joy it is to know him! How delightful to know that he will be honored with the Harold W. Casey Teaching Award.

Sincerely yours,

Marilyn J. Wolfe

MARILYN J. WOLFE, D.V.M., Ph.D.
Pathologist

MJW/sfh

UNIVERSITY of PENNSYLVANIA

The School of Veterinary Medicine
Laboratory of Pathology
3800 Spruce Street
Philadelphia, PA 19104-6051

Dr. Annette Gendron
RARC 127 Biotron
2115 Observatory Drive
University of Wisconsin
Madison, Wisconsin 53706

October 30, 1995

Dear Dr. Gendron:

I enthusiastically support the nomination of Dr. John M. King for the Harold W. Casey Teaching Award. I first encountered Dr. King when I entered the residency training program at Cornell in 1978. During the two years that I spent at Cornell, John proved to be one of my most influential mentors. He was always willing to question the established dogma and he impressed me with his breadth of knowledge of the field of veterinary pathology. He was also always willing to help a resident in trouble (or get them in trouble, depending on what they needed). An example:

One evening around 9:00 pm I was called in to do a necropsy on a horse that had died in the clinic. The clinician was very excited about the case because they thought it was one of the first documented cases of DIC in the horse; although they had been unable to pinpoint a primary disease process. As I was beginning the necropsy Bob Lewis walked through the postroom on the way to his car and gently chided the clinician for failing to have done all of the necessary tests to make the diagnosis of DIC. The clinician then left the student(s) and I alone with the horse. An hour or so later we had found hemorrhages everywhere, but no primary problem.

I finally called Dr. King at home and asked him if he would drive over and take a look. He walked in the postroom and began to sniff the air, mumbling something about goats. As I explained our lack of findings he walked over to the horse, sniffed around, and began cutting into the muscles of the neck. He came upon a black/red area in the muscle and suggested that we culture that area for Clostridial organisms. We later demonstrated Clostridium septicum in the muscle by immunofluorescence and the clinicians eventually published the case, unbeknownst to me, as I had left for the San Diego Zoo. When I finally saw the report in print (Clostridium septicum infection in the horse. Equine Practice, 1979), my name was on it, but there was no acknowledgment of Dr. King's role. I suspect that this is not the only report in the literature that would not have been published without his help or inspiration.

John has been tireless in his devotion to veterinary pathology. He has been an important and regular contributor to the C.L. Davis Foundation and other educational endeavors. This year he successfully organized the first Northeastern America Veterinary Pathology Conference in Cobleskill, N.Y., and I suspect that conference will become an important educational meeting for pathologists and pathology trainees in the northeast.

I can not think of another veterinary pathologist that deserves this award more than John King. If you have any questions, please contact me at (215) 898-4523 or by FAX at (215) 898-0719.

Sincerely

Thomas J. Van Winkle, VMD
Associate Professor
Laboratory of Pathology

Dr. Annette Gendron
Research Animal Resources Center
University of Wisconsin
380 Enzyme Institute
1710 University Ave.
Madison, WI 53705-4098

Dear Dr. Gendron

I am writing to express my enthusiastic support of the nomination of John King for the Harold W. Casey Teaching Award. During my three years of residency training at Cornell I found Dr. King to be an inspiring teacher. Dr. King has a talent for noticing small details about anatomic pathology, especially post-mortem lesions, which is truly amazing to see in action. In addition, Dr. King has an ability to present his observations and theories generated by years of experience in a manner which is both educational and entertaining. While John has a reputation for being cantankerous I would say that side of his personality is reserved for those individuals who 'got no interest', to quote John. For those residents who have a genuine interest and passion for pathology John is always available and always dedicated to teaching in the manner he finds most effective. Dr. King's own passion for anatomic pathology is unsurpassed and I can only hope that I can live up to the expectations he has for all graduates of the Cornell residency in anatomic pathology. I recently heard that John will be retiring in the near future. While this made me glad for John it also made me sad for anatomic pathology. We will be losing the day-to-day interactions with one of the few remaining giants of veterinary anatomic pathology. I have come to rely on John for my occasional telephone calls to discuss difficult cases and I can only hope that he won't mind me calling him at home to discuss these cases after he retires. In closing I would say that John King is fully deserving of the award for which he has been nominated and I can think of no one more appropriate for an award in the teaching of anatomic pathology.

Sincerely,

John M. Adaska DVM, MPVM, Dipl. ACVP
California Veterinary Diagnostic
Laboratory System
UC Davis, School of Veterinary Medicine
18830 Road 112
Tulare, CA 93274

WYETH-AYERST **W** RESEARCH

14 November 1997

Dr. Annette Gendron
Research Animal Research Center
University of Wisconsin
380 Enzyme Institute
1710 University Avenue
Madison, Wisconsin 53705

Dear Dr. Gendron:

I support the nomination of Dr. John King for the Harold W. Casey teaching award given by the C. L. Davis Foundation.

Dr. King is an excellent teacher and diagnostic pathologist. Those of us whom he trained over the years realize he has no equal in the necropsy room or at the microscope. Dr. King was always available to answer questions and to share his knowledge and interest in pathology with his students.

No one would be more deserving of this award. He is the best there is.

Sincerely,

James L. Inhelder, D.V.M.
Diplomate, ACVP

University of Illinois
at Urbana-Champaign

College of Veterinary Medicine
2001 South Lincoln Avenue
Urbana, IL 61801

Department of Veterinary Pathobiolog
217 333-2449
217 244-7421 *fax*

November 16, 1997

Dr. Sam Thompson, Director,
C. L. Davis Foundation

RE: Nomination of Dr. John M. King for the C.L. Davis Foundation Teaching Excellence Award

Dear Dr. Thompson: Sam

Dr. John King's passion is veterinary diagnostic pathology! His professional life has been devoted to the advancement of veterinary pathology through teaching and discovery. A flamboyant showman and demanding teacher, he has taught diagnostic pathology to professional and graduate students, as well as to faculty, throughout his tenure at the NewYork State College of Veterinary Medicine at Cornell University. John has left a legacy of well-trained veterinarians and veterinary pathologists who have made significant contributions to academia, diagnostic laboratories, and industry, particularly the pharmaceutical industry.

While John is a memorable teacher in all aspects of pathology, he will be best remembered for his show and tell, which occurs following afternoon necropsies. John King's vast knowledge, his cocky and self-assured attitude, and his use of diagnostic specimens, often dripping with blood, make him a truly memorable teacher. At these rounds, he calls on anybody in the audience, from the professional student to the senior professor and administrator, to identify and discuss the lesions of the day. Let me assure you, that if you do not know the answer, and he asks someone else or explains it himself, you will never forget the answer to that question! While John's diagnoses and explanations often seem off the cuff and off the wall, one often came across similar explanations when reading less well-known pathology texts.

Not being satisfied with simply teaching in the professional and graduate program at Cornell, John took delight in preparing boxes of kodachromes and glass to send to his previous students and others. He also took a traveling show on the road to adjacent veterinary schools and diagnostic laboratories, hauling buckets of specimens with him. In addition, he took many sabbaticals and leaves to lecture and demonstrate in countries around the world, including Australia, Africa, Taiwan, Africa and Europe. Although John appeared opinionated and hard-nosed, he really had a heart of gold beneath that exterior that was apparent to the people that he worked with. He often took his graduate students and professional students who were interested in pathology on some mad-cap expedition for rock climbing. Different life lessons were learned by this adventure. However, it did eventually catch up with him, he broke both ankles during a fall when rock climbing. Although not politically correct at all times, he certainly got his point across in the language that he used. He has many sayings, including the "kiss principle"--keep it simple, stupid. When you hear hoof beats, think horses and not zebras. John has also been a C. L. David Foundation faculty discussant for more years than one cares to remember; he has taught in C. L. Davis Foundation short courses all over the countryside over many years.

In summary, John can be described as a passionate and inspiring teacher who has left his mark on veterinary pathology around the world. He has been responsible for the training of numerous pathologists who are now scattered throughout the world and in many different careers. I am proud to be one of John's pupils while I was in Cornell's combined residency/PhD program from 1974 to 1977. John King is truly one of the great teachers of veterinary pathology and truly deserving to be awarded the Teaching Excellence Award.

Yours sincerely,

Wanda M. Haschek-Hock, BVSc, PhD
Professor and Head

A:\KING.WMH

WYETH-AYERST **W** *RESEARCH*

14 November 1997

Dr. Annette Gendron
Research Animal Research Center
University of Wisconsin
380 Enzyme Institute
1710 University Avenue
Madison, Wisconsin 53705

Dear Dr. Gendron:

It is with the greatest pleasure that I endorse the candidacy of Dr. John M. King for the Harold W. Casey Teaching Award from the C. L. Davis Foundation. I spent almost 6 years at Cornell University under Dr. King's mentorship. He always evidenced such a great sense of enthusiasm for Anatomical Pathology and more importantly his efforts were always dedicated to teaching the students and residents. Dr. King imparted his enthusiasm to us, and encouraged us to become "lifelong" learners.

Dr. King always made available to us, the opportunity to expand our knowledge of Anatomical Pathology by encouraging independent thought, research into a given subject matter, and the opportunity to publish case studies in various journals.

On a more personal note, Dr. King cared about me as an individual, not just as a resident and senior resident. He helped me to procure employment in the pharmaceutical industry. We have kept in contact over these past 7 years and he still is concerned about me and my career development in toxicological pathology. He is a true friend.

Nobody deserves the Harold W. Case Award Teaching award more than Dr. John M. King. His likes will never be seen again in the area of Anatomical Pathology. Nobody has seen more, traveled the world more to teach and learn and still remained a truly decent individual. I am most privileged to have been one of his residents and I cherish my experience at Cornell with Dr. King.

Your truly,

Wayne I. Anderson, DVM, Ph.D
Pathologist, Anatomic Pathology

CHAZY, NEW YORK 12921 • TELEPHONE (518) 846-7123
FAX (518) 846-6345

Xiantang Li
3024 Bonnie Brae Cr.
Flossmoor, IL 60422
February 16, 1998

Dr. King and Ms King
118 Sheldon Road

Ithaca, NY 14850

Dear Dr. King and Ms King:

Congratulation again on your winning the C.L. Davis teaching award. You deserve it the most.

The Veterinary Medical Diagnostic Laboratory at University of Missouri-Columbia is looking for an anatomic pathologist, with 50% effort devoted toward supervising the immunohistochemistry laboratory and 45% toward diagnostic pathology service. I am very interested in this position and I have given them your name as my reference. If they are interested in my candidacy, they may call you.

Thank you very much.

Truly,

Xiantang Li

Xiantang Li

UNIVERSITY OF CALIFORNIA, DAVIS

BERKELEY • DAVIS • IRVINE • LOS ANGELES • RIVERSIDE • SAN DIEGO • SAN FRANCISCO, SANTA BARBARA • SANTA CRUZ

DEPARTMENT OF VETERINARY PATHOLOGY,
MICROBIOLOGY AND IMMUNOLOGY
(916) 752-1385
FAX: (916) 752-3349

SCHOOL OF VETERINARY MEDICINE
DAVIS, CALIFORNIA 95616-8739

AN ODE TO DR. JOHN KING, THE POET LAUREATE OF VETERINARY PATHOLOGY

The opening scene sets the stage.....Wildlife Pathology course 1977. I am new on campus, having just transferred from the veterinary school at UPenn, and an older student, having spent the last 6 years working in northern Vermont among free-spirited eccentric Yankees which made me a bit disappointed by the reserved academic atmosphere of veterinary medicine. When, in struts John King (this was before the ankle remodeling), armed with those infamous carousels, ranting and raging tales of caribou lesions, worm migrations, toxins, and viruses and death and destruction. It was (professional) love at first sight. I spent the semester in the back row, enjoying the theater of the wildlife disease class and "Show and Tell". But then took the front row (with Boothby, in skirts) during the summer of 1978 when I was one of the student necropsy prosectors hired for the summer.

Although I came to vet school enjoying pathology, any doubts I might have had that this was the career for me dispersed that summer, hanging out as a "Pathology Groupie" with such infamous grunts as Roland ("things take time", "Hey, Jack") Gunther, John ("have you ever thought about driving truck, Jim?") Lay, Jim ("this horse died from terminal politeness") Crisman, Tom Van Winkle, Paul Meunier, Paul ("Hey old man") Frelier and others. Those were grand times with a great enthusiastic faculty. But the greatest and most enthusiastic of all was John King. After 2 years in practice, I had to come back for more.

John King brought pathology and pathogenesis to life ("and then this ole hard fecal ball goes through the narrow pelvis and SQUASHES the prostate causing ..."), made us think probabilities (" I have a cow heart under the table, what has it got Munson?"), inspired us to think critically ("prove me wrong"), to see all lesions, even those that meant "diddley squat", and to use our noses in addition to our eyes ("smells like apples, what is it Munson?"). Taught us how to triage necropsies when they were piled to the ceiling, how to quickly find the main histopathologic lesions (20 slides in 50 minutes), and to have fun regardless of the fact that it was midnight and you were not yet done your biopsies for tomorrow. His service-oriented work ethic should be a model for all University Pathology departments.

No Pathology faculty member that I have known cared more about the education of residents in Anatomic Pathology. No one has devoted as much time to assembling slide sets and carousels, cruising the necropsy room to help the residents, disseminating information by conducting rounds and archiving pathology through gross photography as has John King. Where, but Cornell, is there a full house at necropsy rounds, requiring two showings on Friday? No veterinary student or resident leaves Cornell without John King imprinted in their soul.

X-Sender: huxtable@numbat.murdoch.edu.au
X-Mailer: Windows Eudora Light Version 1.5.4 (32)
Date: Wed, 18 Feb 1998 09:36:21 +0800
X-PH: V4.1@cornell.edu (Cornell Modified)
To: jms11@cornell.edu (Jean M Strickland)
From: Clive Huxtable <huxtable@numbat.murdoch.edu.au>
Subject: Hi there...and a message for JMK

Hello there Eileen

Yes I am still alive and kicking down here at the end of the world and hope all you folks in Schurman are doing well. Actually, I wanted to get greetings through to Dr. King and thought that this would be the quickest way. Could you forward this on to him please.

John

I saw about your teaching award in the C.L. Davis newsletter and just wanted to say CONGRATULATIONS and what a well-deserved recognition. You have made a major contribution to so many people's lives (even when they might have thought you were a real SOB at times!), and have been and will still be one of life's great characters. It has been a privilege for me to have had the benefit of your knowledge and experience.
I hear also that you are planning to retire this fall - please accept my sincere good wishes for a long, happy and healthy retirement for both you and Marie. Enjoy that big boat!

All the best

Clive H
A/Prof. Clive R. Huxtable
Senior Academic in Pathology
Division of Veterinary and Biomedical Sciences
Murdoch University
South St, Murdoch
Western Australia 6150
Ph. 08 9360 2297
Fax.08 9310 4144

West Trenton Animal Hospital, P.C.
JOHN J. KAZMIERCZAK, D.V.M.
568 GRAND AVENUE
WEST TRENTON, NEW JERSEY 08628

OFFICE HOURS
BY APPOINTMENT

TELEPHONE: (609) 771-0995
FAX: (609) 771-1193

September 8, 1997

John King, D.V.M., Ph.D.
Dept. Of Veterinary Pathology
Cornell University
College of Veterinary Medicine
Ithaca, New York 14850

Dear Dr. King:

This letter is a follow-up in regard to a conversation I had with you at the Veterinary School last June. At that time, I expressed an interest in perhaps returning to do some graduate work in pathology. I have been thinking about it in great depth over the summer, and have decided not to apply.

I would however, like to thank you for your encouragement and advice. I have always felt that you were one of the best professors that I ever had. You were an excellent teacher and had a warm personal side. I always felt inspired and comfortable in your classes.

If I am ever in Ithaca again, I would certainly like to stop in and pay a visit. Again, thank you for your time and all your help, while I was a veterinary student.

Warmest personal regards,

John

John Kazmierczak, D.V.M. (72)

JK/blk

Serge Rousselle
D.V.M., Diplomate A.C.V.P.
Pfizer - Centre de Recherche
France

April 8th , 1997

Dear members of the committee for the C.L. Davis' 1997 Harold W. Casey Teaching Award for Pathology,

As a former resident or should I say despite being a former resident in diagnostic pathology at Cornell, I am writing to you in strong support for Dr King's nomination. Three years under his control have been tough and so demanding but what a reward at the end. It really shapes you up as a self thinking pathologist. Some will argue that it shapes you as a King thinker; that's because there are too few poeple of his kind.

Being an extremely demanding teacher does not prevent him from being someone who cares for people. How many faculties regularly take the time to visit students, residents or staff when they are hospitalized. He consistently did.

As for his dedication to teaching it is unequalled in the cursus I've been through, rivaling with Dr Delahunta's in this matter. If he was in town, there was not a single week without his "King's box histoslide seminar", Kodachrome review and the very famous "Show and Tell". When he was asking you questions this show was your worst nightmare in your first year of residency, becoming the treat of the week by the end of the programm, as the diagnostic reflexes settled in. He had no fear of repeating tens and tens of times the "laws of pathology" until even the most slow-minded and idiot of us, whom I probably was, could look as a smart guy to the eye of an outsider.

I won't finish this letter without presenting the following anecdote to your appreciation:
For april fouls, in my first year of residency I had the histolab prepare a slide from a cross section of hotdog sausage. As it was the use among the residents I was passing the slide around for consultation with the history of it being a mass that was embedded in green exsudate, removed from the abdominal cavity of a hyperthermic dog. Most residents spent long minutes scanning the slide in search for clues and most looked up anxiously to me with a very honnest "I don't know" or with a more colorful "what the fuck is this ?". One resident, , who's name I'll keep secret, came up very confident that this was a classic case of teratoma! When you see the amount of necrosis that some of these tumor have, I guess this was not such a bad idea. Our instructor at the time couldn't put his mind away from the idea that this was just "a piece of sheet"; which, as a french gourmet, I could not totally disagree with. Finally, after such a success, the trick had to be tried on our god to us all, the famous Dr King. Without taking the history as usual, he took the slide and examined it for at least 5 seconds, which is exceptionally long for him. He slowly looked up at me to announce:" what is this, a sausage or what?" ... I could not speak! And I saw the light of deity in hese eagle's eyes!

UNIVERSITY OF CALIFORNIA, DAVIS

BERKELEY • DAVIS • IRVINE • LOS ANGELES • RIVERSIDE • SAN DIEGO • SAN FRANCISCO | SANTA BARBARA • SANTA CRUZ

DEPARTMENT OF VETERINARY PATHOLOGY,
MICROBIOLOGY AND IMMUNOLOGY
(916) 752-1385
FAX: (916) 752-3349

SCHOOL OF VETERINARY MEDICINE
DAVIS, CALIFORNIA 95616-8739

AN ODE TO DR. JOHN KING, THE POET LAUREATE OF VETERINARY PATHOLOGY

The opening scene sets the stage.....Wildlife Pathology course 1977. I am new on campus, having just transferred from the veterinary school at UPenn, and an older student, having spent the last 6 years working in northern Vermont among free-spirited eccentric Yankees which made me a bit disappointed by the reserved academic atmosphere of veterinary medicine. When, in struts John King (this was before the ankle remodeling), armed with those infamous carousels, ranting and raging tales of caribou lesions, worm migrations, toxins, and viruses and death and destruction. It was (professional) love at first sight. I spent the semester in the back row, enjoying the theater of the wildlife disease class and "Show and Tell". But then took the front row (with Boothby, in skirts) during the summer of 1978 when I was one of the student necropsy prosectors hired for the summer.

Although I came to vet school enjoying pathology, any doubts I might have had that this was the career for me dispersed that summer, hanging out as a "Pathology Groupie" with such infamous grunts as Roland ("things take time", "Hey, Jack") Gunther, John ("have you ever thought about driving truck, Jim?") Lay, Jim ("this horse died from terminal politeness") Crisman, Tom Van Winkle, Paul Meunier, Paul ("Hey old man") Frelier and others. Those were grand times with a great enthusiastic faculty. But the greatest and most enthusiastic of all was John King. After 2 years in practice, I had to come back for more.

John King brought pathology and pathogenesis to life ("and then this ole hard fecal ball goes through the narrow pelvis and SQUASHES the prostate causing ..."), made us think probabilities (" I have a cow heart under the table, what has it got Munson?"), inspired us to think critically ("prove me wrong"), to see all lesions, even those that meant "diddley squat", and to use our noses in addition to our eyes ("smells like apples, what is it Munson?"). Taught us how to triage necropsies when they were piled to the ceiling, how to quickly find the main histopathologic lesions (20 slides in 50 minutes), and to have fun regardless of the fact that it was midnight and you were not yet done your biopsies for tomorrow. His service-oriented work ethic should be a model for all University Pathology departments.

No Pathology faculty member that I have known cared more about the education of residents in Anatomic Pathology. No one has devoted as much time to assembling slide sets and carousels, cruising the necropsy room to help the residents, disseminating information by conducting rounds and archiving pathology through gross photography as has John King. Where, but Cornell, is there a full house at necropsy rounds, requiring two showings on Friday? No veterinary student or resident leaves Cornell without John King imprinted in their soul.

X-Sender: huxtable@numbat.murdoch.edu.au
X-Mailer: Windows Eudora Light Version 1.5.4 (32)
Date: Wed, 18 Feb 1998 09:36:21 +0800
X-PH: V4.1@cornell.edu (Cornell Modified)
To: jmsl1@cornell.edu (Jean M Strickland)
From: Clive Huxtable <huxtable@numbat.murdoch.edu.au>
Subject: Hi there...and a message for JMK

Hello there Eileen

Yes I am still alive and kicking down here at the end of the world and hope all you folks in Schurman are doing well. Actually, I wanted to get greetings through to Dr. King and thought that this would be the quickest way. Could you forward this on to him please.

John

I saw about your teaching award in the C.L. Davis newsletter and just wanted to say CONGRATULATIONS and what a well-deserved recognition. You have made a major contribution to so many people's lives (even when they might have thought you were a real SOB at times!), and have been and will still be one of life's great characters. It has been a privilege for me to have had the benefit of your knowledge and experience.
I hear also that you are planning to retire this fall - please accept my sincere good wishes for a long, happy and healthy retirement for both you and Marie. Enjoy that big boat!

All the best

Clive H
A/Prof. Clive R. Huxtable
Senior Academic in Pathology
Division of Veterinary and Biomedical Sciences
Murdoch University
South St, Murdoch
Western Australia 6150
Ph. 08 9360 2297
Fax.08 9310 4144

West Trenton Animal Hospital, P.C.

JOHN J. KAZMIERCZAK, D.V.M.
568 GRAND AVENUE
WEST TRENTON, NEW JERSEY 08628

OFFICE HOURS
BY APPOINTMENT

TELEPHONE: (609) 771-0995
FAX: (609) 771-1193

September 8, 1997

John King, D.V.M., Ph.D.
Dept. Of Veterinary Pathology
Cornell University
College of Veterinary Medicine
Ithaca, New York 14850

Dear Dr. King:

This letter is a follow-up in regard to a conversation I had with you at the Veterinary School last June. At that time, I expressed an interest in perhaps returning to do some graduate work in pathology. I have been thinking about it in great depth over the summer, and have decided not to apply.

I would however, like to thank you for your encouragement and advice. I have always felt that you were one of the best professors that I ever had. You were an excellent teacher and had a warm personal side. I always felt inspired and comfortable in your classes.

If I am ever in Ithaca again, I would certainly like to stop in and pay a visit. Again, thank you for your time and all your help, while I was a veterinary student.

Warmest personal regards,

John

John Kazmierczak, D.V.M. (72)

JK/blk

Serge Rousselle
D.V.M., Diplomate A.C.V.P.
Pfizer - Centre de Recherche
France

April 8th , 1997

Dear members of the committee for the C.L. Davis' 1997 Harold W. Casey Teaching Award for Pathology,

As a former resident or should I say despite being a former resident in diagnostic pathology at Cornell, I am writing to you in strong support for Dr King's nomination. Three years under his control have been tough and so demanding but what a reward at the end. It really shapes you up as a self thinking pathologist. Some will argue that it shapes you as a King thinker; that's because there are too few poeple of his kind.

Being an extremely demanding teacher does not prevent him from being someone who cares for people. How many faculties regularly take the time to visit students, residents or staff when they are hospitalized. He consistently did.

As for his dedication to teaching it is unequalled in the cursus I've been through, rivaling with Dr Delahunta's in this matter. If he was in town, there was not a single week without his "King's box histoslide seminar", Kodachrome review and the very famous "Show and Tell". When he was asking you questions this show was your worst nightmare in your first year of residency, becoming the treat of the week by the end of the programm, as the diagnostic reflexes settled in. He had no fear of repeating tens and tens of times the "laws of pathology" until even the most slow-minded and idiot of us, whom I probably was, could look as a smart guy to the eye of an outsider.

I won't finish this letter without presenting the following anecdote to your appreciation:
For april fouls, in my first year of residency I had the histolab prepare a slide from a cross section of hotdog sausage. As it was the use among the residents I was passing the slide around for consultation with the history of it being a mass that was embedded in green exsudate, removed from the abdominal cavity of a hyperthermic dog. Most residents spent long minutes scanning the slide in search for clues and most looked up anxiously to me with a very honnest "I don't know" or with a more colorful "what the fuck is this ?". One resident, , who's name I'll keep secret, came up very confident that this was a classic case of teratoma! When you see the amount of necrosis that some of these tumor have, I guess this was not such a bad idea. Our instructor at the time couldn't put his mind away from the idea that this was just "a piece of sheet"; which, as a french gourmet, I could not totally disagree with. Finally, after such a success, the trick had to be tried on our god to us all, the famous Dr King. Without taking the history as usual, he took the slide and examined it for at least 5 seconds, which is exceptionally long for him. He slowly looked up at me to announce:" what is this, a sausage or what?" ... I could not speak! And I saw the light of deity in hese eagle's eyes!

This true storry says much about who Dr King is as a pathologist: he has seen everything and thinks much faster than most of us, making erroneously his detractors assume that he doesn't think. Those are probably the ones who didn' want to recognize their mistakes in front of him.

Enough nice thinks said about him; let's not be too nice with the guye. He has other characteristics that somehow balance the extraordinnary picture given above. This makes the character that we all know and respect.

With the expression of my recognition for his teaching.

Serge Rousselle.

Whoao, after he reads this I think it might be a good time to ask for a letter of recommendation from him.

THE UNIVERSITY
of LIVERPOOL

Professor D F Kelly
MA, PhD, BVSc, MRCVS, FRCPath
Professor of Veterinary Pathology

Department of Veterinary Pathology
Liverpool
L69 3BX

Telephone: 0151 794 4265/6122
Facsimile: 0151 794 4268/6005
Email: dfkelly@liv.ac.uk

DFK/vh

19th December 1997

Dr J M King
Department of Pathology
New York State College of Veterinary Medicine
Cornell University
Ithaca
NY 14853
U S A

Dear John

I did not get a chance to see you after the C L Davis Awards evening to congratulate you on the Harold Casey Teaching Award. I am writing to do so now because I can think of no worthier recipient of that acknowledgement than yourself. From afar, and through hearsay, I have long been aware of your many contributions to veterinary pathology and I share the Foundation's acknowledgement of that. It was a particular pleasure for me to meet you when you spoke at the European Division Symposium a few years back.

Another reason for my writing is to ask if you can let me know how I can obtain further copies of "The Necropsy Book" that you published in 1989. I would like to obtain additional copies for my Residents and senior students here.

I look forward to hearing from you.

With best wishes for Christmas and the New Year.

Yours sincerely

Don.

D F Kelly

Ref.: pat 12.1

University of Pretoria
Private Bag X04 Onderstepoort 0110 Republic of South Africa
Tel (012) 529-8000 Fax (012) 546-3102

Faculty of Veterinary Science

Department of Pathology
31 March 1998

Prof John King
Veterinary Pathology
New York State Veterinary College
ITHACA
NY 14853
United States of America

Dear John

Thank you for the mock examination papers and the recall from the boards; it does help the locals to keep up to date and on their toes

I have heard that there is a possibility that you and Marie may come to Africa for an extended tour of the local faculties. I should be delighted to receive you here and am looking forward to listen to your pearls of wisdom particularly in respect of macropathology

I have also read about the CL Davis award that you received; I did send an e-mail to the address supplied of the Cornell web page but do not know whether you received it. Once again, congratulations and well done; it is well deserved

Things here in SA are not too bad although there have been a few hiccups - as one would expect in cases where the government is taken over by people who have never governed. We also have just had visit from the American president and his wife - with not too much effect on the day to day happenings

Keep in touch and let me know if there is any help that you may need if and when you come to darkest Africa

Also give my regards to Marie and tell her that there may be time for some birding in the remote corners of SA - not that there may be many that she hasn't seen!

Regards

Nick

Nick Kriek

Admirative letter for John King : Dr. John Edwards

TEXAS A&M UNIVERSITY
Department of Veterinary Pathobiology
The Texas Veterinary Medical Center
College Station, Texas 77843-4467
(409) 845-5941
FAX (409) 845-9231

Dr. John M. King
Department of Veterinary Pathology
NY State College of Veterinary Medicine
Cornell University
Ithaca, NY 14853

11/10/97

Dr. King;

Those who care to do so have been asked to write a letter of testimonial that:

1. You can keep as a remembrance of your day of honor.
2. Provides some anecdotal information of our (you and I- or should I say, you vs me) interactions.
3. Gives some insight into your contribution to the profession and your teaching methodology.
4. Tells you something about what your students feel about you.

I also realize that there's a possibility that there may be as many letters vilifying you as there are honoring you. I wish I could say, "Who cares about the others?" Alas, I cannot, just as you cannot. The problem is such that you care too much and that has been the source of your greatest consternation. **No matter how useless you thought someone was, you kept trying to save their "Pathologic soul".**

This is a good point of departure for our story. One cold January morning in Ithaca in 1977 while Marilyn Wolfe was breaking me in- in swept the already infamous Dr. King. I had figured I would enjoy working with you because Marilyn said, "I love Dr. King." Somehow, our first meeting was quite different from what I had expected. You came in like a good housekeeper does after leaving chores to someone else while on vacation. It was with the air that you knew things would be fucked up and you'd straighten it out. (You had just returned from Taiwan.) But you came in like a windstorm. Cocky isn't strong enough, cock-sure? Condescending? Confident? Concentrated "King" is a tough medicine to take from a standing start. I felt more like I had just walked into a strange bar, and I stood next to the local "prick". I was to be tested and put into my place. You had on a tweed hat and held your head at an angle that said, "Take your best shot." This was at the same time as you said, "Hi, how are you?" We were circling each other and urinating on every vertical object on the famous Cornell necropsy floor (that is in 6" squares).

It got worse from there on. I knew no more than any other new "grunt". Unfortunately, our first "discussion" dealt with a cat with pleuritis. I said it was FIP, you of course said 99/100 of the time it is a ruptured lung abscess. It was the 1/100th case and you were wrong! Note, I still think of it as you were wrong- not I was right. Therein lies the rub. Everyone enjoys it so much when you're wrong. You make it so delicious! By the same token, we lose sight of that fact that we're glad (really) when you're right. You pulled many folks' fat from the fire. Not one of us likes being wrong so often. Then, many (most apparently) don't listen anymore, and, therefore, they don't learn (If they listened, they could be right more often!). Self defeating ain't it.

John King
11/10/97
Page 2

Show and tell was your opportunity to shine in that "golden age" of Cornell. One day, you said, "It could only be X." I piped up and enjoined, "It could also be that you're wrong!" Paul Frelier almost swallowed his dip. Howie Gelberg's forehead fell against the pipe railing of the "bleachers" used to seat the crowd. Sue Beggs shook with laughter, and Mark Walters just sat looking as non-plus'ed as imaginable. Marilyn shifted from foot to foot and Lois was confused. A new meaning was invented for "if looks could kill"! I believe that was when I saw my life pass before me in an instant. It was a religious experience. I realized that I could sit back and criticize all my life or I could listen and learn. If I spent my time generating facts and valid observations, I'd learn and, some day, teach.

Teach? Yes, I often saw your learning style. Did anyone ever say you were kind of "pushy"? You like to push someone to the limit of their knowledge : 1.) thus you learned what they knew; 2.) you can see if it's different in other places and 3.) you can find out if someone is full of -hit. You do accept other people's ideas IF you feel they've done their homework. You are like a sponge when it comes to learning. That brings me to another driving force to your being. Don't lie. You have spent your professional life "looking". I was with you a couple of times when someone said they had checked for something when you knew they hadn't. You never more trusted them, they committed the unpardonable sin- and they never understood why.

"THOU SHALT NOT BULLSHIT THY NEIGHBOR IN PATHOLOGY.

I guess I agree with you on this one too. There's not enough time to unlearn material that is invalid. Once a source is questionable, you have no use for it. It's like unreferenced statements, unrefereed literature and tabloids. It makes for interesting reading (The *Inquirer* last week commented that Elvis sired Diana's dog-faced love child with an alien.) but it isn't reliable. If you treat a dog with antibiotics and steroids do you treat anything but antibiotic and steroid deficiencies?

The atmosphere at Cornell was fantastic. Almost all of us then were like siblings vying for your approval. I never knew how much I'd miss having you around until I went off on my own. I enjoy so much the phone calls and the continuous generosity of your "care packages". Most people do. Almost every place I go I see your pictures. Even your "enemies"-read that "your strongest critics"- use your photographs. Your selfless dedication to our discipline is something to be proud of. You have seeded the world with a number of Pathologists worth a damn.

This letter has gotten too long. Most of our best stories I cannot write for public enjoyment. It would be a betrayal. You took me to my first MacDonald's. You almost got us into a fight at Tweetman's. I so enjoyed your stories at the State Street Diner. You had me with you listening to Dr. Olafson talk in the old museum. I regret that there are so many people who wouldn't "piss in your ear if your brains were on fire". Yes, you have some dissidents in the ACVP. You never realized that some people cannot separate their discipline from their feelings. Once you offend some people (even if you did not mean to do it), you've lost 'em. You never let up. Even some of the people who adored you got handled pretty roughly. We used to bask in triumph when we answered a question correctly. Then, you'd say something like, "There may be hope for you yet, Edwards." If we answered wrong- the world may crash around us. Do you recall telling someone, "Did you ever think maybe you ought to be a plumber?"? Ouch!! You know of course, that sometimes you say things that aren't politically correct? We can say that may have turned some folks off. It can be said that you believe:

"If you're going to make a Pathologist, you have to break a few egos."

Being a King advocate, it has been frustrating sometimes as you alienate people. I've always wanted everyone to like you and listen to you. You continue to turn folks off. In closing, I admit that some people say there's a little bit of your "style" (perhaps that's oxymoronic)- "way of going"- in me. I'll have to take this note I write to you, and take it to heart myself. I recently was informed at a Dept meeting that I was turning folks off too. I all too well know you don't mean to turn hurt anyone and I'm already wishing I was old enough to retire. Still it's like you said, "Shit I wish I could be around forever to see all the new stuff coming!" I hope to be as successful as you in instilling the desire to learn Pathology in some young people. You have every reason to be proud of your contribution to the discipline, and I'm proud to say you are my mentor. Thanks for everything, Boss.

I remain, John

Veterinary Pathology Catechism : John M. King

• Question

Colleagues

I was told, I think, that I have been invited to the December ACVP meeting in Seattle and that I could talk upon any subject of my choice. You have to realize that I have talked too much in general everywhere already so I'll just ask a few questions on this handout concerning pathology that you can take home and answer. Answer twenty or more and send them to me and I'll send you my answers to all of them. I thank you all now for your indulgence.

Most of the questions have been asked over the years of veterinary students, graduate students, some faculty such as Dr. C.G. Rickard, Dr. Ken McEntee and even Dr. Peter Olafson. You are in great company. In traveling to teach, I have been to five continents.

I was told by one professor not to ask such questions of his students without a more experienced faculty member present when asking such questions, but not having one such nearby with more experience you can be sure not many questions have been asked.

Of some interest to you pathlologists in the crowd, there has been a recent four day meeting for veterinary practitioners in Las Vegas with fifty speakers and with only one DACVP listed on this program. What does this tell us of interest in veterinary pathology?

These questions will usually ask why, what, how, etc, but some are not even deep pathology conundrums, but hopefully will make you think. Several have suggested that I am just showing my ignorance with my answers, but being alone here, I do not get a lot of feedback these days.

1- The first question that started it all was asked by my father-in-law who asked me why his dog gulped down any meat it was fed, but chewed the heck out of bread?

2- Question 2 is what is a probable main reason ruminants chew their "cud"?

3- In the late "50s" many cattle in NYS died acutely with enlarged, heavy, wet lungs affecting 80-85% of the lungs and often they had been exposed to Gypsy Moth control contaminated nearby pastures. Some clinicians said many cows inhaled the brown gas at the bottom of newly filled silos similar to the disease in man of Silo Fillers Disease. Except man usually died with chronic respiratory failure of Bronchiolitis Obliterans Fibrosa. So question 3 is Why the difference?

4- What is the primary lesion of these acute respiratory deaths in cattle?

5- The Brown Gas story was initially considered the answer until several cases came to necropsy with the animals not near silos except quite distant TRENCH SILOS (bunker silo) in which the gas, if any, would dissipate during transport to the cows. Now what is the likely answer?

6- How would one suggest a very novel partial answer to this problem using a less expensive ruminant, as a sheep?

7- As it seemed to be a toxic effect, what would be a suggestive treatment be for this acute, fatal wet lung disease in cattle that was suggested by Dr. Robert Kenney which worked if given in time?

8- The same treatment would not work on the chronic cases, but another treatment would and did.

What was that?

9- This question involves the acute death in sheep and dogs that have a large space occupying lesion of the pharyngeal region that was chronically present causing dyspnea, even while asleep, but that die suddenly when anesthetized. Why?

10- What is your explanation for death in sheep, and probably goats, which are very anemic and die without treatment and with no Haemonchus contortus in the abomasum?

11- Sheep are often found with lesions of Overeating Disease (Enterotoxemia) including extremely soft, mushy kidneys as expected, but we have several times now seen this "Pulpy Kidney" lesion in foals, calves and lambs without overeating, but present with a history of IV or per os therapy. What treatment?

12-Working in Switzerland, Argentina and Newfoundland we have sometimes necropsied young sheep, goats and caribou with evidence of large cat bite trauma. What are the two major lesions seen and where located?

13- What is the other consistent lesion one should look for in lambs with hypoplastic lungs?

14- In both cattle and sheep, Johne's Disease affects the bowel in making it much more than just thick and corrugated. What is it?

15- In several species we recognize a very strong uremic odor of a dark, congested colon. What and why does this occur?

16- The common heart anomaly, not usually noted clinically, is the most common heart anomaly of all animals put together. What is it?

17- Being in Australia I saw many fabulous diseases in many species. One I had seen here in NY, but did not know the cause. It is easily recognized in poorly conditioned lambs on pasture, particularly with potato related pastures. What is the internal, quite specific, lesion and cause? On my return, the first lamb seen with the disease was from the largest potato grower in NY.

18- In all species you may see young or old animals with one small and one large kidney. Possibly they could both be hypoplastic, but histopathology of both will hopefully change your mind. Cause?

19- In Australia, and probably throughout the world, sheep, and many other animals, have easily torn skin even with just finger tension of one hand. It occurs also in calves in utero even to the extent of broken bones with marked fracture repair in utero with large calluses. Name the genetic disease.

20- Lambs are sometimes born with severe inguinal hernias with a mecomium filled small intestine. What and why?

21- It is usually seen in large 400-600 pound male swine in good condition that die suddenly with high fever and early rigor mortis. It can also be found in younger swine. Even doing the necropsy may not be immediately diagnostic unless the adrenals are weighed and muscle examined. Cause?

22- A single twist of intestine in an overhand fashion is characteristic for this entity in pigs and woodchucks. Name?

23- Often the young pig is a "poor doer" and during the necropsy, unless the stomach is opened, the diagnosis is lost. One part of the stomach may be completely missing. Diagnosis? Suspected cause?

24- Pigs with this entity are also "poor doers", but are not necessarily underweight because of a greatly distended terminal colon packed full with feces and often distended small lymphatics on the gut surface. The distal rectal mucosa is present and patent, allowing gas passage, but immediately forward of this mucosal surface, the mucosa is absent and gut distended. Name and cause?

25- Small pigs are usually presented dead and necropsy reveals one or more segments of ruptured intestines. Where would you look for the actual cause and why there?

26- Very young cattle are sometimes seen to be walking on their fetlocks. Other lesions may be seen associated. Cause?

27- Primapaste is a probiotic given to foals to start normal organism growth in the bowels. Just one ounce can be fatal. What is the probable cause and what is the organ mainly affected?

28- Gastric rupture in the horse may be seen in horses with pedunculated lipomas, bastard strangles, ileus, etc, but a commonly missed cause is a low colonic obstruction. Why missed?

Where would the most likely inhalation pneumonia locus be located in cases of the following:
29- Horse following tubing?

30- Calf with White Muscle Disease?

31- Cow down with milk fever?

32- Sheep following drenching?

33- Single oat hull ingestion?

34- Excluding therapeutic intubation, Inhalation Pneumonia in an adult horse should make you think of another probable cause and why?

35- Where might you find irregular scars in the horse heart associated with Strongylus vulgaris and how many scars?

36- Where do you find single square scar in the horse heart and no evidence of strongyles?

37- Horses during races may be in a fall and die on the racetrack or shortly after. Stallions sometimes die suddenly after covering a mare and, in these cases, all die with a ruptured aorta. Many have been explained by high blood pressure. However we have seen older horses standing still, relaxed and euthanized by a bullet with a similar aortic lesion at necropsy. Why?

38- Foals and dogs have sometimes been found dead with severe peritonitis or bowel obstruction with a single, small mass of soft, spongy material as the only cause of the obstruction with marked degeneration of the immediate preceeding bowel. Explain.

39- Horses have this lesion with chronic pulmonary illness ending up with a diaphragmatic muscle rupture. Explain.

40- Idiopathic hypertrophy of the distal ileum is a common lesion in the horse sometimes associated with marked hernial outpocketing in the wall. Why? Explain.

41- Subacute fibrinous pleuritis (empyema, purulent pleuritis) is often blamed on a Strep or Corynebacterial infection with the primary cause overlooked. What is sometimes the primary cause and what other infectious agent can secondarily concentrate and surround the initial lung lesion?

42- Foals sometimes are sent to necropsy with a sloughed hoof, often of the front feet. Other limbs may also be involved. What is the likely Chronic cause of this condition not related to ergot, trauma or freezing.

43- Often stallions are found with thick, cloudy, yellow granular material in the kidneys and bladder. What is it most likely?

44- What is a usual cause of fundic necrosis of the urinary bladder in horses and other animals?

45- Careful observation of the renal pelvis may show an irregular enlargement of its lumen with a sometimes pebbly surface to this enlargement. Name and cause?

46- Small or large areas of brown, green or even partially transparent renal medullary degenerate tissue are seen in many species, but mainly in the horse. Cause?

47- Very large areas of the right dorsal colon usually, may be devoid of epithelium with minimal serosal inflammatory lesions. Islands of regenerating epithelium may also be scattered in these areas. Cause?

48- Where are "stretch ulcers" lesions to be found in the horse's bowel?

49- What is the most common form of heaves in horses?

50- What is the major lesion of chronic heaves?

51- What is the primary lesion of foals with NSAIDS poisoning and where does it occur in the body?

52- Almost all the gastrointestinal cases of Salmonellosis we encounter in the world have what diagnostic odor?

53- Classically, and relatively common, large, firm, bilateral masses of material can be seen just under the bulging peritoneal surface of the horse's abdominal wall. Name?

54- Other than the broken or damaged bones, what should you look at specifically to make a diagnosis of rickets or a cause of multiple fractures?

55- Severe trauma, in any species, to the brain, major nerve plexi or spinal cord often results in what heart lesion if they live at least five days? Most of the lesions are subclinical. These lesions of the heart may be seen with renal failure, gastric torsion and pancreatitis, but rarely.

56- Animals can die after prolonged surgery often with a very severe collapsed lung, but without trauma in the lung. Cause?

57- In all species, but mainly in dogs, some pigs and woodchucks, there may be found pronounced, various sized patches of hypertrophied mucosa present of the stomach. Name?

58- We all recognize the serious heart anomaly of a subaortic stenotic ring, but what would you call just half of that lesion that did not cause appreciable disease, if any, and still is the single most common heart anomaly of all animals put together?

59- What is the most likely cause of dark, fluid filled cysts in the dog prostate. Explain.

60- An acute exsanguination hemorrhage of an animal may be the cause of what lesion on the diaphragm itself. Why? I do not know but I point to the sky and say ask God.

61- At the distal end of the esophagus of older dogs one often finds multiple, tiny, dark dots of no significance, which can also be seen in young dogs on hormone therapy. What are they?

62- Tumor aged dogs may also have marked fibrosis and fat clumping of the gastrosplenic omentum which takes close histological examination to find the cause. Name?

63- Many large wild animals that have been in captivity for long periods of time often suddenly die from a large noise. Why?

64, 65, 66- From my experience I would say that vegetative endocarditis is secondary to three major entities. What are they, excluding those of Erysipelas in pigs and mycotoic disease in German Shepard dogs?

67- Multiple swollen areas of spleen may be found at necropsy of young and even older dogs. These are just multifocal areas of blood. Explain.

68- We all recognize the disease of gastric torsion that is easily reduced by simply untwisting the stomach and spleen, but what do you call the stomach and spleen that is twisted, but inside the omental bursa and not easily replaced?

69- What is the cause of gas bubbles in the urinary bladder mucosa of dogs, cows and horses among others, freshly dead?

70- What is probably the best explanation for cats or other species with Nutritional Panniculitis (Steatosis) in which some fat depots are affected and others, in the same animal, are not? What is the often associated odor of the affected fat?

71- Certainly cats and other species can have liver cavities filled with just blood clots, but other cats (only a few cases) will have masses or large areas of parenchyma in which only the sinuses are distended with blood causing the mass and not a single cavity of blood. Cause? One clue we recognize is that we call it Slow Forming Hematoma and each case has a similar etiological history.

72- Where does one find the most Pacinian Corpuscles grossly in cats?

73- Cats have a pigment nephrosis apparently more than other species. Where is most of the pigment found grossly in the kidneys?

74- With aflatoxicosis one of the very first clinical signs in dogs is what and probably why?

75- In evaluating various toxic effects on the dog liver experimentally between different toxins, what is a major external parameter to be considered and why?

76- Calves in Australia died with marked subpericostal hemorrhages of the distal ends of the ribs. What was the diagnosis in numerous calves from the farm? The children like to fish.

77- Anemic and slightly icteric calves were submitted for necropsy which had a history of a few calves bawling in the morning which involved more calves as time progressed. By the next morning all were bawling. The pipes had frozen and a few calves died after restoration of water source. Why?

78- Calves were treated (illegally) with powdered nitrofurazone and started to die about 8-10 weeks of age with marked hemorrhaging of most tissues. Probable pathogenesis?

79 & 80- Cows die acutely from the toxic effect of abnormal feeds they eat as the higher oxides of nitrogen, 3methyl indole, paraquat, moldy sweet potatoes and even perilla mint. How does the toxic products get to the lungs and how could you prove it?

81- A relatively new disease has been noted that kills cattle with respiratory disease characterized by enlarged lungs with definite yellow appearance of the lung stroma. Probable cause?

82- Cattle die with acute septic peritonitis after mechanically assisted calving within 12-24 hours of being assisted. Cause?

83- Cattle are brought in for necropsy after being ill only a few hours or one day to the next. White powder may or may not be found on the pharyngeal mucosa. The animals are usually dry cows or heifers on old pastures that may have been orchards that are long since gone. What is the suspected cause and explanation related to pastures and orchards?

84- Where in the cow's liver will a solitary liver abscess probably be found and why?

85- A small liver abscess may rupture for the first time. What might its effect be?

86- What might its effect be if it heals and ruptures a second time?

87- What might be the effect of a large liver abscess when it ruptures the first time?

88- A liver abscess may heal over with a thrombus produced at the site and small bits of thrombotic debris may shower the lungs, but if a single larger piece goes to the lung, what may happen?

89- If the larger piece blocks a lung vessel which vessel could it be?

90- If this large infected embolus persists chronically and the cow lives, what is a common sequel to cause death?

91- Cattle with acute to chronic pulmonary disease may develop a displaced abomasum requiring surgery and an abomasopexy. After surgery the cattle are acutely ill with lung disease and die. Why?

92- Pathology is a science that tends to use all our senses and this fatal entity of pigs or cattle with its stomach having such a strong odor of apple cider should suggest what entity?

93- Several Guernsey and Jersey cattle in this man's dairy had been coughing now and then, but suddenly worsened one night with a sudden loss of milk production. Two were slaughtered for lung examination. Slight emphysema was noted with scattered green nodules throughout which turned yellow with time. They were turned out to pasture daily. Suspected lesion and cause?

94- Numerous cases of this entity have come from the necropsy floors from animals that have been heavily treated for diarrhea and fluid loss. The primary lesion seen has been well marked thrombosis of renal veins, not arteries. Loss of renal function has not been remarkable though the animals die. Probable cause?

95- Seen in young cattle mainly and first in dwarf beef breeds as Angus and Herefords, but sometimes in Guernseys and Jerseys, the lesions were initially called Dwarf Bones, but later we had to refer to them as Bloat Bones as we saw them in Holsteins that were never dwarfs, but did bloat. We do not know the cause of the bloat so we point to the sky and say "Ask God". Name the bones and where are they found?

96- A very common lesion seen in aborted calves has been a small, to a very large, relatively clear fluid filled cyst that may cause visceral displacements, but only rarely large enough to hurt the fetus by compression. To what organ is this attached?

97- One of the more common lung lesions in the horse is the finding of a single, locally extensive pneumonia that is usually not very septic. It is usually associated with Shipping. What is the cause and why?

98- This next disease occurs in adult cattle that have calved almost 30 days to the day they calved. They die with classical signs and cultures of the disease. Where are the lesions found?

99- We do see Blackleg sometimes in the heart, but our question here, which we do not have the answer for, is why the heart with no preexisting lesion of heart damage is able to stimulate the activation of circulating spores specifically in the heart?

100- In toxicity testing of experimental animals, what might be happening in the liver when some tests begin to return to normal by prolonged testing?

101- What is the lesion of acute higher oxides of nitrogen toxicity in cattle?

102- What is the distribution of BRSV pneumonia?

103- What is the distribution of toxoplasmosis pneumonia in pigs, cats and dogs?

104- Cats, cattle and some Japanese people die with gastric exsanguination. What is the unique lesion that causes it, excluding gastric ulcers?

105- What is the diagnostic finding in the cow's lung with Bovine Farmers lung disease?

106- As a "disease of progress," what is the crucial lesion of Incomplete Hepatic Infarction in cattle and its cause?

107- Grass and Winter Tetany affects what animals and what is the probable cause?

108- Horses are often found down in the stall or pen with a vertebral fracture for no obvious reason. What is a likely cause and why? (Forensic)

109- A <u>four</u> year old ram was brought for necropsy with very hard bones and a <u>parathyroid</u> tumor. It was raised with a large flock of sheep for wool production. Name the cause and probable pathogenesis.

110- Many lambs, even fawns, are brought in for necropsy and we often find hydronephrosis some with and some without renal disease. Cause and why?

111- Where is lateral pressure the highest in an aneurysm, in the entering artery, or in the dilated aneurysm portion or the exiting portion of vessel? Explain.

112- How many bot species, excluding hemeroidalis, in the horse stomach?

113- Roughly how can one differentiate grossly between a splenic hematoma and a hemangioma?

114- Some say an anthrax case may not show rigor mortis. Why not?

115- Often euthanized dog hearts may show discrete swollen small groups of muscle fibers grossly. Why?

116- What do horse ascarids especially and cockroaches have in common?

117- Although the diagnosis of starvation or chronic emaciation may be similar, what should be clinically evident in the history?

118- Dishrag liver is one descriptor for what fatal disease in horses?

119- What is a suggestive cause for aortic valve leaflets having fibrotic paired nodules along their free edges <u>excluding</u> Nodules of Arantius?

120- Many more calves in the north than in the southern USA die with emaciation. What are the four most likely related conditions in various combinations associated with these cases?

John M. King
336 Savage Farm Drive
Ithaca, NY 14650

(H) 607-257-6912
(C) 607-342-4646

Veterinary Pathology Catechism : John M. King 2006

Answers to 120 questions:

1- Dogs are carnivores thus their stomachs and digestion systems should not want to dilute gastric efforts for meat with bicarbonate saliva, but with bread (starches) salivary amylase is needed.

2- Cows need something to neutralize the marked constant acid production of rumina flora and fauna by saliva as produced with chewing. Benefit also is gained by smaller bits of plant ingesta for the flora and fauna.

3- Anti Gypsy Moth sprays, among other compounds, apparently increased the toxic rumen gases that were subsequently inhaled. The initial gas produced is probably high in the higher oxides of nitrogen, D L Tryptophane and others to cause type I pneumocytes to die and type II to proliferate and kill the cattle, but man is usually treated successfully early if exposed to the brown gas at the silo. Initially humans have acute signs, but with time, the weak nitric acids cause Bronchiolitis Obliterans Fibrosa that affects the humans and cattle when inhaled causing Silo Fillers Disease of man and so called AIP (Atypical Interstitial Pneumonia) as Proliferative Pneumonia in cattle mainly.

4- The primary lesion is the degeneration of the type I pneumocytes with subsequent proliferation of type II pneumocytes. The more chronic lesion is the weak nitric acid causing the bronchial fibrosis.

5- Although we had a few cases of Brown Gas from known exposure to it, we have had some cases that only ate silage from more distant "trench silos" with no known brown gas available except possibly from the eructation from the rumen itself.

6- The pathologists told the clinicians this, but initially physiologists had a difficult time accepting the eructated rumen gas idea until we proved normal sheep would go to sleep when anesthetic ether was pumped into the rumen, but not in sheep with a tracheal canula in place, as they could not inhale any rumen gas, so did not go to sleep.

7- Atropine therapy was used at the suggestion of Dr. Robert Kenney to, in effect, dry the heavy secretion of serum causing the wet, heavy lung effect helping to kill the affected animals. If given in a timely fashion, early on, it was the major successful treatment.

8- In chronic cases, the use of corticosteroids was the effective treatment to hinder bronchiolitis with fibrosis.

9- Apparently, large clinically apparent abscesses, cysts, etc in the pharyngeal region do not cause suffocation in <u>conscious</u> animals <u>if asleep</u>, but can certainly suffocate the <u>unconscious</u> animal because the gagging reflex is lost.

10- Even without treatment the Haemonchous parasite may "leave the sinking ship," the abomasum, and apparently be digested downstream in the now different environment.

11- It is suggested that with IV "sugar" treatment, the kidney load of glucose is sufficiently increased to allow an increase of autolytic digestion now that it has the energy source of glucose to enhance the process, even after death The pulpy kidney, in effect, is an artefact.

12- Large cats will usually bite the throat area to kill, but often hind limb or other trauma will be found in addition as it helps to catch the prey.

13- The finding of congenitally underdeveloped lungs in the lamb fetus is sometimes seen with congenital brain lesions.

14- In some cases of severe Johne's, the bowel is also so fragile that just grabbing the bowel will allow the brittle removal of fist size pieces, not ragged pieces. Probably due to the destruction of collagen and smooth muscle.

15- The large bowel is another organ that attempts or allows the elimination of urinary wastes in cases of renal failure and also allows the intestinal microorganisms to breakdown urea to ammonia, etc.

16- In most domestic animals, the single most common heart anomaly of all animals is the Incomplete Subaortic Stenotic Ring. It is most often not clinical.

17- White Liver Disease causes an easily recognized liver lesion of periportal fibrosis and round cell accumulations. It is due to a cobalt deficiency associated with potato farming with their need for increased cobalt in fertilizer.

18- One should always histopathologically examine both the small and large kidney for evidence of the cause of the initial renal disease in <u>both</u> kidneys such as renal poisoning, bilateral infection, etc, but not hypoplasia.

19- Dermatospraxis is a genetic defect of collagen structure allowing easily torn skin and weak, stretchy ligaments and tendons.

20- Lambs sometimes develop inguinal hernias because of meconium distended blind anomalous bowel that its great distension interferes with fetal passage from the dam at birth.

21- The adrenal glands of these affected animals usually weigh only ¼ to 1/3 of normal, which at this age should weigh about 35-40 grams, but may look normal in these animals with Porcine Stress Syndrome.

22- Intestinal Knotting with a single overhand knot.

23- Such a usually small, underweight piglet will commonly show epithelial loss of the esophageal portion of varying amounts even to complete loss of stratified squamous epithelium of that entire portion of the stomach.

24- Another case of an anomalous loss of epithelial surface is to be found at the distal end of the colon leaving the last 6-8cm of rectal mucosa <u>still present</u> and not affected. The lost epithelial area will be markedly distended because of the lack of protective mucosa. Another example of a congenital epithelial defect.

25- Traumatic bowel amputation from being stepped on by the sow usually has the evidence of traumatic edema and hemorrhage to be found in the flank area which is softer than the rest of the body and tends to trap the sow's foot if she thinks it is soft feces she is stepping in.

26- Collagen defect of the tendons throughout the body allowing stretching of limb tendons.

27- Liver damage in the newborn from a toxic agent that is in the probiotic itself. Some think it's a mycotoxin from the mold present and others think it's a toxic iron compound as part of the supplement.

28- Certainly the easily seen causes of obstruction are often involved with a ruptured stomach, but there are many occasions when lower bowel obstructions are easily overlooked by the severe peritonitis that may been seen mixed with fibrin and ingesta and you already have a cause of death you believe, the ruptured stomach.

29- Locally extensive lesions usually cranioventral.

30- Again, locally extensive lesions in cranioventral regions due to gravity following swallowing problems with the degenerate muscles of deglutition.

31- Cranioventrally depending on downside at time of inhalation.

32- Sheep are usually placed on the rump and leaned backward for drenching so lesions may easily be in both dorsal diaphragmatic lobes.

33- May be anywhere in the lung.

34- Other than tubing, the most common reason for inhalation in an adult horse is CNS disease affecting muscle control for swallowing.

35- As strongyles ascend in the intima of the aorta and affect the aortic arch, the debris may go to any coronary branch and scar the heart muscle with more than one cicatrix that can be of any shape.

36- The usually square scar is almost always in the center of the right atrial wall only and is a single lesion. Its cause is not known, but a problem with the vascular supply to the atrial wall is suspected.

37- Certainly racing horses may have high blood pressure, as do mating stallions, to cause aortic ruptures, but older horses standing relaxed just before euthanasia do not. In all these instances they all fall hard onto their chest to possibly kink the aorta at high systole to cause the rupture.

38- The elastic spongy mass compresses easily and may not be forwarded during peristalsis allowing for the bowel muscle to exhaust itself or ulcerate.

39- The cause with the lung is chronic heaves. It is while muscle cells thicken and strengthen with work the adhesive force between fibers is not strengthened, as is noted with the uterus being much more fragile when pregnant than when not pregnant.

40- Same reason given for question 39.

41- Most cases I've seen associated with empyema in animals have been the result of a ruptured local septic process in the lung, as a foreign body abscess that is not easily found in all the purulent debris without careful palpation of the entire lung. Pneumocystis carinii infection may surround the bacterial reactive site in the lung.

42- Make sure the foals feet are all palpated for temperature and the history checked for a chronic infectious process and high fever in the recent past with peripheral vasoconstriction and core temperature gangrene as a result.

43- Stallions especially among horses often have clumps of cloudy granular material of normal urinary sediment in their bladder and kidney that is often considered erroneously as purulent debris. It is often seen in rats and guinea pigs.

44- Fundic necrosis of the bladder in any species is usually the forced inability of the animal to urinate caused by lack of nervous control caused by spinal cord disease or urinary obstruction. Other bladder ruptures elsewhere in the bladder may be from trauma to a normal full bladder. Not necessarily in the fundus.

45- Irregular enlargement of the renal pelvis area itself is often the result of Postnecrotic Cavitation associated most commonly with NSAIDS damage to the medulla. It may be small and easily missed.

46- The variation of active renal medullary necrosis from NSAIDS is often green or clear. This lesion is also seen in other species less commonly.

47- Right dorsal colitis in horses due to NSAIDS is the cause and again is a commonly overlooked lesion and one often has to flush the mucosal surface to see it.

48- Stretch ulcers are limited to the actual areas of denuded right dorsal colitis caused by NSAIDS.

49- The acute lesion probably due to moldy feed in horses is the bronchiolitis fibrosis which is diffuse and most common..

50-Diffuse emphysema (COPD) is the major lesion of chronic heaves.

51- Foals, as different than mature horses, have the lesions due to NSAIDS in the duodenum and stomach while the lesion in adults is in the right dorsal colon. This has been shown to be due to the difference in prostaglandin production in both ages.

52- Salmonellosis almost anywhere in the world of animals smells like a septic tank.

53- The large masses of necrotic fat in the retroperitoneum of horses is called bilateral abdominal fat necrosis. Its cause is not known.

54- The very consistent lesion of animals with multiple broken bones (excluding trauma) is the white zone, the osteodystrophic line, at the distal ends of rib bones.

55- Five days after severe trauma to the brain, spinal cord or major nerve plexi, white degenerate foci of heart muscle, Brain/Heart Syndrome, or Neurogenic Cardiomyopathy, is a common finding, but not clinically important in itself.

56- Without known trauma involved, prolonged anesthetic surgery sometime results in fatal lung collapse due to failure to inflate the lungs immediately post surgically with air and its non-absorbable Nitrogen content.

57- In all species, but mostly in dogs, pigs and woodchucks, there is sometimes found this patch of hypertrophied mucosa is called just that and no known cause exists.

58- This single most common heart anomaly is just under and beside one or the other side of the aortic valve opening and is called an Incomplete Subaortic Stenotic Ring.

59- Probably the dark cysts, often mislabeled as prostatitis, are the result of very hard feces as from dietary dehydration compression of the prostate by fecal passage.

60- The diaphragmatic hemorrhages on either side of the diaphragm are not explained as yet, but are seen with severe exsanguination deaths.

61- These tiny spots in the distal esophagus of dogs are common and called Dilated Esophageal Gland Ducts. The cause is not known, but they may be seen in young dogs on hormone treatment.

62- Malignant Fibrosis of the Gastrosplenic Omentum which necessitates careful histological search of the fibrotic masses to find the malignant cells of the pancreas or intestine usually involved.

63- Large animals primarily in captivity are the most likely animals to die suddenly with greatly reduced size and/or weight of adrenal glands due to Disuse Atrophy.

Of about equal occurrence, the three entities for vegetative endocarditis are:
64- Congenital Heart Anomaly - 30%.

65- Chronic Septic Joint or Tendon Infection - 30%.

66- Chronic Infection anywhere in the body - 30%, with the other 10% due to Erysipelas in pigs and mycotic heart disease in German Shepard dogs and Streptococcus viridens in Opossums.

67- Blood swollen foci in the spleen of essentially normal dogs are considered terminal findings of Unequal Expulsion of Blood and are not considered significant.

68- Gastric torsions are easily reduced surgically or necroposy, but Gastric Inversions into the omental cavity are difficult and must be emptied and everted to get the stomach and spleen freed.

69- Gas bubbles in fresh necropsies are almost always associated with glucose therapy per os or intravenous and with natural cases of diabetes mellitus.

70- All depots of fat apparently are not metabolically similar and often have a fishy odor of cod liver oil.

71- All the cats we have seen with large areas of liver being markedly enlarged with blood only in distended sinusoids and not as lakes of blood as may be expected with hepatic hematomas. All these distended sinusoid cases have been associated with being laid upon, usually under pillows by children at play. The livers look like those of laying hens liver lesions that we call Slow Forming Hematomas.

72- Pacinian Corpuscles in the cat, although commonly seen by most histopathologists in the pancreas, are to be seen more easily by stretching the mesocolon grossly.

73- Clumps of pigment are commonly found distending the renal pelvis as friable dark masses in suspected cases of hemobartonella or other blood breakdown entities in the cat.

74- One of the first signs of aflatoxin poisoning seen in dogs that would die was anorexia, even before liver lesions were noticeable histologically.

75- Dogs, rats and probably any other animal used experimentally should all be tested with the many "tests" within a definite time frame to say one test is better than another.

76- Lead poisoning from motor scooter batteries in Australia killed many calves with well marked subperiosteal hemorrhages of the ribs.

77- The frozen pipes were helpful in diagnosis, but the reason some died was that when the COLD water flowed and the calves drank excessively, its absorption caused the blood to hemolyze and caused the anemia. Human marathon runners drinking really cold water often urinate red urine for the same reason.

78- Calves eating nitrofurazone, which is illegal for use in calves in the USA, would die in abut 8-10 weeks of multiple hemorrhages. The bleeding was due to bone marrow damaging effect of the chemical related to bone marrow damage of megakaryocytes to produce platelets. Platelets have a half life of 8-10 weeks so their loss from the marrow allowed the hemorrhaging. Fistulated ruminants lose weight if a fistula is not closed with some kind of plug.

79- It has been shown now that when rumen gas is eructated, up to 80% is inhaled allowing toxic gases to be absorbed from the rumen. Without the toxic gas, the gases from the rumen are often of essential nutritional value.

80- Ether gas put into the normal sheep's rumen would put the sheep to sleep, but if put into a sheep with a tracheal canula, preventing the sheep inhaling rumen gas, nothing would happen.

81- Moldy red clover silage made both the farmer and cattle have difficult respirations and, at sacrificial cattle necropsies, the lungs were inflated and the stroma was distinctly yellow with eosinophils to allow a diagnosis of Bovine Asthma.

82- These cows dying within hours of assisted calving from septic peritonitis as the result of pulling the calf through the pelvic canal in which a loop of bowel, usually small bowel, is also present, plus the calf pulled easily through the slippery uterus while both organs were in the pelvic canal at the same time. With the mechanical pulling of the calf the loop of bowel was squeezed and ruptured into the pelvic cavity. One had to get a good history to prove it in the cases seen.

83- The dead patches of grass scattered in the pastures used to be the location of the many sheds housing the toxic herbicides of fifty years ago that fell apart to allow the paper bags of arsenic, nicotine, etc to dissolve and soak into and remain in the ground for the animals to lick and die.

84- Often when a single abscess is found in the liver it is usually near the hilus as it is the entry port for venous return from the bowels to the liver.

85- A small abscess in the liver that ruptures for the first time may not have much effect except multifocal, tiny granulomas in the lung easily tolerated by a big cow and palpated at necropsy of a cow dead for other reasons.

86- A second time rupture of a small liver abscess may however cause an acute anaphylactoid lung reaction with marked edema, but also one may palpate the previous granulomas. The hilar area of the liver should be searched diligently for the abscess.

87- A large liver abscess rupture for the first time may physically block both pulmonary arteries and their branches. Pus may actually be seen in the pulmonary vessels.

88- A large liver septic thrombus may embolize to the lung and cause a sudden death or may first get trapped. An infarct may occur from the blocked entity bed, but due to the lungs dual blood supply it usually will not cause infarcts. Older areas of infarctions may be recognized by their brown/tan color.

89- The septic embolus may now continue the septic collapsing lung of surrounding parenchyma as it grows. With time the septic process may erode through a thicker major airway and with the continued blood pressure behind it cause fatal exsanguination.

90- Massive hemorrhage of epistaxis is the usual outcome with blood spread in front of the cow or, if not a large vessel is involved, some animals will swallow the blood fast enough so the blood may not be seen clinically except for an anemic animal.

91- Some cattle can live with various forms of cranioventral pneumonia for years as not all die from that entity. However some may be subjected to a surgical procedure, as for an abomasopexy, involving being placed on their backs. Purulent debris from the previously affected lobes can now drain from what were ventral airways into the now ventral airways and Secondary Inhalation Pneumonia may develop with severe emphysema.

92- Pigs usually, but cattle too, may bleed massively into their stomach or abomasum which will give off a strong characteristic odor of "apple cider" to the surrounding area or necropsy room.

93- Insecticide "face fogging" for flies incidentally was inhaled and killed the lungworms in the Guernsey and Jersey dairy cows, with Holsteins more resistant, that responded with coughing, respiratory distress and marked drop in milk production.

94- The only probable cause suggested, as in man, is that all the cases are related to heavy electrolyte therapy and/or diarrhea that affects both pigs, calves and man, especially very young or aged, allowing the efferent renal vessels to develop thrombi.

95- Initially we saw the bones only in Herefords, Angus, Jerseys and Guernseys that were dwarfs, but now we see them in Holsteins, also, that are bloated, but that are never dwarfs. The bones in the affected animals are in the skull and are the Wing of the Orbito sphenoid (WOS) and the Posterior Intraoccipital Synchondosis (PIOS).

96- The cyst referred to is considered to be an anomalous ventral mesenteric cyst on the liver.

97- One of the more common lung lesions of the horse causing focal pneumonia is called Shipping Fever due to the horses haltered head being tied up during shipping preventing the horse from SNORTING to rid its respiratory system of dust, etc during transport. It is often accompanied by somewhat proliferative nasal mucus which is not very septic whereas inhaled ingesta or dirty fluid can be very septic.

98- Postpartum Blackleg as a disease is known to occur 30 days postpartum in the muscles of the perineum apparently associated with trauma at the time of birth.

99- We also note a discrepancy in thinking that Blackleg in heart muscle only can be found without any previous or active extraneous damage to the heart muscle as thought to be causative.

100- Providing the experimental animals live long enough to develop regenerating liver cord cells, some of the liver function test being used, as prothrombin time, can return to normal even with the continuance of the same toxic dose to the regenerating cord cells as they may be resistant to the original toxins genetically.

101- Alveolar epithelial proliferation of type II pneumocytes in over 80% of the lung. Some call it atypical interstitial pneumonia which we believe is erroneous as it is the lining epithelial cells that are the targets of the toxic effect and NOT the interstitium which is only for structural support of the lung parenchyma, nerves and vessels .

102- The distribution of the BRSV lung lesion is a multifocal one, not diffuse or locally extensive, but if, for instance, a cranioventral pneumonia is already present one may certainly find the BRSV virus involved, but not associated directly with the preexisting cranioventral lung disease and lesions.

103- Toxoplasmosis in pigs, cats and dogs usually causes a diffuse lesion.

104- The usual finding in the affected stomach is a single arteriole just under the mucosa which has ruptured and most consider it an anomalous lesion.

105- One will be able to palpate the small multifocal nodules of granulation tissue with the mycotic cause of Polymicrosporon faenii present.

106- Considered a "disease of progress" because it follows the replacement of a displaced abomasum by allowing the release of trapped stagnating thrombi to embolize to the liver, but not causing true infarcts as they are in veins not arteries.

107- It has been published that both sheep and cattle can die with higher magnesium levels than others with lower levels still standing and normal. Almost all the animals have probably been eating green grass or pasture. Beef cattle with Winter Tetany on farms with richer owners again probably feeding better Vit A quality hay. These two types of hypomagnesemia can be prevented by magnesium therapy. It is thought that the excess Vit A levels interfere with the function of Vit D which is active absorption of calcium which then allows magnesium and other minerals to be absorbed passively if available.

108- Often when euthanizing horses with electricity, the animals die instantly followed by the noise of the vertebral column fracture which the severe electrical muscular contractions caused.

109- One should consider the extremely hard bones, as tested by hand breaking a rib against its curvature, plus a tumor of the parathyroid gland as related to the excess dietary calcium in the diet of the young ram eating the same diet as the milk producing ewes.

110- Most of the cases of various degrees of renal pelvis hydronephrosis are related in young animals that are orphaned and thus without their dams to stimulate urination and defecation for whatever reason. It is also the reason pouched animals do not live in a septic tank. The dam keeps them clean as the baby animals void wastes only when stimulated by the dam's warm, wet tongue.

111- Highest pressure would be at B according to Bernoulli's theorem that the water (blood) fluids, would be moving fastest as air does along an airplane top wing surface or curved away from the wind boat sail also It would also explain why you tend to swerve towards the truck that you are passing on the highway.

112- Close observation will usually show Gasterophilus intestinalis in the pyloric area of the stomach and G. nasalis in the duodenum.

113- The hemangioma is more likely to have renewed blood vessel growth.

114- The blood of such cases clots too fast and incompletely and just seems not to clot at all.

115- The chemical causes multifocal muscle swelling apparently.

116- They both have the same odor en mass apparently of female hormones.

117- The investigator should be aware that one is intentional and the other not intentional, for instance, ignorance or a bad tooth.

118- This term dishrag liver defines the horse's liver with Theilers Disease necrosis.

119- With age the structure of the heart changes to allow the valve leaflets to rub together as "kissing" lesions.

120- A calf or lamb that is cold (1) and wet (2) and maybe not being fed properly (3) standing in a windy (4) area, is a common cause of emaciation.

Cornell Webpage

Dr. John M. King's Necropsy Show & Tell

https://secure.vet.cornell.edu/nst/nst.asp

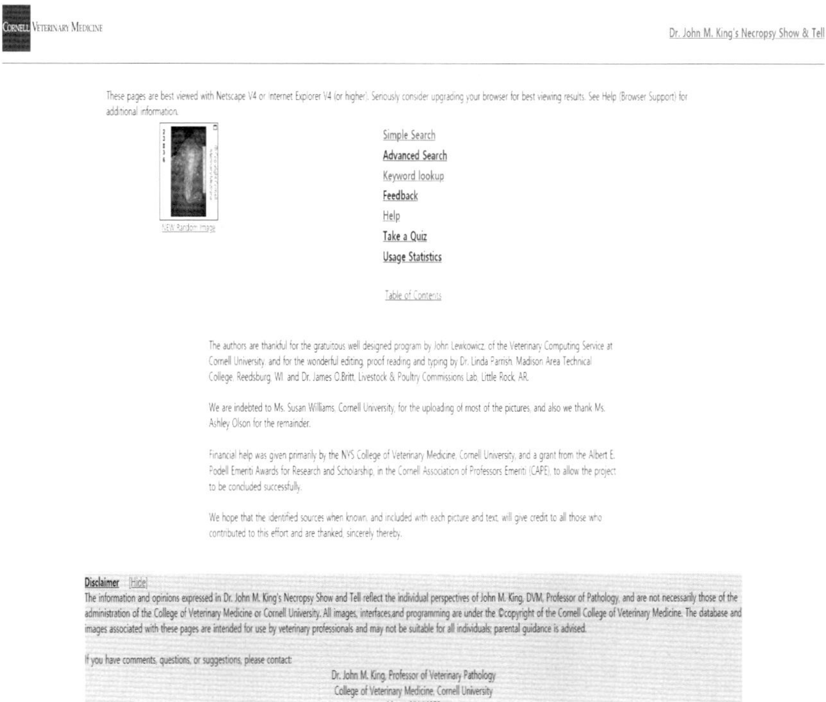

Cornell Veterinary Medicine

Dr. John M. King's Necropsy Show & Tell

These pages are best viewed with Netscape V4 or Internet Explorer V4 (or higher). Seriously consider upgrading your browser for best viewing results. See Help (Browser Support) for additional information.

NEW Random Image

Simple Search
Advanced Search
Keyword lookup
Feedback
Help
Take a Quiz
Usage Statistics

Table of Contents

The authors are thankful for the gratuitous well designed program by John Lewkowicz, of the Veterinary Computing Service at Cornell University, and for the wonderful editing, proof reading and typing by Dr. Linda Parrish, Madison Area Technical College, Reedsburg, WI. and Dr. James O.Britt, Livestock & Poultry Commissions Lab, Little Rock, AR.

We are indebted to Ms. Susan Williams, Cornell University, for the uploading of most of the pictures, and also we thank Ms. Ashley Olson for the remainder.

Financial help was given primarily by the NYS College of Veterinary Medicine, Cornell University, and a grant from the Albert E. Podell Emeriti Awards for Research and Scholarship, in the Cornell Association of Professors Emeriti (CAPE), to allow the project to be concluded successfully.

We hope that the identified sources when known, and included with each picture and text, will give credit to all those who contributed to this effort and are thanked, sincerely thereby.

Disclaimer [Hide]
The information and opinions expressed in Dr. John M. King's Necropsy Show and Tell reflect the individual perspectives of John M. King, DVM, Professor of Pathology, and are not necessarily those of the administration of the College of Veterinary Medicine or Cornell University. All images, interfaces,and programming are under the ©copyright of the Cornell College of Veterinary Medicine. The database and images associated with these pages are intended for use by veterinary professionals and may not be suitable for all individuals; parental guidance is advised.

If you have comments, questions, or suggestions, please contact:
Dr. John M. King, Professor of Veterinary Pathology
College of Veterinary Medicine, Cornell University

Disclaimer

The information and opinions expressed in Dr. John M. King's Necropsy Show and Tell reflect the individual perspectives of John M. King, DVM, Professor of Pathology, and are not necessarily those of the administration of the College of Veterinary Medicine or Cornell University. All images, interfaces,and programming are under the ©copyright of the Cornell College of Veterinary Medicine. The database and images associated with these pages are intended for use by veterinary professionals and may not be suitable for all individuals; parental guidance is advised.

If you have comments, questions, or suggestions, please contact:

Dr. John M. King, Professor of Veterinary Pathology

College of Veterinary Medicine, Cornell University

Ithaca, NY 14853

jmk31@cornell.edu

The authors are thankful for the gratuitous well designed program by John Lewkowicz, of the Veterinary Computing Service at Cornell University, and for the wonderful editing, proof reading and typing by Dr. Linda Parrish, Madison Area Technical College, Reedsburg, WI, and Dr. James O.Britt, Livestock & Poultry Commissions Lab, Little Rock, AR.

We are indebted to Ms. Susan Williams, Cornell University, for the uploading of most of the pictures, and also we thank Ms. Ashley Olson for the remainder.

Financial help was given primarily by the NYS College of Veterinary Medicine, Cornell University, and a grant from the Albert E. Podell Emeriti Awards for Research and Scholarship, in the Cornell Association of Professors Emeriti (CAPE), to allow the project to be concluded successfully.

We hope that the identified sources when known, and included with each picture and text, will give credit to all those who contributed to this effort and are thanked, sincerely thereby.

John King's Collection of Antique Veterinary Instruments

Started in 1975, this author, to remind the public what little the veterinary profession had to work with initially compared to the present, has collected ten to fifteen thousand veterinary instruments and paraphernalia for cleaning, wire brushing, waxing and mounting into museum quality glass fronted wooden display cases with individual identification of name of the item, probable manufacture source and use, if not self explanatory. The name of the veterinarian or person who donated, used or informed me about the items is typed on acid free paper and laminated for protection and mounted on or near the items.

Twenty-odd cases are mounted on the wall along the corridor near the Cornell veterinary library. The original cases were designed by Dr. Roger Panciera, Oklahoma State Veterinary College, Stillwater, Oklahoma, and Dr. Bruce Calnek, Cornell University. These multiple display cases have been registered with the American Veterinary Medical History Society with the continued efforts of the Secretary-Treasurer Susanne Whitaker.

These boxes, and subsequent boxes, have been made by J.M. King and are constructed of wood boards salvaged from a barn on the Elmira Road out of Ithaca. These boards came from a now disintegrating barn which in 1946 housed some dairy cattle that died from Bovine Virus Diarrhea ten to fourteen days after the ambulatory clinician, Dr. Frances Fox, and his students accidently transmitted the first known cases IN THE WORLD OF THIS DISEASE.

The latter boxes with many instruments and paraphernalia, as can reasonably be displayed within, have been donated to many small town museums and historical societies that would take them. A few larger cases have been donated to several larger museums such as the New York State Farmers Museum in Cooperstown, New York,

The American Museum of Veterinary Medicine outside of Philadelphia, PA and the new Veterinary Museum at the school in Stillwater, Oklahoma. Some of the many duplicate instruments have been donated to individuals who have indicated their desire to build showrooms for such.

The multiple Cornell display cases have been registered with the American Veterinary Medical History Society with the continued efforts of its Secretary-Treasurer, Susanne Whitaker.

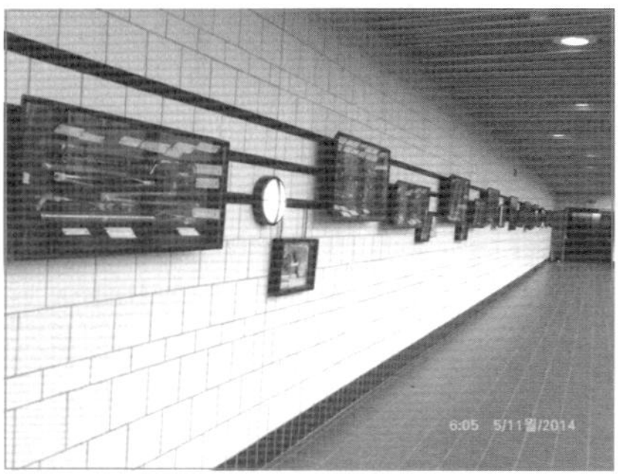

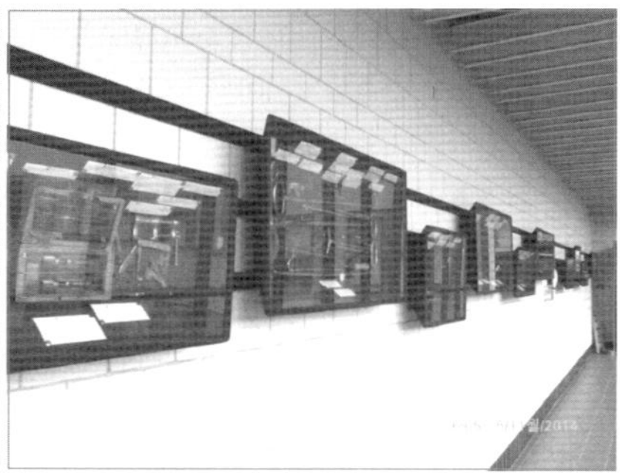

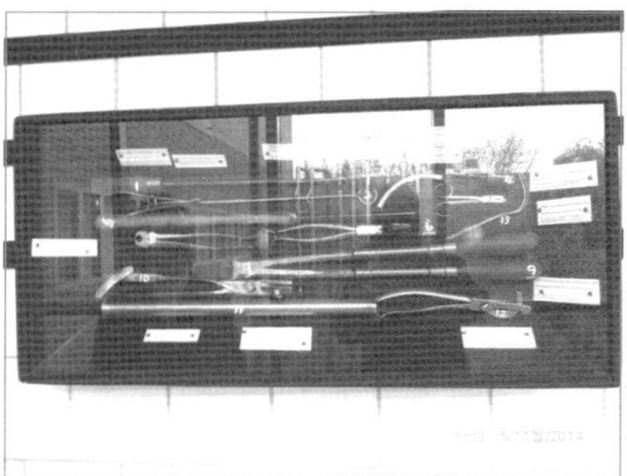

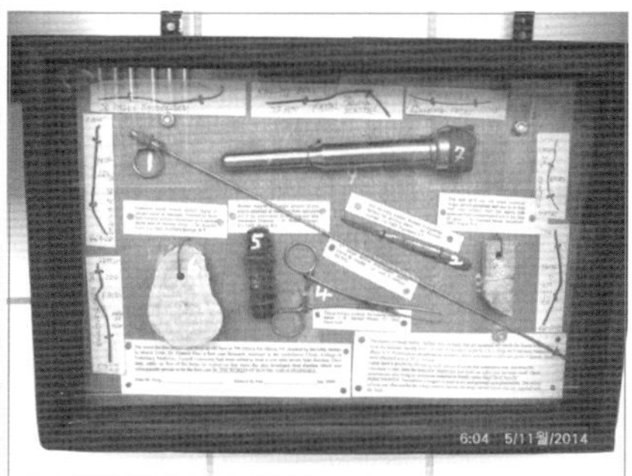

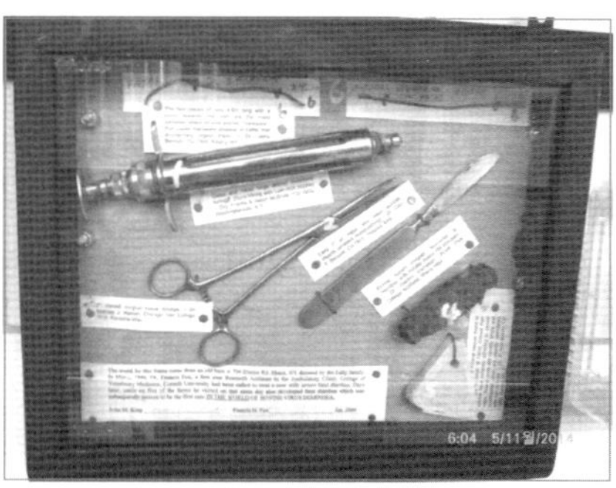

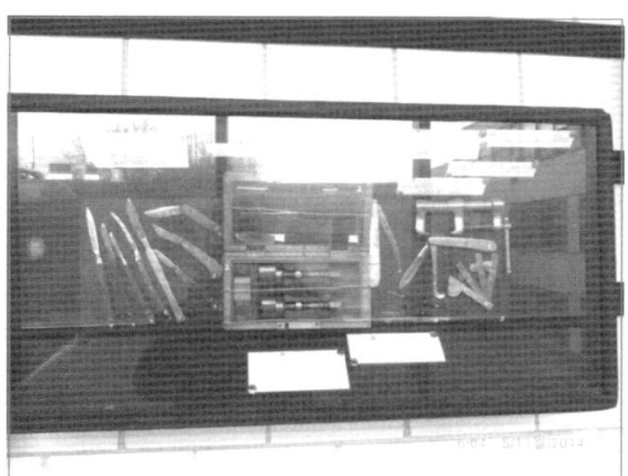

Special Issue of C.L. Davis Newsletter, June 2016 : Bruce H. Williams

C.L. DAVIS/S.W. THOMPSON DVM FOUNDATION
A TAX-EXEMPT, DONATIVE, PUBLICLY-SUPPORTED CHARITY
FOR THE ADVANCEMENT OF VETERINARY AND COMPARATIVE PATHOLOGY

Senior Editor: B. H. Williams, DVM   Managing Editor: V.S. Carreira, DVM, PhD

June 2016   Volume 43 Issue 5b

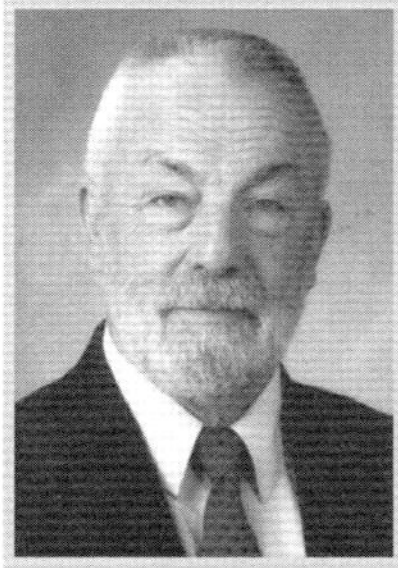

In Memoriam: John M. King, (1927-2016)

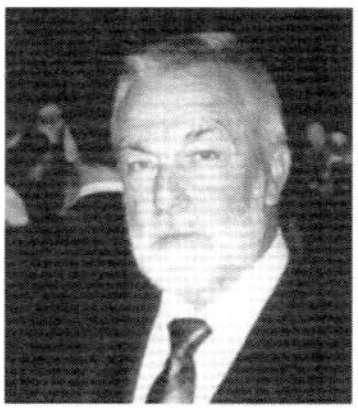

A giant's heart was stilled recently and its silence will reverberate forever within our profession. It was far larger the most, filled with a love of pathology, a love of learning, of students and of teaching, and a love of challenging both young and old minds alike. It was a heart whose generosity filled our textbooks with his observations without the need for recognition, that filled our lectures with his images without the need for attribution, and whose "Necropsy Book" - the best-selling volume ever written for veterinary pathologists - raised money not for his pocket, but for the education of veterinarians around the world.

John M. King's peers called him a "legend" or a "pillar of pathology", but he was so much more. John was beyond larger than life, he was mythic. His childhood in an orphanage where his only shoes were a pair of rubber boots, his service in as a U.S. Army paratrooper in Nazi Germany and his life-long love-affair and 70-year marriage to his darling Marie - even without veterinary pathology, it was a magical story.

Everyone who knew John has stories of him to tell, and some are probably even true. Some of us were blessed to know John a bit more than just his public persona, and our stories can only paint a pale picture of the influence he had on our lives and careers. But knowing John, he would rather have me impart story or two, rather than perform a dry-as-dust recitation of accolades from his amazing career.

I said that without the pathology, his story would still be amazing - but oh, the pathology! John was the unrivalled master of observation and perhaps the finest pure pathologist our field has ever known. His library was the necropsy floor, and his books were the endless stream of autopsied animals divulging their secrets to his knife or the knives of his students under his watchful eye. For 50 years, he saw with those crisp blue eyes alone what most pathologists, backed by the steady progress of technology, could or would not. Unlike most of us, who have assimilated the mass of our professional knowledge from books and the work of others, John learned it all on the necropsy floor. Although few of these discoveries were published at the time, they populate textbooks today, largely through the hundreds, maybe even thousands of his students around the world, who learned from him and later proved them to be true during their own careers.

John's curiosity was his defining feature. but perhaps even more important was his unflagging questioning of literally everything. He was not someone to accept an explanation simply because it was in print or was cited by a prominent pathologist. Seeing John's hand go up in the middle of one of your lectures meant that the podium was about to become your hot seat, much to John's and the audience's delight. More importantly, he imbued this truth-seeking into his thousands of students, encouraging them to challenge even what he was teaching them. I believe that it is this simple trait which has resulted in so many of his graduate students becoming renowned teachers on their own, as well as professors of veterinary pathology, outstanding researchers, and leaders of our profession.

In his later years, he wouldn't interrupt your lecture but he would let you know at the end. On a lecture trip I made with him to Korea a number of years ago, I thought I was doing pretty well until a week later when I received a 24-page handwritten letter from John of all of the things I had "gotten wrong". I felt terrible about it, until another more senior teacher than I admitted he had gotten one of 26 pages. (It isn't as bad as it sounds – John's handwriting was "unique" at best and try as he might, he could only fit about 10-12 lines onto a sheet of lined paper.) I still have that letter and it is one of my fondest possessions.

The necropsy room was not only his library, but it was also his theater. He was a master showman, always playing to packed houses. Even at 5PM on a Friday afternoon, at his "Show and Tell" sessions, the risers were always packed and it was standing room only. This wasn't just a Cornell phenomenon – "Show and Tell" toured the country as well. Each spring he would pack a truck with grad students and barrels of tissue in Klotz solution, sloshing his way down the East Coast and the South hitting every vet school from Ithaca to finally Texas A&M where the tissues were frayed and broken from the thousands of exploring hands they had encountered in between.

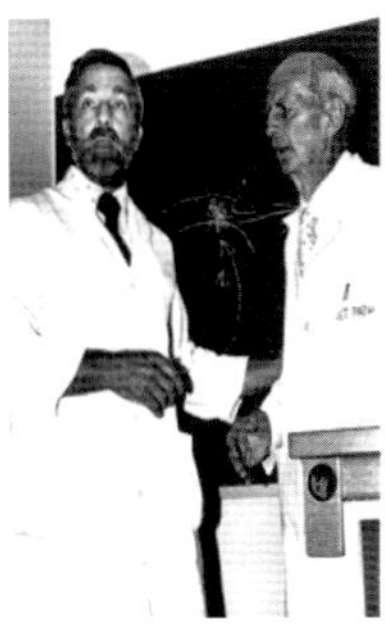

Many pathologists who only knew John from afar were put off by the size of John's personality. For those of us who were able to know him, we knew John's bluster to be far more a part of his myth than grounded in any truth. One of my favorite stories about John concerned his mentor Dr. Peter Olafson, who had "owned" the Cornell necropsy floor before John. When John took over that responsibility, each Friday afternoon he would help the frail and nearly blind Dr. Olafson to a seat at the edge of the necropsy table in front of a hundred or more students and faculty. John, an amazing pathologist by now in his own right, would simply describe the lesions for Dr. Olafson, who would either comment on the case, or wave his hand for John to describe another lesion. John never offered a dissenting opinion, and his kindness and obvious love and respect for Dr. Olafson was not lost on a packed house.

Later in his career, John was the driving force in instituting the Olafson Medal, an award given to pathologists around the world who have made distinguished contributions to the field in the combined disciplines of diagnostics, teaching and research. After many years, and only after stepping down from the committee, he was unanimously given the award for which he had steadfastly refused to allow himself to be considered.

To see John with the students was to see the real man. Students loved John and he loved them back. No question was beneath him, and his time was always theirs. John had some rough edges to be true, but they were necessary as a defense for the softest, kindest heart imaginable. Passing years were not always kind to John's unfiltered nature; however, the tremendous diversity of those in our profession who love him shows that good people will always triumph over progressively narrowing sensibilities. Sadly, on this day, I would rather hear one of John's "Williams, just what good ARE you?" than a compliment from anyone else I know.

God, John loved to teach – anywhere and anyone. My glass tabletop still proudly bears scratch marks from when he would hold court with non-pathologist dinner guests and my kids, showing them bezoars, blister beetles, and other bits of magic from his "Black Box" - a battered old suitcase with a chain leash for a handle into which he had piled a career's worth of portable oddities and treasures that didn't require fixation.

One of John's favorite pastimes was giving young (and old) booksmart pathologists the "pathology catechism"...over a 100 questions about veterinary pathology that aren't in any textbook. I took it several times, always failing miserably (and later pretending to after I had memorized a copy he left lying around) to his great delight. While a correct answer would bring a twinkle to his eye and a paternal smile, he loved wrong answers best, because he knew a spirited discussion was in the offing. John loved the argument, because in his later years, when he was no longer in the necropsy room, that was where he would learn something new (not that it would change his long-held views on pathology, but he delighted in learning new things almost as much as he did in teaching). At the 2012 ACVP meeting, where he was invited to talk as a "Pillar of Pathology", rather than recounting the high points of his unrivaled career as expected, John decided to give the assembled guests a part of the "catechism" instead. The ACVP learned that day what we all had known for so long – you never know what John was going to say, but it was always entertaining.

John didn't know everything, and he was the first person to tell you this fact. There were few questions he probably had never considered, and he knew the ones that had him stumped. When you asked him one of these, he would just smile and simply raise his index finger to the sky and say "Ask him". And his later years, he would tell me "Ask him yourself, because I'm too close to doing it for real".

Now that my friend John is gone, I know that God is going to be busy for a while.

...Bruce H. Williams, DVM (JPC)

A Very Short Biography (which John would still say is too long...)

Born January 16, 1927 in Boston MA, John attended public school until his family separated in 1935. As a seven-year-old, he attended Hillside School (a farm home school) in Marlboro MA until 1945. It was at the Hillside School, under the tutelage of a visiting veterinarian, where he gained his lifelong interest in veterinary medicine. In 1945, John joined the US Army and served in Germany for a year. In November 1947, he married Marie Ryan, whom he had met at a dance during the war at Aberdeen Proving Ground. (The state still required John, an Army paratrooper at the time, to obtain his mother's permission to marry). Following the completion of four years in the military, John worked a year for Delaware Power and Light Company as a lineman before attending the University of Delaware for two years in pre-vet studies. Using his GI bill, he went on to Oklahoma Agricultural and Mechanical College (now Oklahoma State University) for a year prior to entering veterinary college (where John admitted to getting a "D" in clinics because of his "cocky" attitude).

In 1955, John came to Cornell (replacing Kenneth Jubb) to begin a Ph.D under the renowned Peter Olafson, and remained for 50 years in the College of Veterinary Medicine, performing, in his own estimation, over 120,000 autopsies. During his teaching career at the NYS Veterinary College at Cornell he spent all of his sabbaticals in foreign countries to which he was invited to teach and do applied research. While many of his discoveries went unpublished due to his unflagging interest in the necropsy room and teaching his students, they populate veterinary textbooks today, thanks to those hundreds of students who verified them in their own subsequent practice.

John's own best-selling work "The Necropsy Book", published with Lois Roth and David Dodd, has sold more copies than any other pathology text, and his "Show and Tell" catalogue of over 20,000 images is used around the world by every teacher of veterinary pathology.

John and Marie were married for 68 years, a union that over the years continually served as an inspiration to all those around them. John and Marie had a son Jon David ("J.D"). in 1954, who passed away in 2002. J.D. (who studied business and hotel management at Cornell) and John built houses together on weekends, and shared a wonderful relationship. In a 1996 interview, when asked if he had any regrets, John said "...Only that I wish I had taken more time for family."

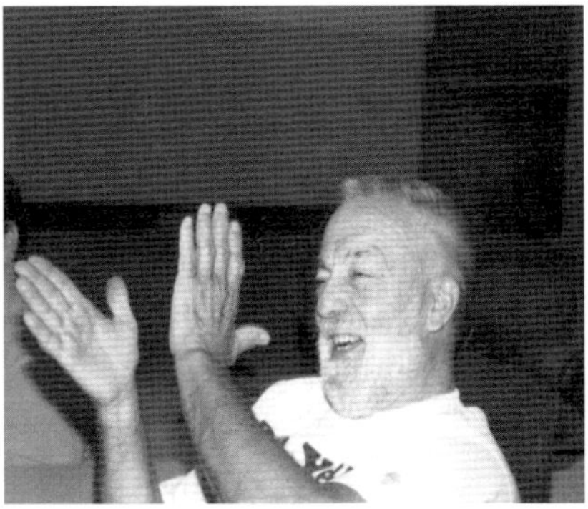

Dr. John King passed away Thursday April 14, 2016. John is survived by his beloved Marie Ryan King of Ithaca; a sister Ruth King of Florida; nieces and nephews. John is interred in Pleasant Grove Cemetery, Ithaca.

From Roger Renne (Tox Path Consultant):

I only knew John King for a relatively short time, at the CL Davis course meetings, the course he and other staff at Cornell offered to people studying for the ACVP boards, and at an occasional ACVP meeting. But I remember envying those who knew him better and worked with him. I found him to be an excellent, caring mentor and an interesting person to talk with about veterinary pathology or anything else.

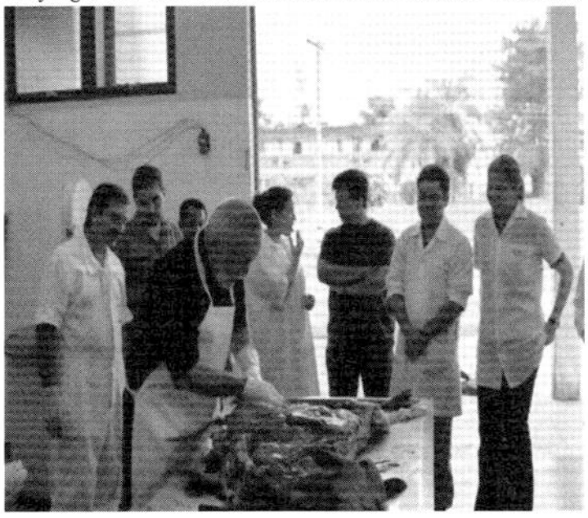

John on a visit to Brazil in 2003 – always teaching. (Image by Raquel Rech)

While at the Cornell course in 1973 I asked him for some wet tissues, blocks or slides from some lesions in large animals, since as a military vet in the preceptorship program I had limited experience and opportunity to look at slides from farm animals. He enthusiastically agreed to do so, took me into his office/lab and gave me a large number of these tissues/blocks/slides. I still have them, haven't looked at them much lately but whenever I see those boxes of slides I remember John King, his generosity and his willingness to help others.

From Wanda Haschek (Univ. of Illinois)

I arrived from Australia in June of 1974 as a naïve and overwhelmed student in the combined residency/PhD program. I was immediately given coveralls, boots, a knife and thrown into the necropsy room. There a loud brash cocky American held sway. Dr. King ignored me for a while before proceeding to demonstrate necropsy procedures at lightning speed but with great attention to detail. He asked "Are you married?". I replied "No" – he said "Pity". A man of few words but lots of questions – always questions - to find out what you didn't know! A stern look but a twinkle in his eye. Luckily I had George Apple, Claus Buergelt, Jim Inhelder, and a few others to help me survive and thrive during this "reign of terror".

Dr. King enjoyed putting me, his first female resident, through the rigors of pathology training. If I got responses to his questions wrong – it was "Bull---" or "Baloney!". If I got the answer right – it was" Not bad for a girl". His KISS (keep it simple sir/stupid – depending on the audience) principle – also stated as "If you hear hoofbeats think horses not zebras" was always in play.

But to really be initiated into the program you had to prove yourself by rock climbing. I did do so several times but that was enough for me. However, others like Lois Roth and Jeff Everitt accompanied John frequently. John managed to break his ankle in a failed belay but this did not deter him from continuing to rock climb.

A few other remembrances – Rattlesnakes in his office! Washboard music!

As my training progressed, the number of corrections on handwritten reports decreased – although they remained virtually illegible - as were his later letters. Punctuated by a shout of "coffee!" or "lunch!", John would take me and any other poor souls in the immediate area out to the donut shop for coffee or to lunch – but no handouts.

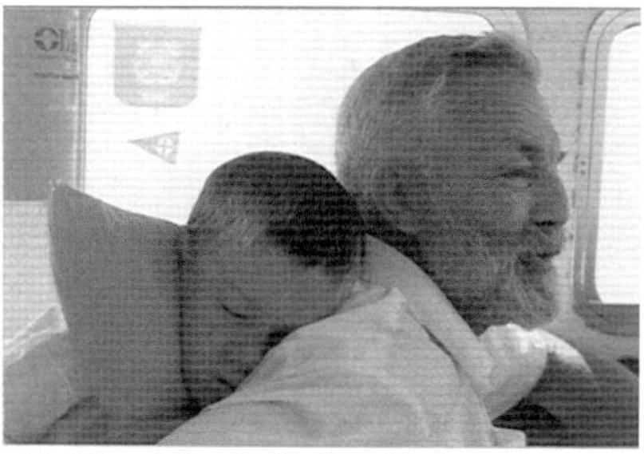

Antonio Fernandez Jr. and the King forever in our hearts and in our teaching "knives". From Canaries with LOVE , our FAMILY. See you again ¡¡¡¡ (1994) Image from Antonio Juesus Fernandez Rodriguez)

I dreaded seminar and Show and Tell – as you felt his gaze fall on you, a pit opened in your stomach. As Helen Han Hsu so aptly put it – we all got our daily dose of humiliation. However a mistake made was never repeated (especially if it involved "dumpster diving".)

John always kept you honest. Diagnostic choices were

- The answer according to the gospel of John
- One of his "off the wall" "theories" – these were based on his own observations and/or obscure publication(s) often from the medical or experimental literature
- Hands in prayer position signifying "only god knows"

One of these so called theories was the "brain-heart syndrome" – a syndrome that actually was based on published experimental work – Lois Roth and I did get a paper out - **King, J. M.**, L. Roth, and W. M. Haschek. (1982) Myocardial necrosis secondary to neural lesions in domestic animals. J.A.V.M.A.* 144-148.

John was responsible for my career specializing in tox path:

- Introduced me to Dr. Lennart Krook for my PhD research - on Vitamin D toxicity
- Introduced me to Don Lisk in Food Science to provide pathology support on some toxicology studies
- drove the residents to New Jersey to Sam Thompson's CL Davis Foundation lectures in industrial pathology

A credit to John's training, many residents, including me, passed ACVP boards first time round. John and Marie took pity on me and often had me out to their home for a meal. He was the emcee at my wedding in 1976 which was held in the Annabel Taylor Chapel. Jay Georgi and his oompah band played the night away at the reception. Guests included Lennart and Nancy Krook, Don Lien, Don Lisk, Jeff Everitt, Anne Merson, Bob and Hilda Riker. As I was finishing my training, Don Meuten, Marilyn Wolf, Chuck Wimberley and others arrived to join the newly constructed residency program ---.

After leaving Cornell, I went to Oak Ridge National Laboratory in Oak Ridge Tennessee and then to the University of Illinois. I visited with John at meetings and during a few return trips to Cornell, including his retirement in 1998. He participated in a CL Davis Course I ran at the University. One day he showed up in the path seminar I was running without any notice. He gave me a pathology goodies box that included blister beetles, enteroliths, a mouse skeleton stained with Alizarin red. He had made the box from an Ithaca barn that housed the first recognized BVD infected cattle.

John gave many of us a superb grounding in pathology. While tough on the outside - and certainly not politically correct by today's standards – he had a heart of gold. A true teacher and life long learner himself – he gave of himself across the world. Truly a pathology giant. He will be greatly missed by all of us in the veterinary pathology community.

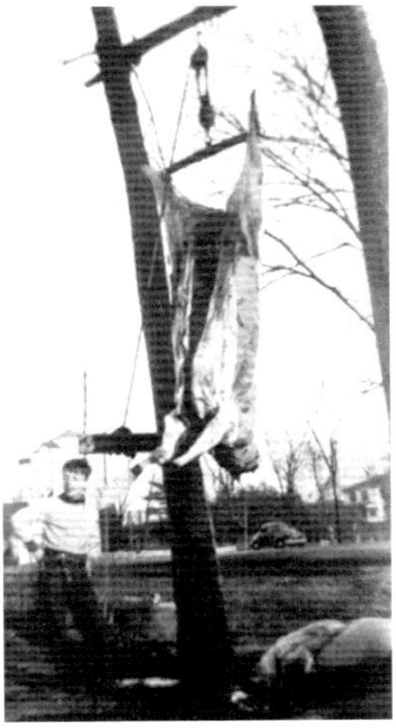
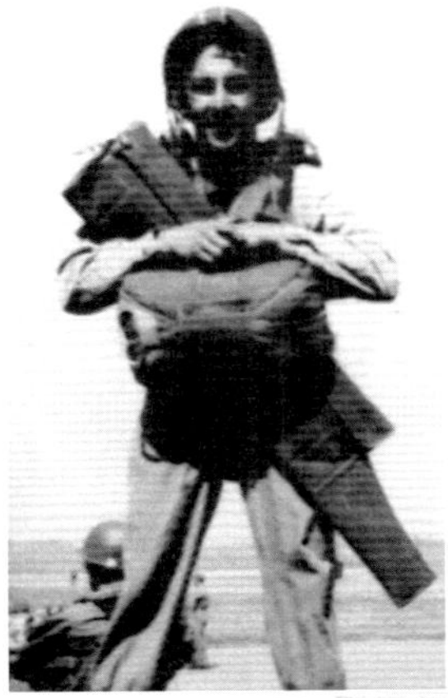
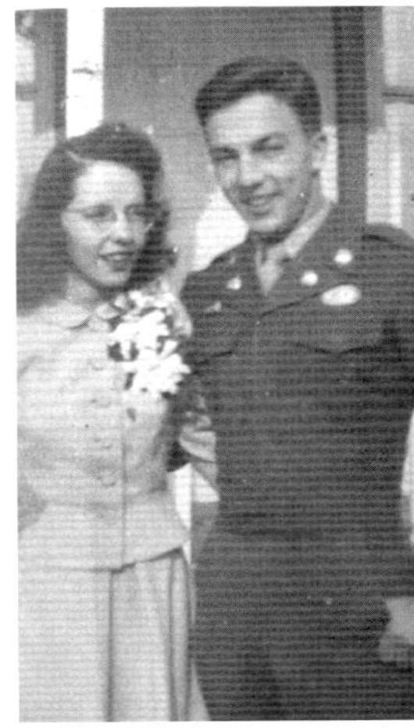
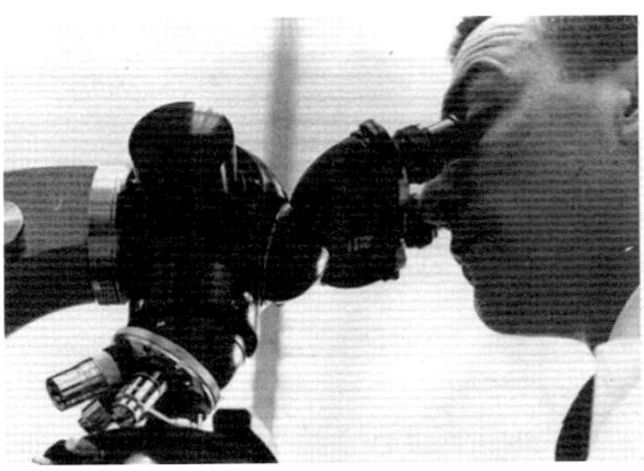
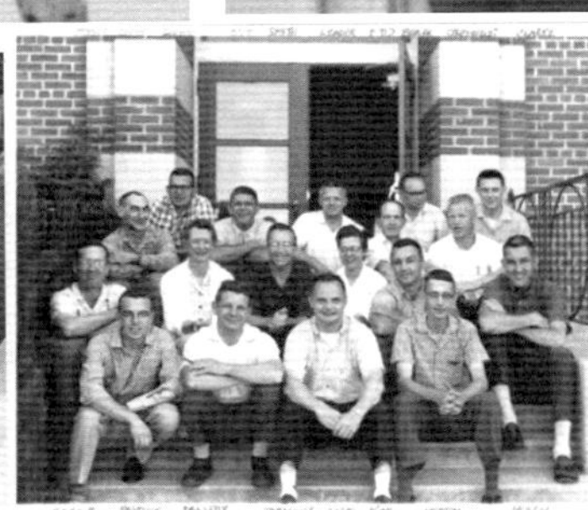
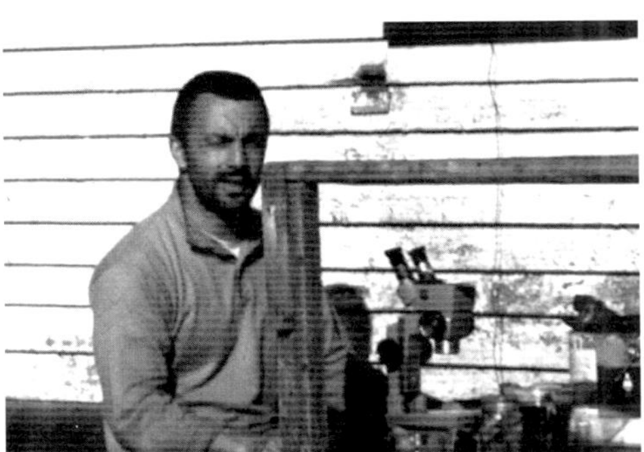

Top row: (Left) John (circa 1938) at the Hillside Farm home for boys. A ten-year-old John was both assistant vet and butcher for the farm animals at the school. (Center) In 1944, John enlisted and became an Army paratrooper with the 82nd Airborne Division. (Right) On Dec 14, 1947, John married Marie Ryan, a union that would last almost 70 years.
Center row: (Left) A young pathologist at Mellon Institute's Bushy Run Laboratory. (Right) A group photo at a 1961 WSU neuropath course with other notables including Don Cordy, Bob Leader, John Gorham and David Dodd.
Bottom Row: John in the field in Newfoundland in 1963 studying caribou mortality and associated diseases.

From Nelva Bryant (Centers for Disease Control)...

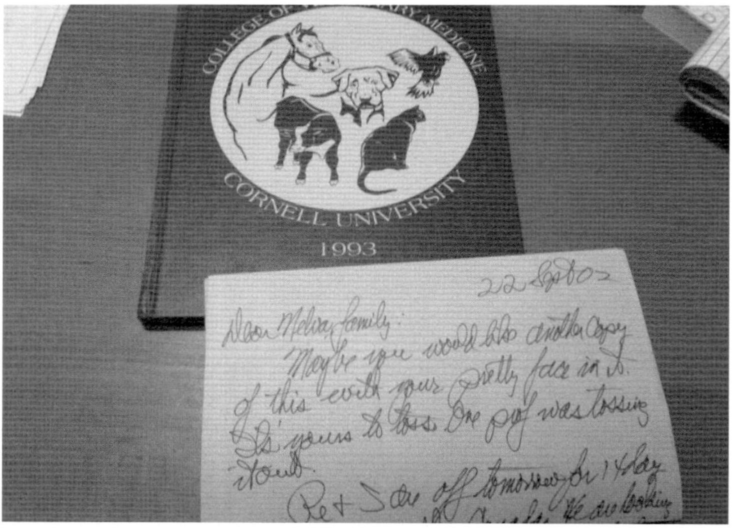

I'm proud to say that Dr. King was my mentor!!!

As a student, I was initially terrified of him. His teaching style was different, and sometimes he'd put you on the spot and would challenge you. Many students avoided him because of that. But something inside me knew that he cared deeply and he wanted his students to learn. I remember trying over and over to identify a "lesion" while performing necropsies. I would call him over to ask "Is this a lesion?" And he'd say "No", and then explain why it wasn't. Then finally, after numerous requests for him to see the "lesion".......I actually identified one and he smiled and said....."Bryant, I think you got something there!" If only he knew how happy that made me!

I am so fortunate to develop a close bond with him as a veterinary student, a member of the Necropsy Crew (Summer 1991), and as a veterinary pathology resident. He looked out for me on numerous occasions. After graduating from Vet School, I decided to pursue private practice in Atlanta, GA. I remember him tracking me down through my mother to see how I was doing. He wanted to know if I was happy in practice, and I wasn't. So he said get your application together to apply to become a pathology resident. That suggestion from him changed the course of my life and I'm so thankful. Throughout the years, we kept in touch. I'd send him photos of lesions, and I'd share with him my personal/professional ups and downs.

Back in 2002, I received a package from him. Inside was a 2 page letter and my class yearbook. I was so honored that he even thought to send it to me. Dr. John King meant the world to me. I'm going to miss him, but he's not gone. A part of him still lives inside me. He influenced my life and guided my career path. I will always cherish him. He was my mentor.

From Jey Koehler (Auburn Univ.)...

I met John King a few years ago when our Wednesday Slide Conference guest moderator stints lined up back-to-back and I allowed a few extra days on my trip to meet the legend. To be frank, his reputation as an outstanding gross pathologist was rivaled only by his reputation as a sexist, insensitive boor. I fully expected to be impressed by his knowledge, and appalled by his behavior.

But as is generally the case when we set aside our preconceived notions for a moment and approach people openly and without prejudice, what I encountered instead was a personality much more nuanced and sympathetic than I could have anticipated. During his seminar, as he rifled through his famous Black Box (as he must have done hundreds of times), he lit up with the puckish joy of someone engaged in doing the thing they love most in life. His pure delight in teaching was infectious and inspiring, and it was clear that he was able somehow to not only *deliver* the material in a way that felt fresh to the students in the room, but also to actually *experience* it himself as if it were the first time. This was the wonder of John—he was the consummate showman, but it was never just an act.

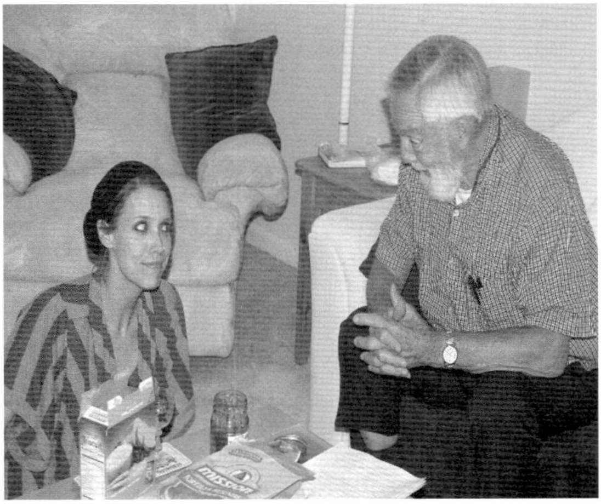

At the traditional post-conference happy hour, we ate and drank and listened to his stories of growing up in a Boston boys' home. For me, a mother of boys and a member of a bubble-wrapped generation and a privileged socioeconomic class unaccustomed to the kind of Depression- and WWII-era danger, deprivation, and sacrifice he experienced, these stories were heart-crushing. John delivered them with the nonchalance of someone reading a grocery list as almost everyone at the table struggled to inconspicuously dab the tears at the corners of our eyes.

When we took a trip to the special collections room in the National Library of Medicine, I watched the reverence and wonder on his face as he gently turned the pages of a hide-bound notebook from the Roman era detailing the various ailments of horses as they were understood at the time. Later, at Bruce's apartment, I showed him gross images of various interesting cases I planned to share with the residents, including one he had never seen before. He expressed genuine excitement, after which he tested me on the "catechism" and told me I was "pretty smart for a broad". Did he make this and other tone-deaf comments? Yes. But I don't think I'm being an apologist or a self-loathing feminist when I say that despite these flaws, the world of veterinary pathology (and the world in general) was greatly enriched by his being in it, and I feel privileged to have spent a little time with him.

From Wayne Anderson (Wyeth-Hoechst):

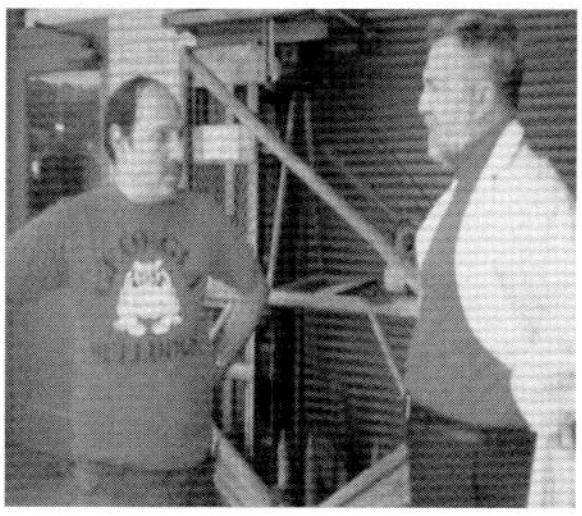

On a very snowy, and blustery weekend afternoon in Ithaca, I received a telephone call from John. I was not on service at the time. The phone call was direct and to the point. It went something like this. "Hey a__hole!" (John's nickname for me) We have some great shit down here in the postmortem room, I've only seen this 3 times in my career, you will never see it again". With my great fondness for snow and winter driving, I was presented with a real dilemma. Should I go down to Cornell, brave the unplowed roads, or stay at home in the warmth and comfort that I was experiencing. Knowing John's enthusiasm for teaching, I got into my Dodge Ram Charger SUV, and headed to Cornell. The 2.5 mile trip took some 25-30 minutes to get there, as the vehicle did not want to navigate the Ithaca hills very well. When I arrived in necropsy, John greeted with "It's about time you got here. What took you so long?". There was a big bull opened upon the table. John told me to have a look, and "tell me what you see" I looked the carcass over, and found nothing obvious, but did see 3 calculi in the pancreatic duct. I told this to John, his response "damn right, that's the good shit I was talking about". I still have the kodachrome that John gave me of that lesion, and he was right, I never saw that finding again.

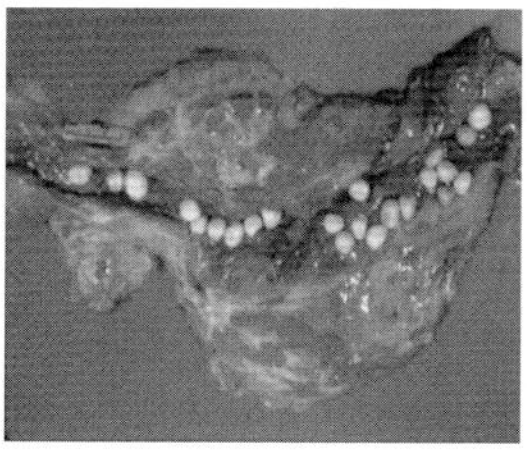

I think this speaks so well for John's enthusiasm about Veterinary Pathology, and teaching, wanting you to see and learn everything that you could . In my year's at Cornell, I received many after all calls from John. They summoned me to Cornell at all times of day or night, mostly to look at slides one on one with him, slides that he received from different parts of the US, and other countries in the world. Some of these slides became parts of his round robin boxes. I was fortunately, the beneficiary of this intense, but individual attention, and I became a better veterinary pathologist because of this. I will always be grateful to John for showing interest in me, and taking the time to share the wealth of his knowledge with me, in a very personal way. His likes will never be seen again, and I think all who trained with him owe a great deal to him. He certainly gave a running start to our careers in veterinary pathology. His wisdom, and the unique way that he looked at postmortem specimens, and microscopic sections gave us a very strong foundation on which to build our careers.

Dr. John King

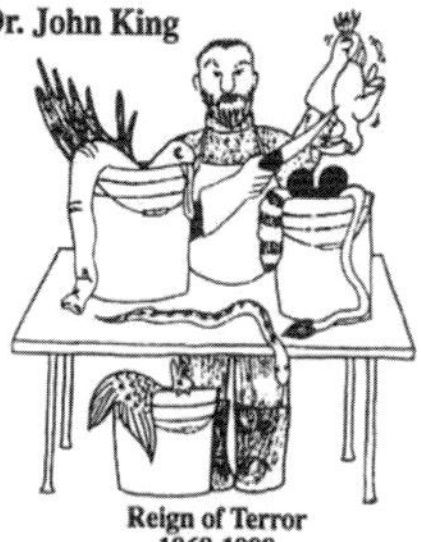

Reign of Terror
1968-1998

From Howard Gelberg (Oregon State University):

In the spring semester of 1969, John taught the entirety of Special Pathology. He opened his lectures by having us turn to a designated page in Smith, Jones and Hunt. His lectures consisted of going page by page through the book and correcting what was wrong...

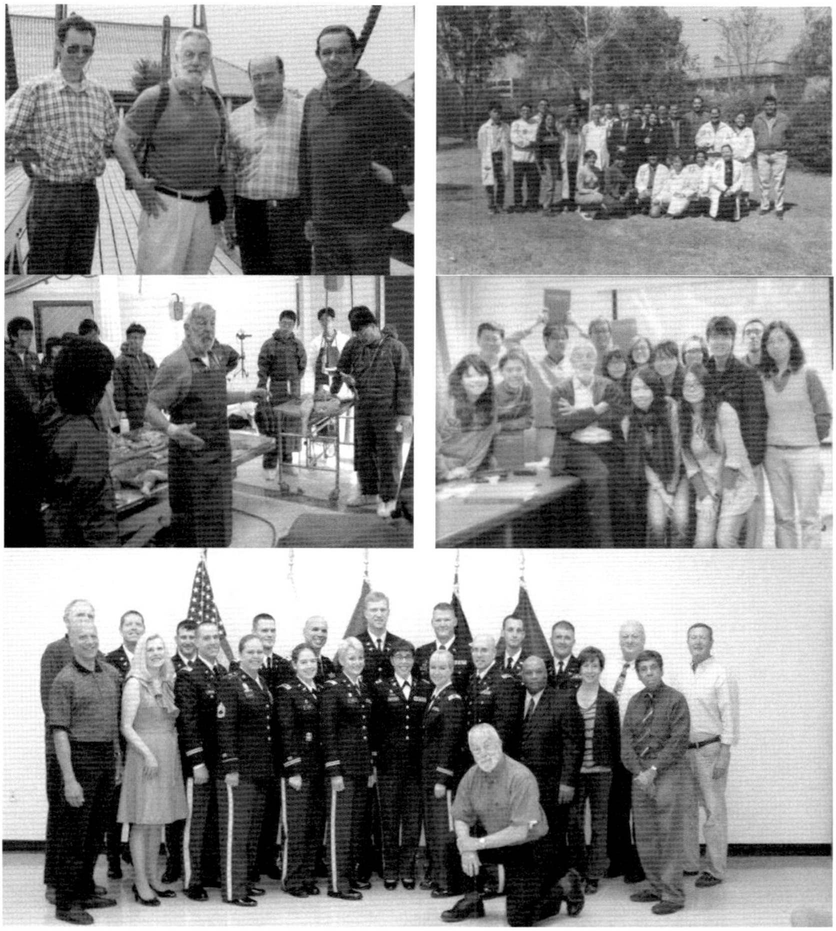

Top row, left: John visits Buenos Aires in 1995. L-R: Dr Gabriel Traveria, Dr King, Dr Julio Loureiro and Dr Enrique Costa Mundo Marino, San Clemente del Tuyu. Top row, right: John and the staff and graduate students of the Pathology Department University Nacional Autonomia Mexico, 1998.

Center row, left: Conducting a necropsy lab at KyungPook National Universityin 2008 with Dr. Il-Hwa Hong at left. Center row, right: John and the students at the National University of Science and Technology, Ping Tung, Taiwan. John had given many short courses on the pathology of swine here over the years.

Bottom row: John with the staff faculty and residents of the Joint Pathology Center, 2013. John loved the Army, and the Army loved him back.

From Jeff Everitt, DVM (Cornell Class of 1977)

I began my association with John King while an undergraduate student at Cornell in the 1970's when I was privileged to have him teach me rock climbing. Actually he taught me confidence and how to believe in myself as well as a bit about ropes and knots and rock. Oh and those memorable trips to the "Gunks" traveling in the pickup camper. When I entered veterinary school I got a job cleaning the necropsy room and assisting John. I learned so much pathology at his side in that position that I didn't appreciate until much later in my training. As I observed John's relationship with Peter Olafson, I learned how important it is for a student to have a mentor. John served as a pathology mentor for me throughout my training, despite the distance. I learned that it was never too late or inconvenient to call him when I had a vexing case. Knowing that John was in the background as a consultant did wonders for the confidence and ability of a young pathologist. I remember vividly a really difficult diagnostic case when I was at University of Pennsylvania. John remotely and correctly diagnosed "hairy vetch" toxicosis in a group of cattle.

John was tough and gruff on the outside but had a heart of gold and a kindness that touched all of his students. Throughout my training he sent me kodachromes and glass slides and covered the postage as he knew I had limited funds. He encouraged me, while all the time keeping me honest, and humbling me along the way. I remember the ACVP meeting in 1982 as it was my first with a "diplomate badge", having just passed my board examination. John abused and humbled me in that way that only he could, in that bright red jacket. It makes me smile every time I think of it. I think we should all now strive to perform the Lord's work as I know he has his hands full up there!

From Melissa Behr (University of Wisconsin)....

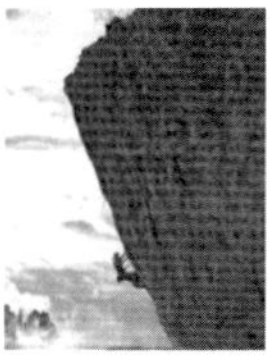

Doc liked to rock climb (a lot; he kept doing it even though he fell and broke both his ankles; he would go on trips to the Shawangunks, which are mountains south of Ithaca and a famous climbing destination, with a whole bunch of students and trainees; I think that it was on those trips that we referred to him as "Doc", and the name stuck); and then the "don't go away mad" quip that he used at nearly all rounds, which was really hilarious, and still makes me laugh. "But don't go away mad, because here we have another calf lung".

I was also at quite a few of the sessions where Dr. Olafson was propped up on a little stool and Doc would ask him for his opinions on the cases. Sometimes, Dr. Olafson would say something like "Well it shudda had a gastric ulcer!", and Doc couldn't help but smile - he was usually pretty serious during rounds because that was the place where he picked fights with Dr. Lewis or really anyone - I think he would say preposterous things on purpose sometimes, or corner a student or resident knowing perfectly that they wouldn't know the answer, and then state: "And of course that is exactly the wrong answer!" - all very serious - but Dr. Olafson was the rare person who made Doc smile.

Surely you also know that Doc liked to study mnemonic devices. He would sometimes try to explain how he was able to recite the genus and species of every possible lungworm of every animal for example. It had to do with alphabetizing them, and somehow associating the parasite with the letter. So A was for Dictyocaulus, and B for Protostongylus and so forth; I never did understand the system and I was too afraid to ask him to explain it, so I had great difficulty remembering things, and still do.

When he retired, Doc sent everyone a box of kodachrome slides. I still have mine somewhere. It was really great that he also scanned them in, and that they have been available on the Necropsy Show and Tell (NST) website. I use NST for my teaching, and go to it as well when looking for ideas. I hope it's available to us for many years to come. NST is written in the understated, concise style that Doc favored, and it is a real treasure.

John King – The Educator Par Excellence…. By Eric A. G. Blomme (Abbvie)

Having spent two years as a resident trained by the legendary Dr. John King, one can imagine that I would have abundant memorable anecdotes and stories to relate here. However, as I am thinking about Dr. King's impact on my career as a veterinary pathologist, two themes are paramount.

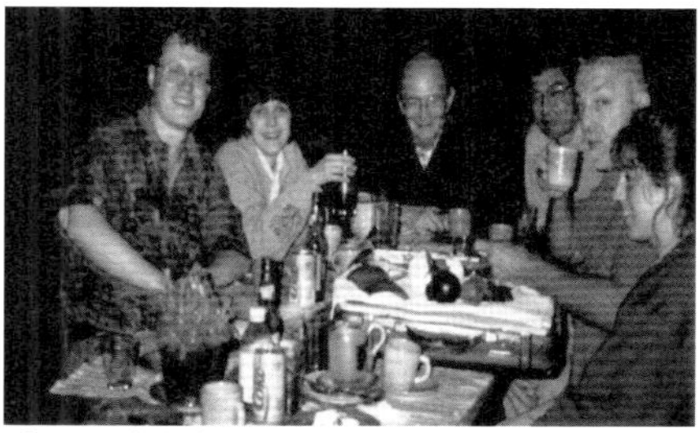

From a road trip dinner at New Bolton Center with L-R: the author, Dr. Magali Guffroy, Dr. Bob Kenney, Prof. Toshi Masegi, John King, and an unidentified student at far right.

The first one is passion: Dr. King was not teaching from the books, he was teaching from the heart, and by doing so, was developing in his students scientific curiosity and a passion to not just learn, but discover, question and comprehend. For Dr. King, no book (with the exception of his small pocket-size grey necropsy book of course!) could beat hours in the necropsy room, attention to details (like the small "hepatoma" in the liver of a woodchuck that was once again missed!), the countless unusual or classic lesions in his slide box sets that he shared with everybody interested, or the discussions during the morning rounds when he was on necropsy duty (which seemed to be every rotation, as I don't think he ever took vacations).

The second one is sharing: knowledge obviously, but also small stories, friends, good times and the history of his beloved country, the United States. I was fortunate to enjoy two of Dr. King's road trips along with other resident mates. The final destination of the trips was Tifton, GA for the annual slide conference. During these trips, while driving from one veterinary school to another, Dr. King would share with us the history behind the places we would drive by: the Suwannee River while singing Stephen Foster's song, the events of the American War of Independence, the cat fish industry in Mississippi… Every evening we were hosted by his generous friends, typically former students or colleagues. To name a few of these well-known hosts he loved so much to argue with: Bob Keeney at the New Bolton Center, Talmage Brown and Don Meuten at North Carolina State, Dave Slauson and Linda Munson at Tennessee, Cory Brayton in Manhattan, Claus Buergelt in Florida, or Charles Capen and Steve Weisbrode at Ohio State. This was the time for good story telling (often using his famous black box), regional meals (crawfish in Baton-Rouge, BBQ in Florida) and for some impromptu fiddle concerts. The morning was dedicated to Dr.

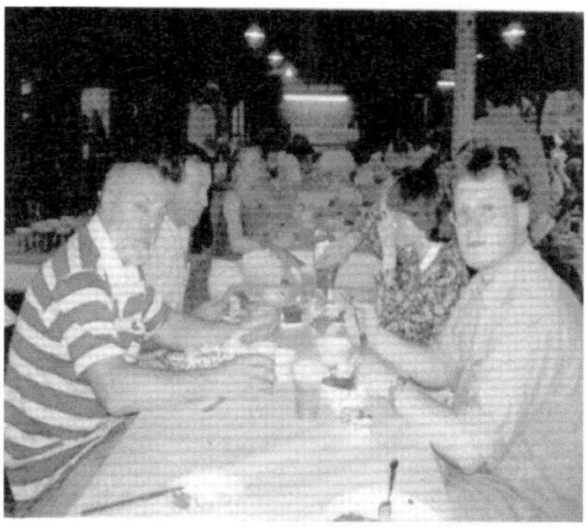

The author at right with John King at left at the annual veterinary pathology meeting in Tifton, Ga.

King's Show & Tell at the institution being visited using the necropsy specimens he collected for a couple of months beforehand in his magic Klotz solution. Obviously, the Show & Tells were the opportunity for heated arguments around the cause of various diseases or lesions (remember atrophic rhinitis, unilateral renal shutdown, or calf pneumonia!), for many "God said so" or "Ask Him" (pointing his finger to the sky), and for residents to consider a career move as truck drivers. Besides the inconvenience of long trips and the smell in the van, these trips were one week of unmatched education, fun and discovery.

There are many ways to educate veterinary pathologists. Dr. King 's approach was certainly unique and provided many opportunities for education, humor and argumentation. Trainees of Dr. King were participants in an educational style that was "atypical", but with proven success. It probably would not fit today's standards and I am not too convinced that this is a good thing. Dr. King's passion and dedication to students and veterinary pathology were real and enormous, he was a man with a big heart and with high expectations for his students, and these traits made him the veterinary pathology educator par excellence. I am so grateful to have been a John King's "wannabe" and for the opportunity to share these precious memories in tribute to this exceptional mentor.

From Cory Brayton (Johns Hopkins University)

Despite his words I was fortunate to recognize Dr. King's great heart, and his love of pathology, teaching, and Cornell early in my veterinary education. I am grateful for the time and effort that he offered to any and all who were interested, even for the hard times that he gave some of us.

Pathology is Fun and Fundamental. Gross photographs should be beautiful and informative, not gross. Knives should be sharp. Scalpels should be avoided.

I am fortunate and proud to be a part of this larger family that love pathology and the Kings.
will miss his stories that made pathology memorable even to those who expected to have no interest in pathology, his enthusiasm for a great case, his unconventional approach to actively searching and researching causes of disease, his black box museum pieces, his inscrutable letters, current case concerns, and thought provoking questions.

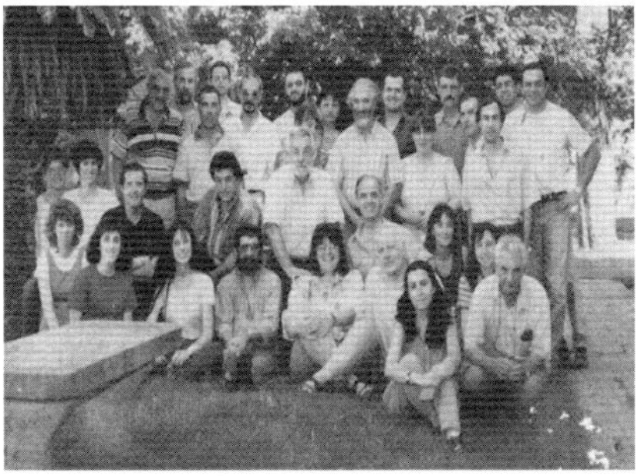

Dr. King in Argentina, 1995. Prof Eduardo Gimeno on his immediate right.

THANK YOU, John and Marie King.

From Don Meuten ... (as spoken at Dr. King's memorial service in Cornell's Sage Chapel on May 12, 2016).

I told those gathered I may need to read this or I will falter. I am only one of the many students that learned from THE LEGEND. There are more articulate and accomplished colleagues in the audience or that will come to this podium that can pay tribute to my teacher, a Cornell icon. He was our Secretariat, our JFK, and our CSI before we knew that term, and he was a character, larger than life itself. He truly stepped to the beat of his own drummer. Stories abound. His heart was the size of Secretariat's but in the end not even a heart full of students, passion for pathology, love for his wife and pride in his art could beat forever. And now we are gathered to tell Marie, his colleagues, his students and maybe him, what we should have said over the years.

I thank Marie for letting us return to her life for these few days. We should have returned more often, it is something I regret not doing for him, he would have loved a visit. He absolutely loved his students, sometimes he withdrew that love for moments or months but he gave it back as long as we worked hard. He rewarded those that worked hard. If I visited I would have gotten his quizzes wrong and he might say, "Maybe you should have been a truck driver after all, Donald." I think I disappointed him by studying cancer, which was not a big enough challenge for him. And Marie, we all thank you for sharing Dr King with veterinary pathology for so many years. He loved you and your son but you let him spend hours and hours, years, with us doing what he loved to do, teach and solve diagnostic cases. He was always in the lab.

I called their home when I heard how sick he was and Marie gave me a memory we can all smile about. *"He is in and out of consciousness but when he checks away from me he rambles on and on about pathology."* That is our teacher, talking pathology. I thank Bruce Williams, he does an excellent job at whatever tasks he is given, and sadly saying goodbye and writing eulogies for legends and heroes of veterinary pathology has befallen him. He mixes facts with lore and humor and reminds me, *"Go light, Don and just tell some King stories... there will be plenty of wet eyes."* I also thank Cornell. I want to be very clear - Dr King loved Cornell... yes, the road had some bumps, but he was proud to be a Cornellian, remembrances of him should be told here. He was a student of history and he knew of the individuals that walked our halls and built the reputation of Cornell – Olafson, Jubb, McEntee, Rickard, Krook, Fox, Kirk, Dr D, Tasker, Bentick-Smith, Evans, Habel, Bruner, Carmichael, Roberts and more and now he is one of those. You should not have to die to be a legend.

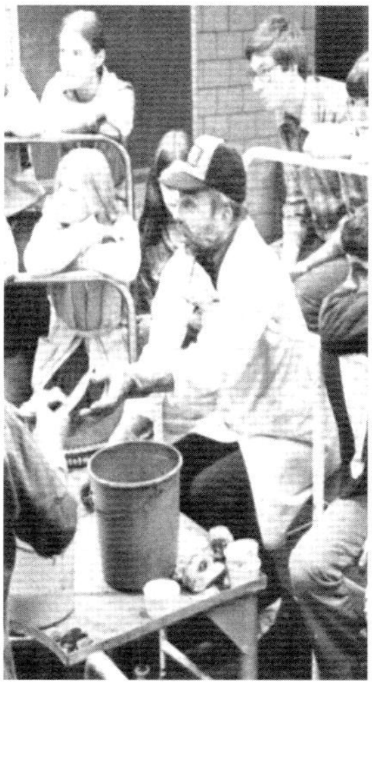

As Dr King aged he became softer,.... he only had that direction to go. People, old friends and history were now as important to him as the necropsy room and his students had been. Years ago, he gave me a gift of gift was a wooden framed collection of old (antiquated) veterinary medical instruments -tthe fact he gave me something of the history of Cornell, a present he made with his hand (he and his son liked to work with wood) is something I cherish. It came from the man, a pathologist that we all respected and we hoped we could earn his respect in return. I am certain that Cornell will do something that honors him, the pathologist that gave so much to all of us, and a University he loved and respected. Dr King deserves that.

On the lighter side – I composed a list of "*Dr King-isms*" last night, the things he did or the phrases he coined that were a fun part of him.........NO GREAT SHAKES, BALONEY, BUNK, Unilateral renal shutdown, right dorsal colitis, brain-heart syndrome, rattlesnakes on the necropsy floor or in his office, rock climbing, climbing silos!!! He did have a few loose screws, Marie – such as the 1500 lbs of blood guts and glory packed in a van with American and foreign grad students and residents travelling the east coast from NY to Florida for the JOHN KING SHOW and TELL! Who else would do something like that?

Dr. King did not tolerate fools, the necropsy lab was HIS, it was his theater and he ruled it, he was tough and he said he was tough on us so WE WOULD LEARN. He did not quote Kahlil Gibran, and perhaps I should not, but part of his quote about a teacher reads, *"If he is indeed wise he does not bid you enter the house of his wisdom, but rather leads you to the threshold of your own mind."* That is what Dr. King did through example and questions.

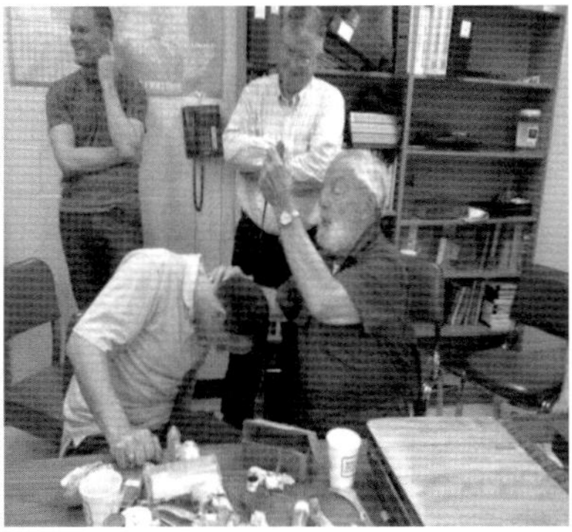

Dr. King demonstrates how to kill an ox using the next best thing – a handy student. (Photo by Dr. Cindy Driscoll)

One of my learning experiences took me to the threshold instead of the necropsy cooler.......I was sent ***dumpster diving.....*** for the limbs of an angus cow that had died with anemia, icterus, splenomegaly but its urine was yellow and not red or brown. Well, Dr King was not on duty, but that did not matter, I was the resident and when he came in, he quizzed me. "Well, Meuten what did you see?" I told him and then..... "Well what was the cause?" ......I had to say we did not know the exact cause but these were my differentials. "Not only do you NOT KNOW THE EXACT CAUSE Meuten, you do NOT know the CAUSE AT ALL!. Listing possibilities doesn't help anyone, (a few expletives) and... you FAILED. Did you look for anaplasma in the blood?" "It was dead, Dr. King and there was no CBC performed." "I know it was dead, they are all dead in here and you will be soon if you don't go get me a leg from one of the barrels." "Yes sir.!"

We made the slide and I took it to Dr Bentick-Smith who commented on the quality of the film, and I WAS NOT about to tell Dr King his slide was not up to the standards of *Clinical Pathology*, Dr. Bentick –Smith stained the slide and of course he and Dr Tasker showed me dark dots on the RBCs - anaplasmosis. HE WAS RIGHT and it does not take many of those cases for the LORE and the LEGEND TO GROW. It is also a good example of how a series of events and words with Dr King can be branded into your memory for 40 years!

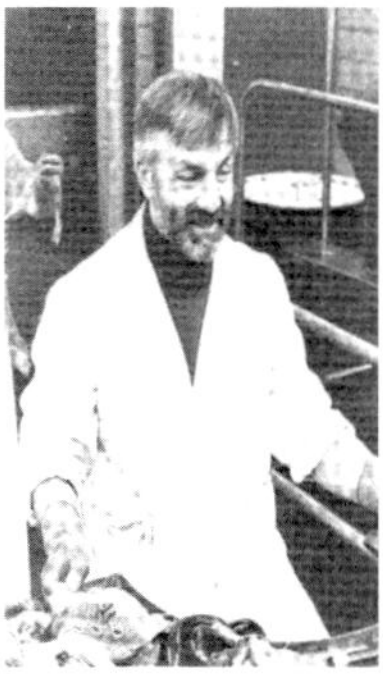

I will conclude with this. In 1996, Bruce gave me the honor to interview Dr King on tape for the first in a series of interviews for the Foundation on "Legends in Pathology". The interview went for hours and yesterday, Bruce gave me a copy of the tape. It was great for several reasons – I saw and heard the Dr King we all remember – bigger than life, wry smile, facial twists, strong, dynamic, a little full of himself – all the features we want to freeze in time. He was back for that moment, I never had to see him grow old or weak, and he will be forever strong to me. At the end of that three-hour interview, I asked what he would like to be remembered for professionally and personally- what he might like to hear said on this day. He thought for a moment and said, "Professionally...for all of my students." He was very proud of us. He loved teaching, and using the necropsy lab to teach from. I was pleased that of all his many accomplishments, that was the one he singled out. He was the finest diagnostic pathologist I will ever know and I suspect that is true for many of you reading this. On the personal side, he said – "I'd like to know my son loved me and my wife."

Goodbye, Dr. King - my teacher.

...From Evelyne Polack (Biogen-Idec)
....a school report on John by her 8th grade daughter Keni

The Life of John McKain King

During the Great Depression, a boy with no money living at a boy's school wanted to be with his friends at a local football game. The game was at a high school three miles down the road, but there was a small fee that he could not afford to pay. The only solution he could find was to pretend he could play the clarinet. Although he could not play a note, the band still accepted him with a uniform and free entrances to all games.

When talking about his childhood, John King makes an effort to point out that the boy's school he attended was not a reform school. John's father was an alcoholic, while his mother had to give up her son and three daughters because most of the time she did not have a home for them to live in. John's three older sisters went to live with relatives, but for an eight-year-old boy the only proper place for an upbringing was the boy's school. He was born on January 16, 1927, in Boston Massachusetts. From 1935 until 1944, John lived at the boarding school. There he went to school and had chores. He was probably the only boy that actually liked to take care of the sick animals in the farm. It was at that time that he decided he wanted to be a veterinarian. Again he did not have any money, but he never doubted he was not going to be able to afford college. He also did not doubt himself in school. He questioned just about everything and he wanted to learn about all that was offered. Many of the adults would say to him "John you are a cocky boy" but it never stopped him from going out and getting what he wanted.

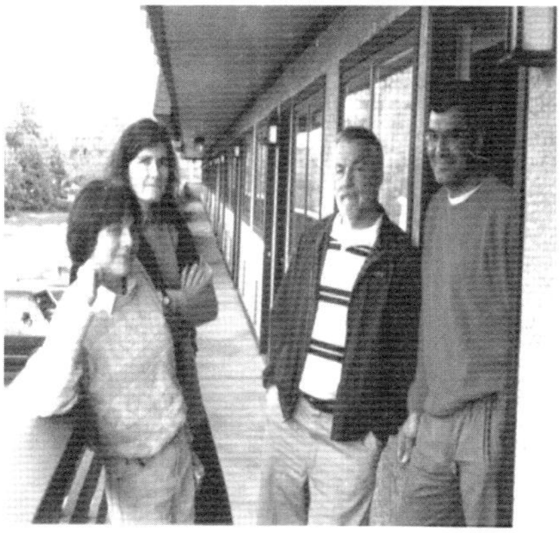

From a 1997 Road Show with Magalie Guffroy, the author's mother, Evelyne Polack, Dr. King, and Adel Hanson.

The best thing that ever happened to John was in 1944 when he volunteered to join the army. Like many seventeen year old boys, he was curious and thought he was immortal, otherwise he would not have gone. Luckily when he went to Germany, the fighting there was over although the war was still on. While in the Paratroopers John had a great time. He enjoyed seeing the new machines and different places, he met a girl named Mary, she was an E.T.O. (European Theater of Operations). The couple moved to Delaware, where months later they married and had a son, Jon David King known as JD. There John attended the University of Delaware for no charge as one of the benefits for serving in the war. He was also offered fifty dollars a month to help his new family. From there he went to Oklahoma State University for his DVM. The army no longer paid full price for that, so John took up many odd jobs to pay the rest. He is proud of all the jobs he did which ranged from a wheat harvester to a cop at the race tracks. When he was done with vet school he wanted to take care of everybody's sick pets. But soon enough he found himself being a "Jack of all trades but master of none". He did not have answers to all of his questions. So he came to Cornell University and in 1960 he finished a PhD in veterinary pathology. John got a job in Washington state doing what he studied to do, but what he enjoyed the most were his rock climbing adventures that came to an end after he broke both of his ankles twice and his hip bone. He came back to Cornell in 1968 as a professor of pathology, which is the title he still holds. This job allowed him to travel to many countries, not as tourists but as residents learning all sorts of new things.

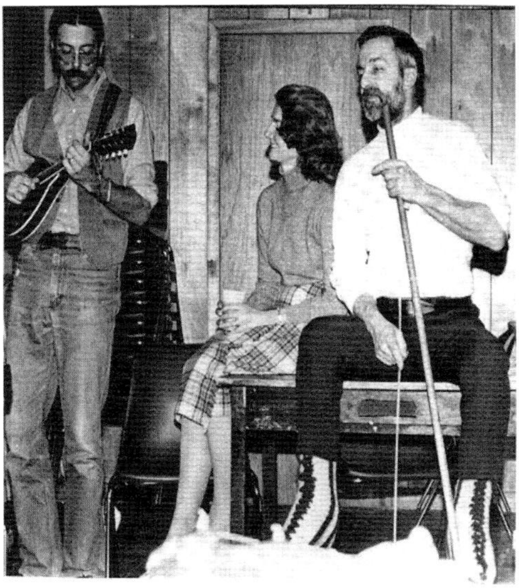

John has a career in vet pathology, but at the age of seventy he still does not know what he wants to be when he grows up. A few years ago when he bought a house he found an old violin in the attic. He fixed it up and took a few lessons just for fun. When walking around Shurmann Hall at Cornell some familiar tunes might be coming from his office. It might not be the best of sounds but it's good enough for him. Playing the violin was just one of the many things he wants to do. His interest in just about every field keeps this seventy year old younger than many teenagers.

John likes to take things as they come. He has enjoyed every place he has been to, and he would do it all over again. Right now he is very close to his son. He works with JD, who builds houses. They joke around with each other and go to movies together. While JD was growing up John was always busy with his work, but he is glad he got a second chance to know him. He is also very thankful that his wife allowed him to pursue all of his interests. This December they are celebrating their fiftieth anniversary with a cruise through the Panama Canal. In 1998, John King plans to retire, but he will be an emeritus professor. This allows him to stay in tune with his profession, but gives him enough time to go after all of those jobs and hobbies for when he "grows up".

...From Ana Alcaraz (Western University)

There has been nobody who has trained more pathologist than John King. He was the faculty who helped the residents the most, and as such he gained the respect of all us. We are all blessed for having had him as part of our life.

He was legitimately interested in the development of his students. He was generous and had a good heart. John was honest, direct and responsible. He was a true champion and now he is a legend. He did for veterinary pathology more during his lifetime than anybody I know. It is for all of this, that we all found in John the best mentor.

Path stories:
• Emphasis on gross observation
• Coconut theory
• Equine pulmonary fibrosis
• bloat line bloat bones
• brain heart syndrome
• three reasons to have valvular endocarditis
• hypercholesterolemia associated with diabetes or hypothyroid
• Regeneration vs hepatomas
• Adrenal cortical adenomas
• What is the shape of the wire that killed the cow?

His Phrases:
• "Ain't firm, ain't pneumonia"
• WET THE TABLE!
• All animals on the left side
• Do not read the history (until afterwards)
• "God said so and everybody agrees"
• You need to know how to sharpen your knife
• "Mickey mouse stuff"
• "Maybe you should have been a truck driver"
• "Baloney!"
• Could it be a meteorite?
• "Drop dead as a doughnut!"
• No interest

Who does not remember his black box or his penmanship?

He shaped the professional identity of many of us. All of us should continue with his legacy. Let us keep using his website and lets us keep reading his words and his comments. Like he used to say "you do not have to agree with me but if you do not have a better explanation than mine, then use mine"

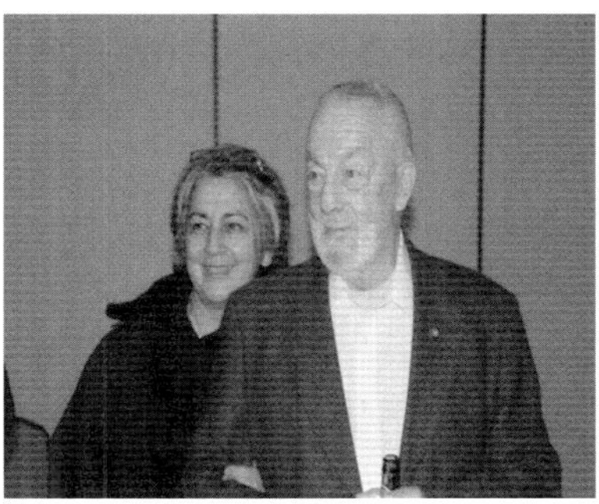

From Stephanie Muller, (IDEXX)

I met John in 2004 at the University of Bern, Switzerland when I started my residency in anatomical pathology and while he spent his 8 months sabbatical there.

Before our first necropsy duty together, he gave me a copy of his Necropsy Book telling me that I should learn it by heart. He convinced us that his book contained the optimal autopsy technique, and he was fond of saying, "The faster the necropsy is completed, the faster one can drink coffee". One day, we were brought a cow found dead in the fields. It had been dead for a couple of days, and the body showed an advanced state of decomposition. From a distance, he said "This is a case of blackleg". Bacteriology subsequently confirmed the diagnosis.

I also remember his wonderful macro sessions; his "Show and Tell". We learned a lot of important things… how to say "pneumonia" [noo-mohn-yuh, -moh-nee-uh, nyoo-] and quite often, "Because God said so". At the traditional post-necropsy coffee, we spoke of many topics other than pathology, such as his experiences as a GI., the landing in Normandy and the arrival in Berlin where the German ladies were frightened by the advancing GIs, having never seen black soldiers.

One day he asked us to accompany him a restaurant because his host – Maia Suter - had guests. He had found a restaurant in Bern which served ribs. On this occasion, he told us how much he he missed his wife Marie, because she had not accompanied him to Switzerland this time, as well as stories of their meeting at a dance during WWII. I will always remember this wonderful man, the great Dr. John King, as well as his stories, his knowledge, and his many kindnesses to us, his students.

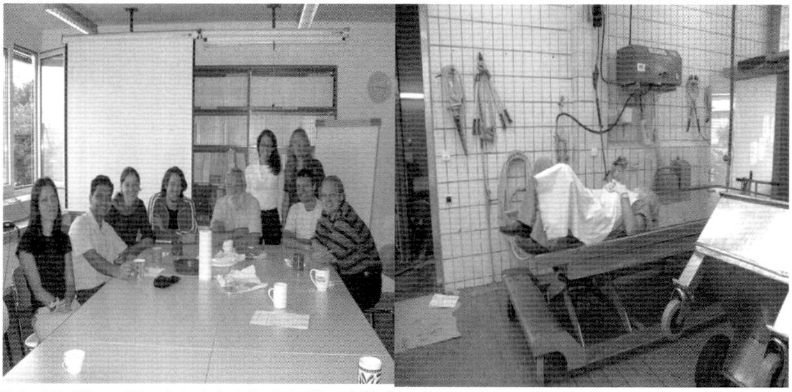

Left: John King and the students (and faculty) of Bern (with the author on his immediate right).
Right: A clean autopsy table makes for a good place to stretch your back (or take a quick nap) between autopsies.

Farewell, But Never Goodbye

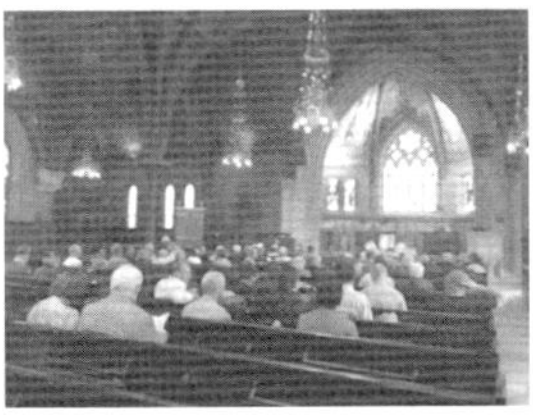
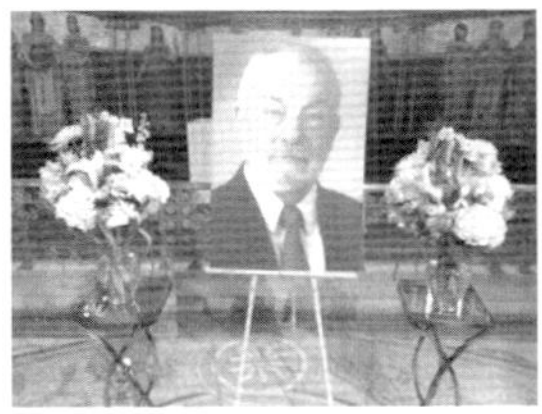
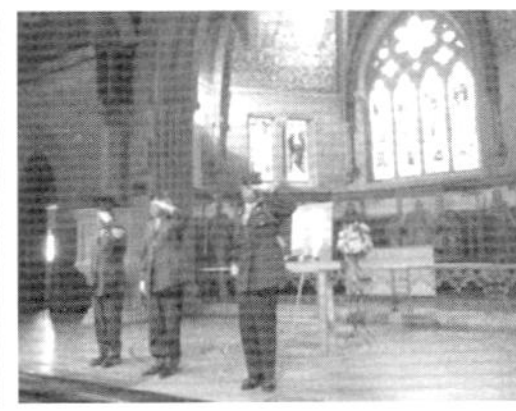
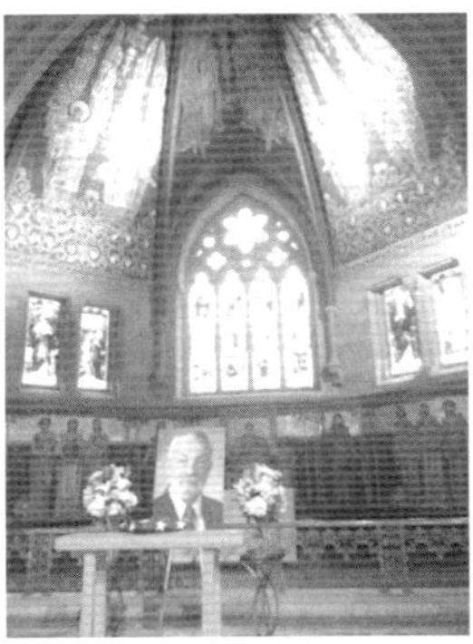
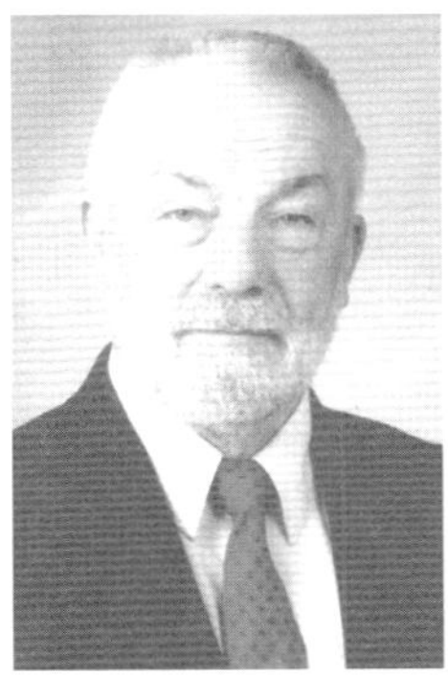
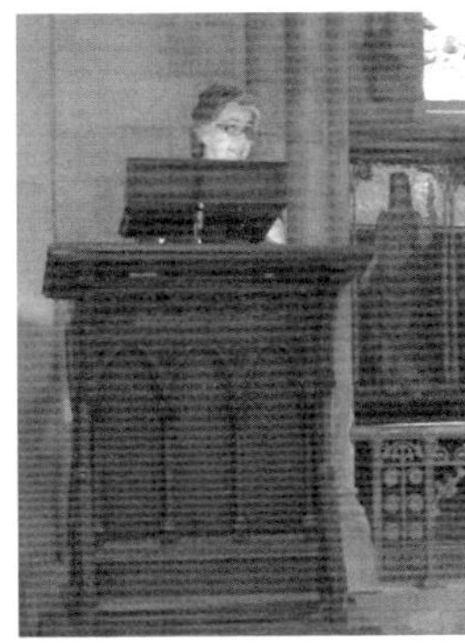
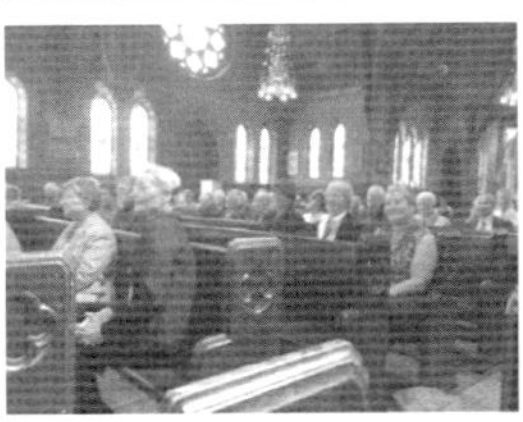
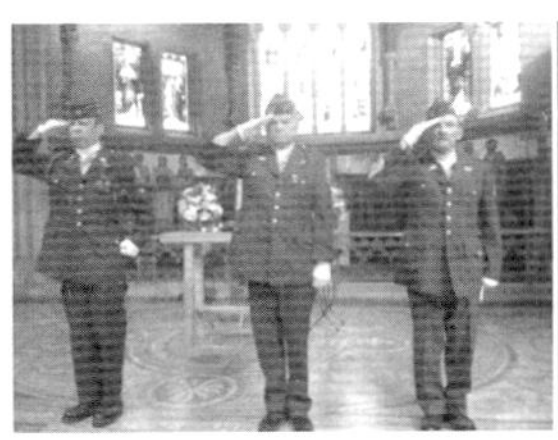
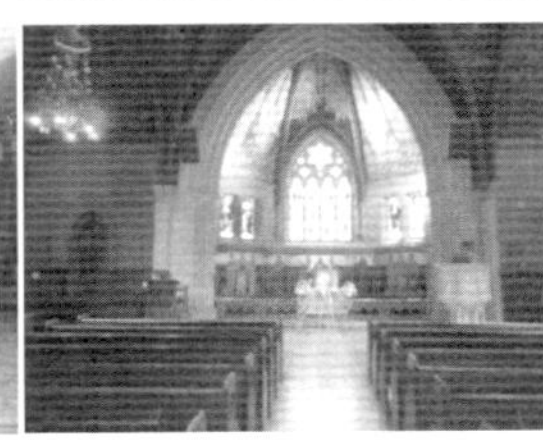

Thank you, Dr King.

Books Written by John King

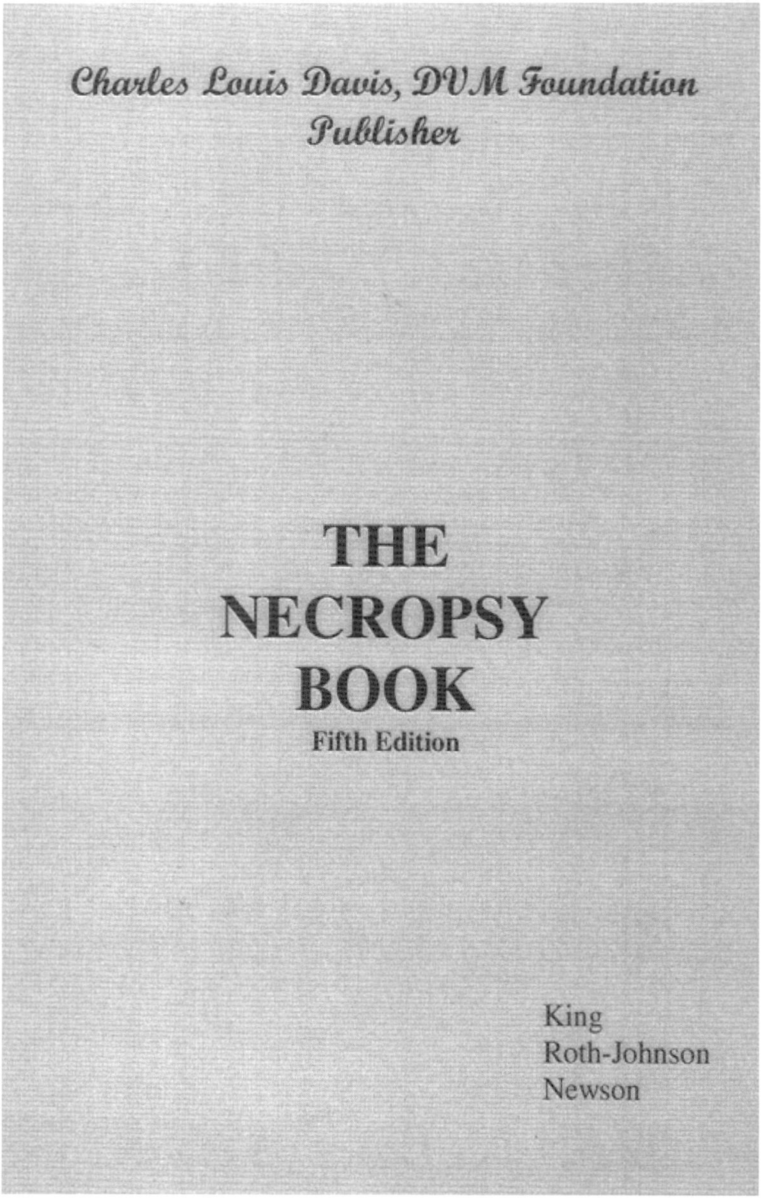

THE NECROPSY BOOK

A Guide for Veterinary Students, Residents, Clinicians, Pathologists, and Biological Researchers

Revised January 2007

John M. King
Lois Roth-Johnson
Marion E. Newson

Reportable Features of Most Lesions

Location
Color
Size/Weight
Shape
Consistency
Number (#) or Percent (%) Involved
Content
Odor

There are many common lesions but never any normal ones

Morphological descriptions and interpretations of lesions may include the following:

Distribution:	Organ(s) Unilateral-Bilateral Focal - Multifocal (Disseminated) Locally Extensive-Diffuse Whole Body - Localized Generalized
Time :	Peracute – Acute – Subacute – Chronic - Chronic Active
Severity :	Minimal Moderate Marked Slight Severe
Cause:	Verminous – Bacterial – Chemical – Viral - Traumatic – Protozoal – Mycotic – Toxic - etc.
Type:	Croupous - Hemorrhagic – Purulent – Fibrinous – Fibrinopurulent – etc.

John M. King
N.Y.S. College of Veterinary Medicine
Cornell University
Ithaca, NY 14853
jmking31@aol.com

Lois Roth-Johnson
2955 Herring Brook Rd
Eastham, Ma 02642

Marion E. Newson
304-1234 West 14th Avenue
Vancouver BC V6J 2J4
Canada

Dedicated to

Marie King

Jon David King

This booklet could not have been written with out the teaching by great teachers

Dr. John Bentinct-Smith

Dr. Lennart Krook

Dr. Wendell Krull

Dr. Kenneth McEntee

Dr. Peter Olafson

Dr. Roger Panciera

Dr. Charles Rickard

Table of Contents

Table of Contents

Table of Contents **Page**

INTRODUCTION

A necropsy is an autopsy performed on an animal. A method for doing a necropsy, using the horse as a model, is described. Since the use of the horse may be questioned we could merely reply that we had to use an animal and the horse is ubiquitous. Another reason, not usually expressed, is that the horse not only has a single stomach as does the pig, dog, and cat, but also has large fermentation chambers equivalent in function to the rumen of the ox and sheep.

The actual procedure of doing the necropsy is one of many used by veterinary pathologists and its practicality and adaptability have been demonstrated. We make no claim for the superiority of this method over others, but from considerable experience with it ,we know it can be used with facility on any species under consideration; by adhering to it, no organ will be and no lesion should be overlooked. No special equipment or instruments are usually required. Any phase of the procedure can easily be modified to suit the prosector's special needs or interests. We stress, however, that having acquired facility and speed with one procedure, it is unwise to change it capriciously; a different method usually takes more time and may cause one to forget a necessary part of the procedure. A change in technique may also preclude instant recognition of an absent or displaced organ or otherwise familiar abnormality. For instance, the pylorus and first part of the duodenum are always close to view when the abdomen is opened by this technique and, if not directly in view, one should immediately consider a twist or displacement of the stomach. The first kidney observed is the right kidney, and if it is the only one with the cranial pole infarct, this can be remembered more easily if one necropsies all animals with the right side up. Except for the GI tract , all tissues and organs are examined as they are removed to prevent gross contamination of the carcass. This portion of the technique is quite different than that done in the human field of removal of all viscera *en masse*.

We have not gone into many areas, such as organ weights, because as general pathologists, we are more than likely to recognize organs as being too small, or too large, or too thick, or too thin. Average weights are given in many texts or reference books. However, several weights have been given. For instance, the cat's heart is normally under 17 grams, and knowing this helps make one specific disease more recognizable.

Although it takes time, a thorough necropsy is probably the best use of time overall. The vast majority of lesions, especially significant ones, will be uncovered. At a later date, the pathologist will know that he/she had looked at all of the significant tissues and organs without thinking — " Did I or didn't I" ?

In the same vein (no pun intended), the worst disservice a teacher can do to a student is to say: "Go ahead and do the necropsy and if you run into a lesion or find that you have a problem with one, call me and I'll be right there to help you out." How about the seventeen great or even insignificant lesions or non-lesions causing interpretation problems that the student did not recognize as being abnormal? The least the instructor must do for a trainee in any area of diagnostics is to review every carcass, tissue, and organ before it is discarded or destroyed.

This booklet is intended to be used at least in part with the pictures of actual tissues to be found on the Cornell Web page:

https://secure.vet.cornell.edu/nst/nst.asp

From this page, in order to locate a particular slide, click on Advanced Search and type the WP number of the slide into the Image ID box.

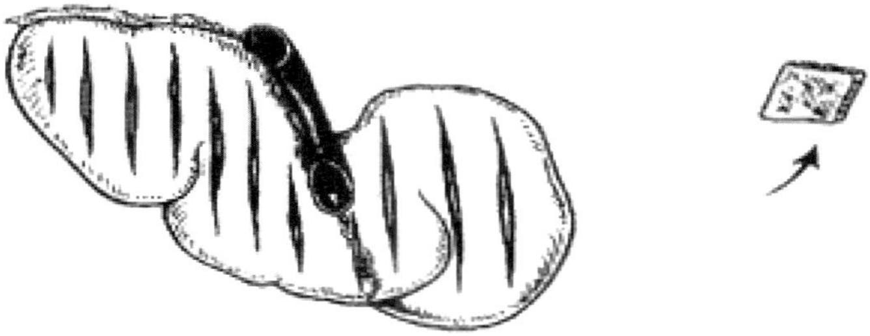

Remember: All sections for fixation should be less than 1/4" (0.5 cm) thick. Caution: Do not scrape or squeeze sections to be taken for histological examination. Always take sections of all tissues with a sharp knife, never with a pair of scissors.

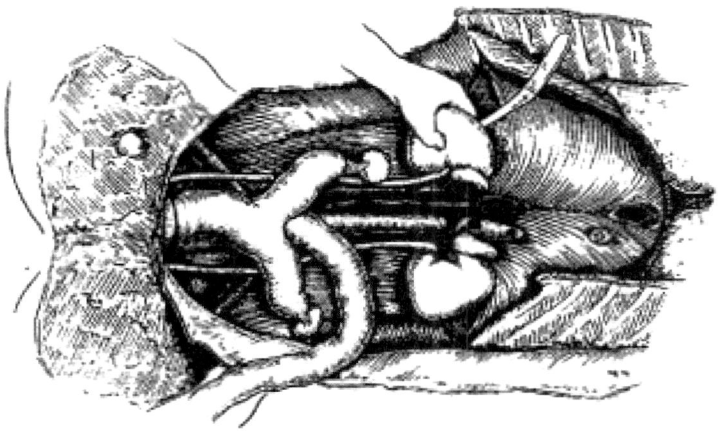

Remove kidneys separately after examination of adrenals. Leave ureter attached to kidney and bladder. Care must be taken when removing the kidneys, ureters, adrenals, and uterus not to damage the aorta and vena cava located dorsally and close to them. In most species, the adrenal glands are found just in front of the kidneys or just medially to the cranial pole of each kidney.

ABDOMINAL VISCERAL REMOVAL

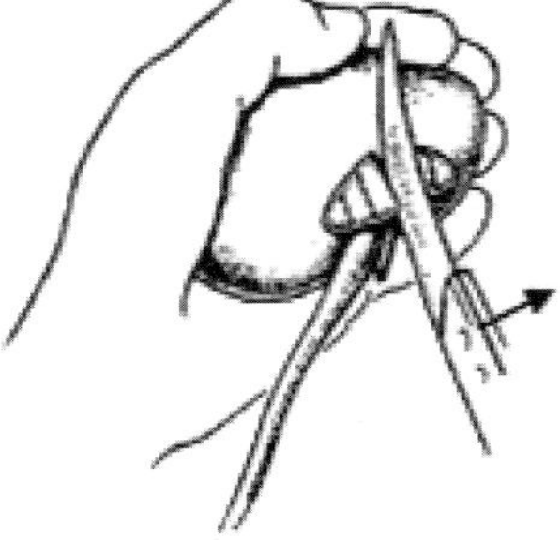

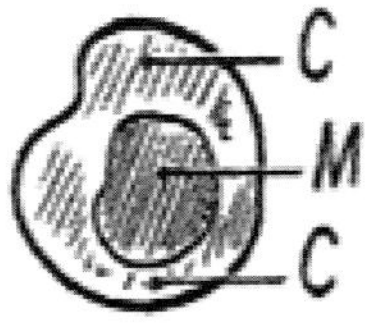

The ratio is roughly 1:2:1 in this example.

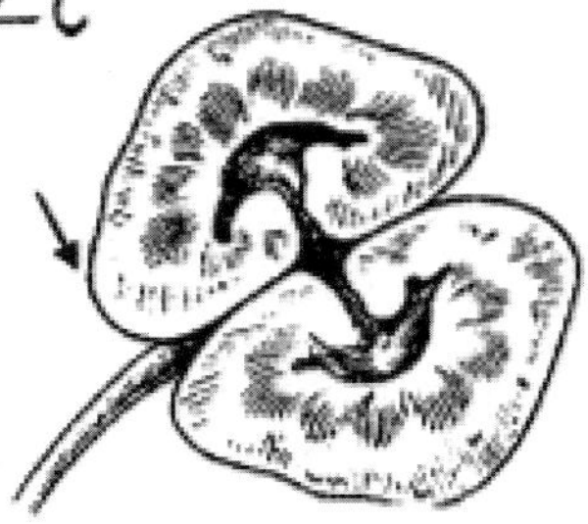

Do not hold the adrenal itself. Incise the adrenal. Note the cortex-medulla-cortex (CMC) ratio.

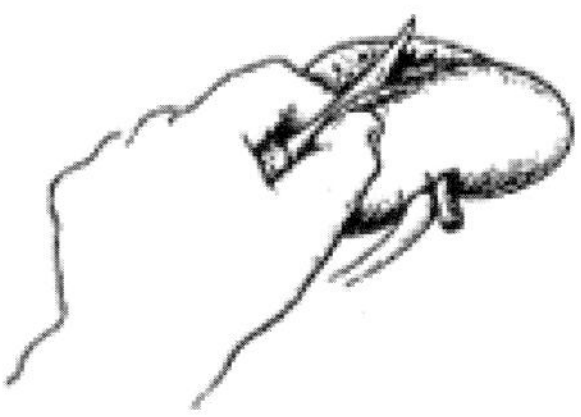

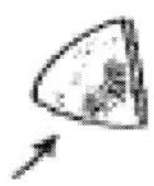

Cut each kidney longitudinally to pelvis. Leave each kidney attached to the bladder to allow the ureter to act as a third hand when handling the small slippery tissue.

Peel away the capsule. Take a tissue cross section to include the cortex, medulla, and pelvic epithelium. Make multiple transverse inspection slices through the organ.

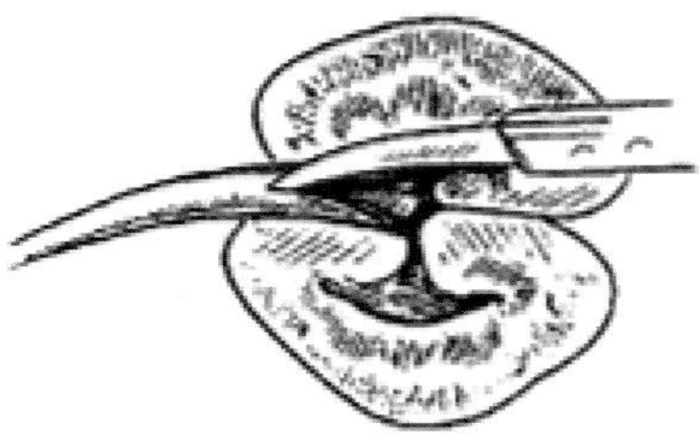

Cut down ureter by pulling slightly on the kidney to straighten the ureter and to allow a sharp pointed knife to cut it open to the bladder

The Necropsy Book, Fifth Edition

Updated and now pocket-size for use in the necropsy room. Price includes shipping.

List Price: $45.00

Your Price: $30.00

You Save: $15.00 (33 %)

Detailed Description

THE NECROPSY BOOK FOURTH EDITION

By Drs JOHN M. KING, DAVID C DODD & LOIS ROTH

and profusely illustrated by MARION E. NEWSON, BETSY UHL, & MIKE SIMMONS

Released January 1st 2006, as a permanently bound, "pocket size", 242 page book weighing 8.9oz. This book is a valuable reference and guide for every clinical veterinarian and veterinary pathologist who has any requirement to perform a necropsy on any species of animal. 243 pages covering:

Necropsy Request Form:Necropsy report, necropsy descriptions and write up, sample report

The Pneumonias

The Necropsy Technique

Line Drawings for Necropsy Lesion Localizations

Greek and Latin Combining form word list

Nonlesions (68 entities you might mistakenly report as a lesion)

A. General and External Findings (13 entities are described)

B. Spleen (4 entities are described)

C. Liver and Gall Bladder (4 entities are described)

D. Endocrine (5 entities are described)

E. Kidney and Urinary Bladder (7 entities are described)

F. Respiratory (8 entities are described)

G. Cardiovascular (8 entities are described)

H. Bone ((1 entity described)

I. Central Nervous System (2 entities are described)

J. Fetus (2 entities described)

K. Gastrointestinal (14 entities described)

Addended Notes

A. The Smells of Pathology (20 entities described)

B. Brief Comments on Neoplasia

C. The Time of Death (7 indicators discussed)

D. Decomposition

E. Miscellaneous Comments

Representative Stages of Post Mortem Lung Inflation

Rough Sketches and Comments on Lesions

Lung (47 pages); Liver (21 pages); Kidney (17 pages); Heart (28 pages)

AN ATLAS OF GENERAL PATHOLOGY

VOLUME Ⅰ AND Ⅱ

BY

J.M. King, D.V.M., Ph.D.

R.C.T. Lee, D.V.M., Ph.D.

A Special Publication of the
Council for Agricultural Planning and Development Executive Yuan
and the
Pig Research Institute of Taiwan
Republic of China
and
Cornell University, Ithaca, N.Y. USA
March, 1983

First Printing, March 1983
Printed by
Shen's Art Printing Inc.
Taipei, Taiwan, Republic of China

In Dedication To

Peter Olafson

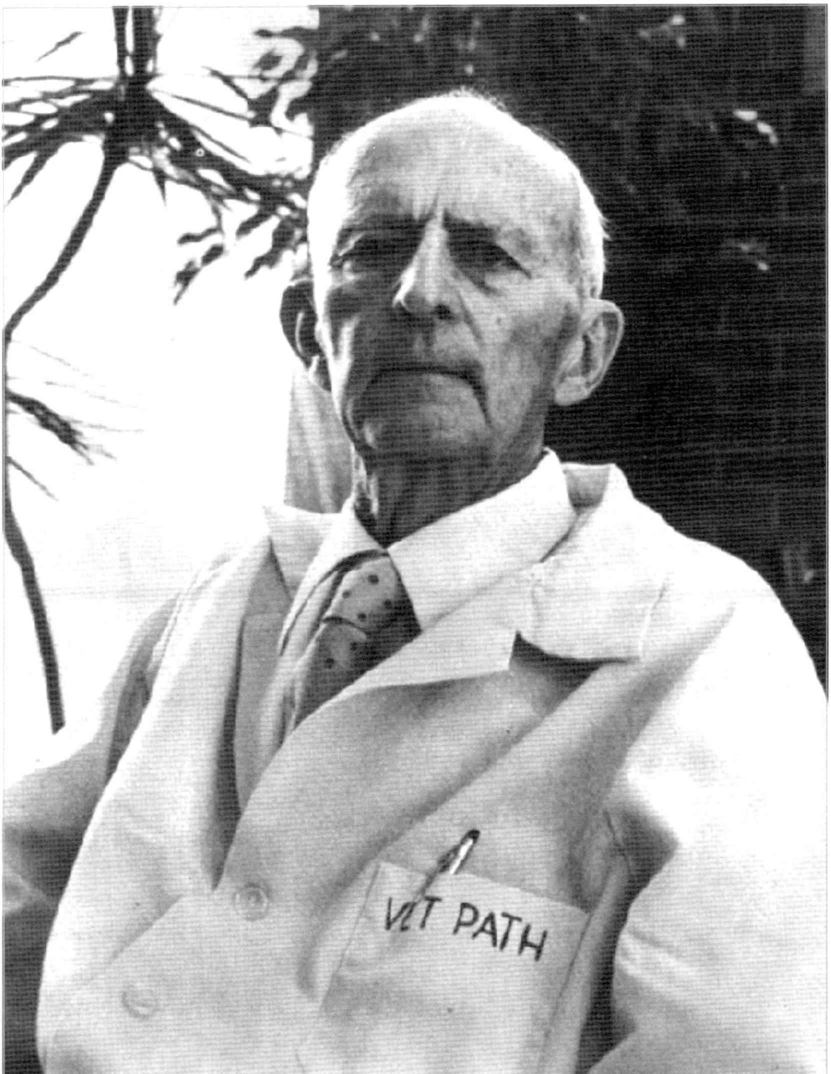

John king's mentor Dr. Peter Olafson

Preface

The present work is intended as the second volume of an Atlas of General Pathology, of which the first was published in May 1976; it includes a large number of common lesions not found in the previous book, though a few are reprinted here for various reasons. The first volume focuses on pig lesions, but the second deals mostly with lesions seen in other species and includes swine specimens as well. Both diagnostic and incidental lesions and findings are covered. It is indeed quite frustrating for a pathologist to record a lesion without being able to interpret it because no such picture of it has been ever seen before. Nevertheless, this volume together with its forerunner should greatly enhance pathological studies.

The same general format has been followed in presenting the cause of the findings in the order of congenital defects, normal structures and findings commonly misinterpreted, artefacts, functional and physical changes, bacterial diseases, viral diseases, protozoal, fungal and parasitic diseases, and neoplastic problems. Exceptions to the aforementioned order occur, however, as when efforts are made to emphasize the value of some special lesions.

All pictures except those which carry the names and locations of the individuals who either supplied the pictures or had a part in their interpretation are ours, good or bad, and all captions for the pictures are also written by us.

It is our hope that no major errors have been made but we also expect that there will be discrepancies in the interpretation of some lesions. Part of the idea of this atlas is to stimulate pathologists to think of alternative possibilities in interpretation.

We are deeply indebted to many for helping with this book; they include Drs. F.M. Wu, C.I. Liu of the National Chung Hsing University, and Redmen Chu, S.J. Du of Pig Research Institute Taiwan, Republic of China. Our thanks also go to the Council for Agricultural Planning and Development, the Pig Research Institute of Taiwan, and the New York State College of Veterinary Medicine of Cornell University for their support, without which this publication will not be made possible. A special kind of thanks goes to Dr. Lois Roth who did the major amount of final proofreading under some duress of speed as well as to Mrs. John M. King who did the initial proofreading and the typing of the manuscript.

John M. King, D.V.M., Ph. D.
Professor
New York State College of Veterinary Medicine
Cornell University
Ithaca, New York, U.S.A.

Robert C.T. Lee, D.V.M., Ph. D.
President
National Chung-Hsing University
Taichung, Taiwan
Republic of China

Contents

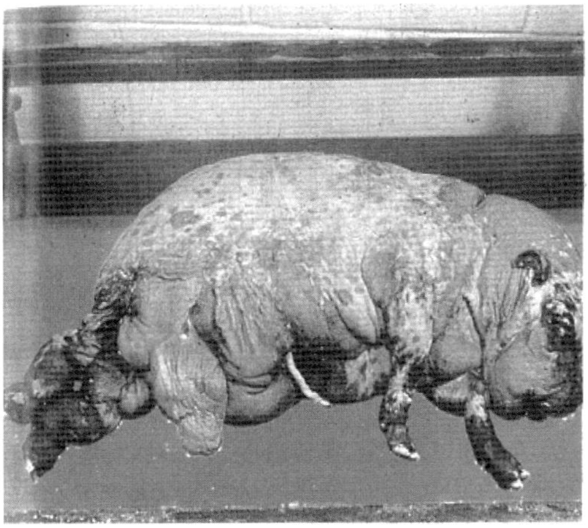

PLATE 1: GENERALIZED ANASARCA

This lamb fetus weighs about 20 kilograms but should weigh only 3 or 4 kilograms. The cause of the excess weight can be seen to be the marked edema that was present throughout the body. The cause of this Anasarca is not really known but some consider it due to malformation of lymphatic vessel drainage of the skin.

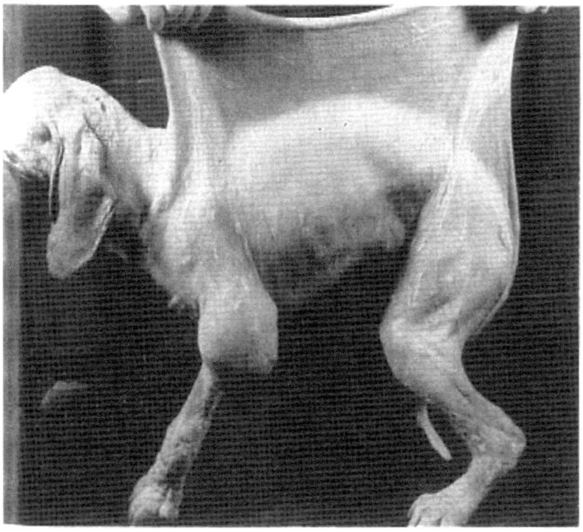

Dr. R. Minor, Cornell, USA

PLATE 2: CUTANEOUS ASTHENIA (DERMATOSPARAXIS)

The marked Asthenia shown by this dog's skin is a congenital disease caused by a defect in the formation of collagen. Several different species have similar skin lesions but they are not all necessarily due to the same defect in the collagen. Asthenia (meaning weakness) is also to be noted by the large rounded mass which is filled with fluid over the dog's elbow. This, a greatly distended bursa, is the result of trauma to the skin and underlying soft tissue over the bones in this area. The term Dermatosparaxis has been used for the condition in cattle but some think it is a better term for the entire group of similar diseases in all species. Collagen in other tissues may also be affected.

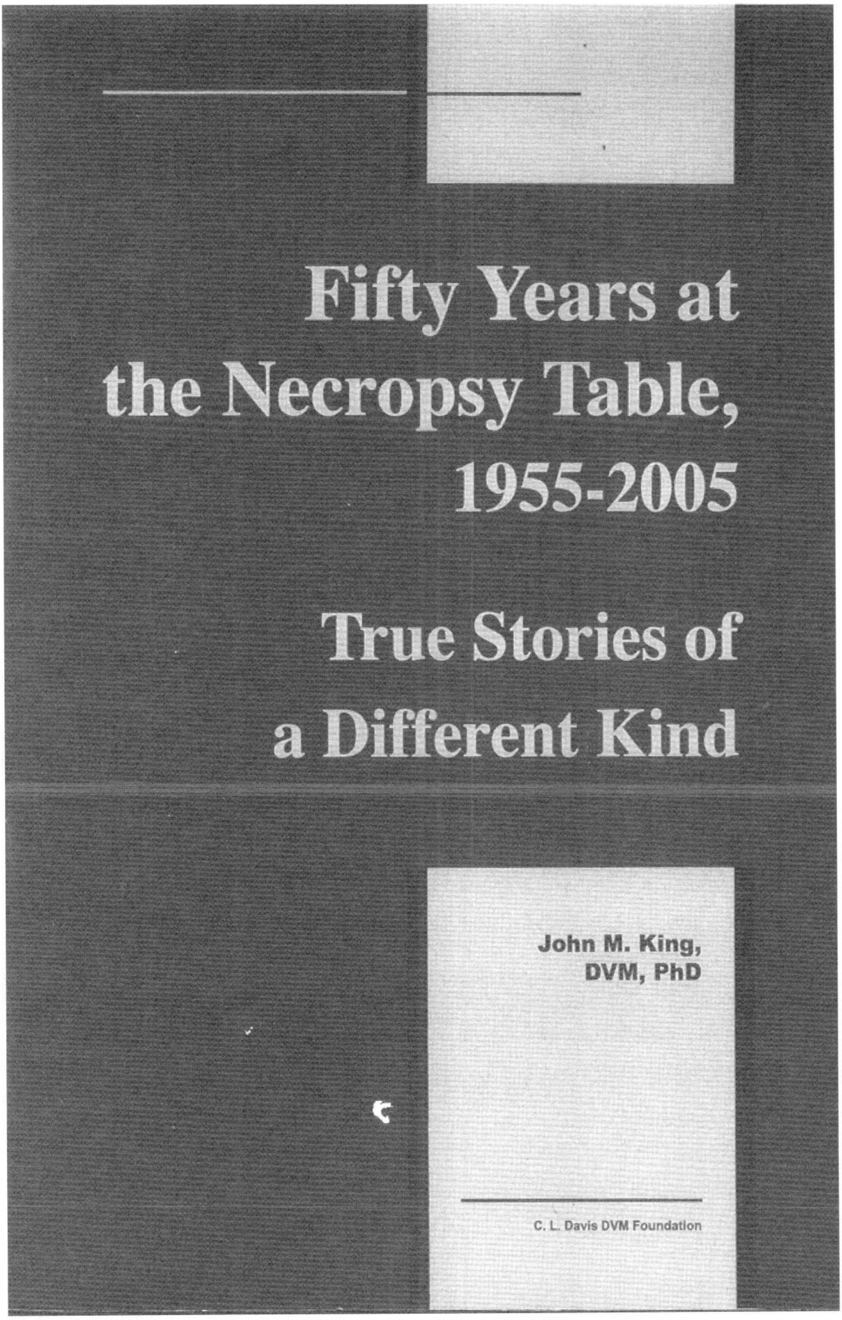
Fifty Years at
the Necropsy Table,
1955-2005
True Stories of
a Different Kind
John M. King,
DVM, PhD
C. L. Davis DVM Foundation

Fifty Years at the Necropsy Table, 1955–2005

True Stories of a Different Kind

John M. King, DVM, PhD

Professor Emeritus of Pathology

N.Y.S. College of Veterinary Medicine

Cornell University

Charles Louis Davis DVM Foundation

Available from the
Charles Louis Davis DVM Foundation
6241 Formoor Lane
Gurnee, Illinois 60031-4757

ISBN 978-1-4507-4562-8

This collection of stories is dedicated to my son,

Jon David King.

He liked hearing these stories and said you would also.

CONTENTS

II. Canine

III. Feline

IV. Equine

V. Miscellaneous

VI. Porcine

VII. Ovine and Caprine (Sheep and Goat)

PREFACE

These true stories are based on the thousands of necropsies performed on many species of animals during the fifty years from 1955 to 2005, mainly in the necropsy room at the Veterinary College, Cornell University, Ithaca, New York. Also, many were necropsied in various countries throughout the world, where the author spent months to years during sabbatical leaves or leaves of absence from Cornell at the request of the various countries and teaching faculties involved. The history for each case was obtained from the animal's owner, veterinary clinician, or during actual farm visits by the author and students assigned to necropsy room services during those years.

The majority of cases were subjected to a complete necropsy including the brain, and histological study of all tissues for each case as needed. Blood work or other clinical pathological studies, parasitological examination, and chemical studies were all done at the various ancillary laboratories by their personnel.

All conclusions and comments, including errors, are the author's alone if not mentioned otherwise.

It is estimated that thirty or more percent of final diagnoses can be significantly aided by an investigative farm or other involved type facility visit by the pathologist, who having performed the necropsy, can make a more definitive final diagnosis.

The necropsy would allow for the more specific direction of the visit for instance to find the partially buried, many stranded, wire cable causing the "hardware" disease outbreak; to learn that the calf was indeed pulled by extreme mechanical traction rupturing the cow's small intestine in the pelvic canal at parturition; that the foal with fractures was exercised "outside" only at night for its eight months of life; that the suspect dogfeed was stored in a leaky roofed shed containing '1080' chemical for rat rodent control. Such histories may not be on the necropsy request form but only ascertained by these visits to the premises.

Most of the stories are grouped by species in which they are mainly seen. Several groups include other species in which a similar condition can also occur and is so stated.

Following each of the stories, WP (Web Page) number references are given from the Web site **http://w3.vet.cornell.edu/nst/** to illustrate at least some of the conditions, with pictures of the lesions as described.

I. Bovine

B-1

Double-Notched Bones

Again lucky to spend another sabbatical in Brazil and Argentina in 1995, I was able to pick up, in several veterinary facilities, four defleshed bones of about the same size and shape that had been obtained from the rumen or reticulum of cattle. All the bones measured about five to seven inches in length by two to three inches in width. They were suspected bovine metacarpal bones, each having a well-formed V-shaped notch at each end, an inch or so in depth. One of the four was a very shiny-surfaced bone while the other three were just dry bones.

The diagnosis made in all these cases from the various schools in Argentina and Brazil was botulism. The cases were thought to be related to a nutritional problem causing "pica," a craving of abnormal food such as bones, for the mineral value in them. In eating and chewing the bones, the animal incidentally releases the spores of *Clostridium botulinum* from the prolonged protection of the bone marrow. The organisms are still in the unopened bones even years after the owner of the bones has died. Sir Arnold Theiler worked on this clostridial entity problem in the late 1800s.

The diagnosis of botulism in cattle is a difficult diagnosis to make in most cases and very difficult to prove. In warm countries, it is made with more difficulty because of the often severe postmortem changes that occur quickly after death. The actual cause of death

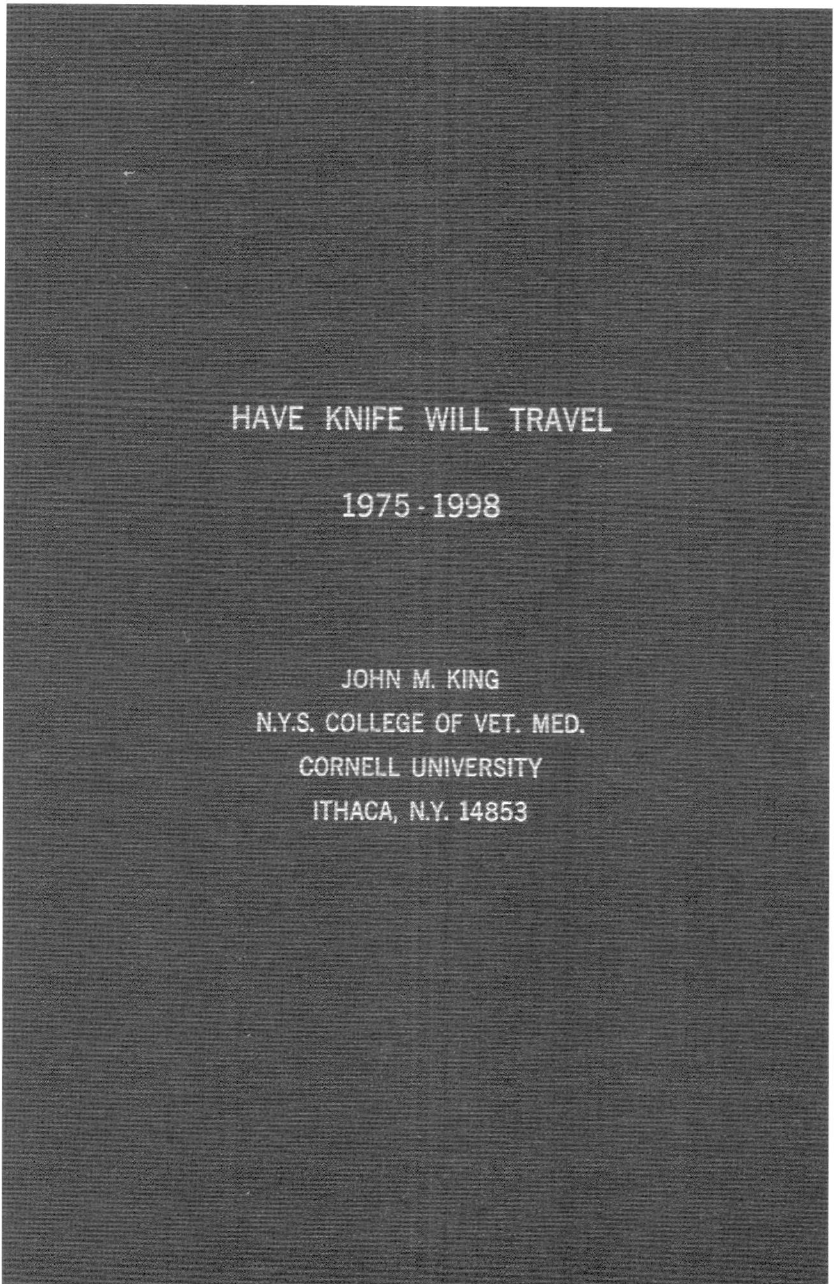
HAVE KNIFE WILL TRAVEL

1975 - 1998

JOHN M. KING

N.Y.S. COLLEGE OF VET. MED.

CORNELL UNIVERSITY

ITHACA, N.Y. 14853

Have Knife Will Travel

Sabbatical

1975-1976
1979-2010

John M. King
N.Y.S. College Vet. Med.
Cornell University
Ithaca, N.Y.
14853

Countries Visited

Taiwan I June 1975-March 1976

Hong Kong
Thailand
India
Kenya
South Africa
Israel
Finland

Morocco September 1979
Taiwan II March-May 1981
Australia August 1983-July 1984
New Zealand July 1984

Switzerland I September 1989

Egypt November 1989
Lichtenstein February 1990
France February 1990
Germany March 1990
Italy April 1990

Brazil I March-June 1990
Greece November 1992
Spain I November 1992
Spain II November-December 1995
Argentina I August-December 1996
Brazil II December-Christmas 1996
Chile January-February 1997
Brazil III March 1997

Trinidad & Tobago April 1997

Mexico January-February 1998
Brazil IV July-August 2003
Argentina II August-September 2003
Switzerland II April-September 2004
Peru September-October 2005
Peru 2008
Korea April 2008
Taiwan III April 2010

John M. King's Penmanship

6 May 09

Dear Son;

Another note to go with all the stuff I've already sent. Hope it suffices as there is not much else.

I make a special request however when and if you decide to say anything about my webpage HTTP://W3.VET.CORNELL.EDU/NST that you please put in a comment with it that; The author of the webpage is everlasting thankful to Dr L. Parrish, Wisc., and Dr. James Britt, Arkansas for their gratis, typing and editing, of most of the texts and descriptions, of the over 26,100 pictures from the poor handwriting submitted to them.

I cannot think of anyone who had done more to help make the webpage possible. John Leibowitz who designed the program and Susan Williams who loaded the Kodachromes also are to be thanked.

Just wanted to make sure they get credit for the tremendous work they did in helping me.

So for now

Best

John

6 May 2009

Dear Son,

Another note to go with all the stuff I've already sent. Hope it suffices as there is not much else.

I make a special request however when and if you decide to say anything about my webpage http://w3.vet.cornell.edu/nst/ that you please put in a comment with it that: The author of the webpage is everlasting thankful to Dr. L. Parrish, Wisconsin and Dr. James Britt, Arkansas for their gratis, typing and editing of most of the texts and descriptions of the over 26 000 pictures from the poor handwriting submitted to them.

I cannot think of anyone who had done more to help make the webpage possible. John Leukovitz who designed the program and Susan Williams who loaded the kodachromes also are to be thanked.

Just wanted to make sure they get credit for the tremendous works they did in helping me.

It for now.

Best, John

Distribution of Most Pneumonias :

John. M. King

Distribution of most pneumonias-

By:: Dr. John M. King

General: Palpation is a required aid for these efforts and if it is not firm, it's probably not pneumonia.

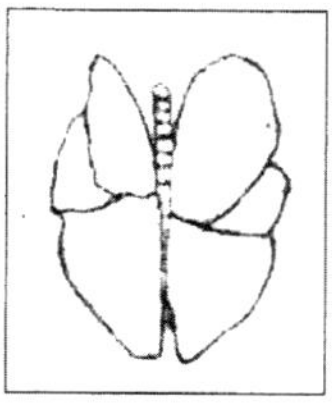

Anatomic Patterns of Distribution

Focal
Multifocal
Locally Extensive
Diffuse

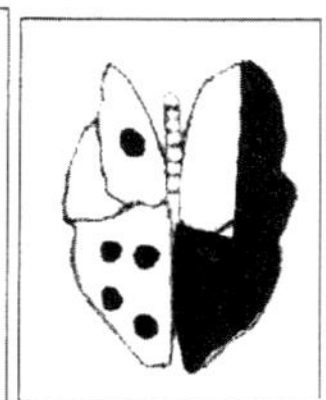

1.. Pig-large, locally extensive area of bloody and fibrinous areas scatteed but not always in cranioventral lobes, soon fatal; *Actinobacillus* pneumonia

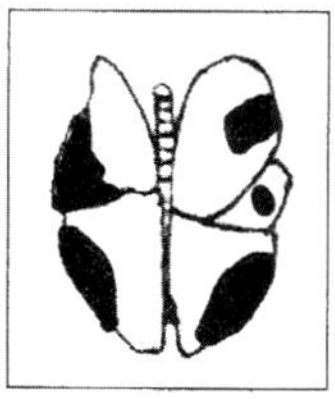

2. Pig-red, cranioventral areas of locally extensive pneumonia; acute *Mycoplasma* pneumonia; same distribution but pale, white lesion=chronic *Mycoplasma* pneumonia

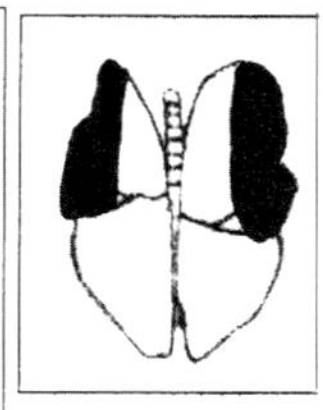

3. Most species-greatly reduced size of entire lung in animal recently subjected to gas anesthesia in which animal's lung is not filled with air but only oxygen; Anesthetic gas/lung machine atelectasis

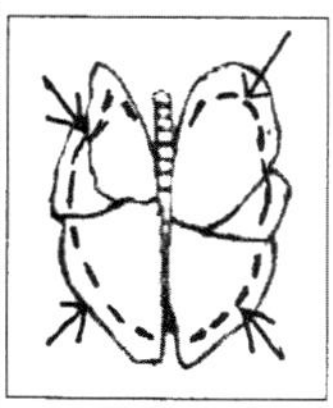

4. Inhalation pneumonia-single dirty foreign body (oat hull)

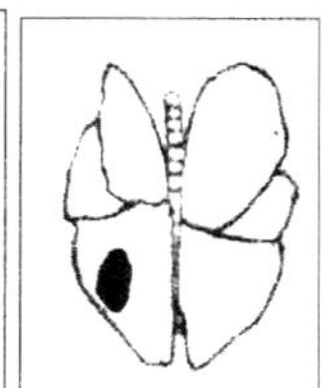

5. Downer cow-one side regurgitation inhalation; calf-inhalation of milk, fluid, medicines induced by white muscle disease of muscles of deglutition; iatrogenic, medicines

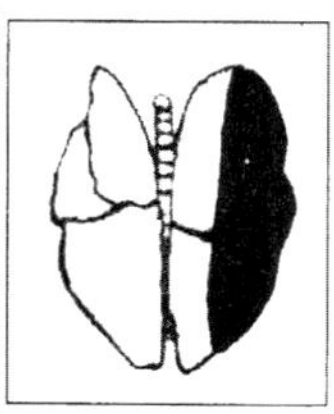

6. Calf-enzootic pneumonia; Cow-Shipping fever (*Mannheimia*); fibrin, firm

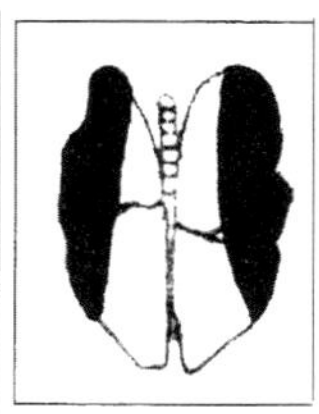

7. Cow-*Histophilus*-high fever, fibrin, acute death, often not cranioventral

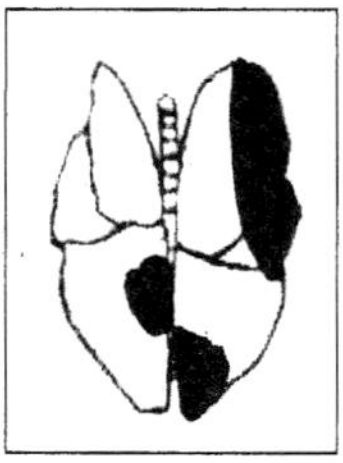

8. Calf-30 days after septic cranioventral enzootic pneumonia, they die with secondary proliferative pneumonia, unknown cause

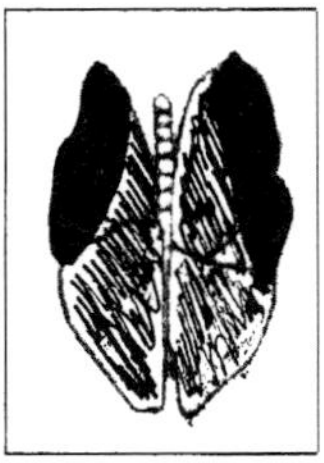

9. Adult cow with chronic cranioventral pneumonia turned on back for displaced abomasum surgery. Gravity effect of bronchial debris to now ventral diaphragmatic lobes and secondary inhalation pneumonia with often serious emphysema

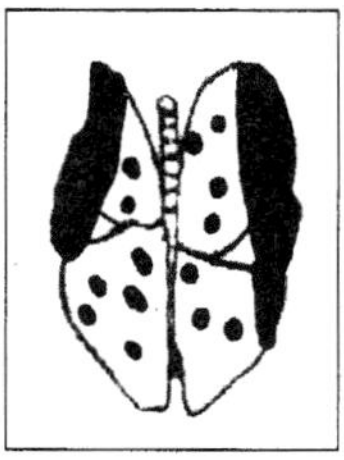

10. Cow-diffuse, firm, heavy, maybe tan. Alveolar lining cells are proliferative, rare hyaline membranes; cause-3-MI, moldy sweet potatoes, Perilla mint, paraquat, etc; Tx-high doses of atropine; proliferative pneumonia aka Fog Fever or atypical interstitial pneumonia

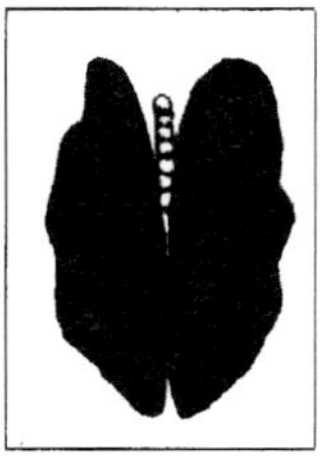

11. Cow-chronic stage of proliferative pneumonia with bronchioles plugged with connective tissue; silo fillers disease from brown gas at bottom of newly filled corn silage silo

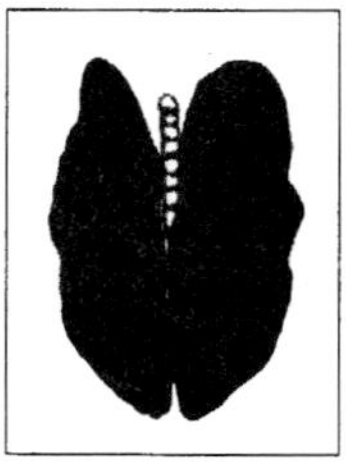

12. Cow-diffuse, edematous, heavy, wet lung, not firm. History of BAR vaccine, others; drying off cows-allergic response to milk letdown prior to milking; chronic heart failure when tan with heart anomalies.

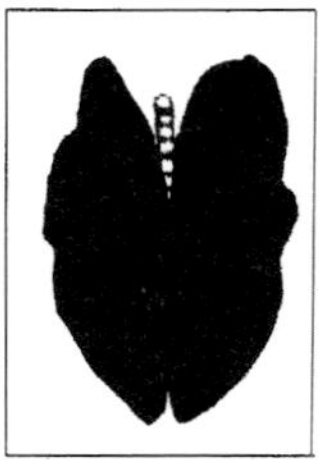

13. Cow-heart failure with multiple palpable nodules throughout from ruptured liver abscess or embolic shower from heart, etc. septic joints, udder, liver, etc

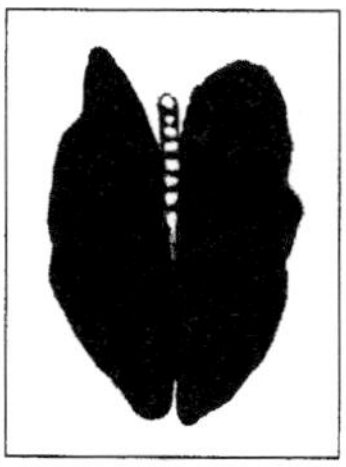

14. Cow-Bovine asthma-yellow nodules of eosinophils around airways, eating moldy red clover haylage, mostly Jersey and Guernsey cattle; Farmer's lung of cattle-inhalation of *Polymicrosporon faeni* in hay dust, palpable and visible granulomas

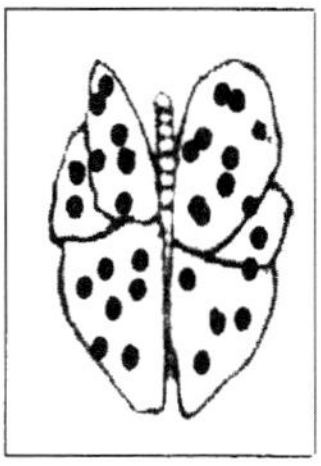

15. Cow-multiple, yellow to green, variably-sized nodules in Jersey's and Guernsey's lungs with visible dead worms (*D. viviparous*). Post-fogging pneumonitis (dead worms).

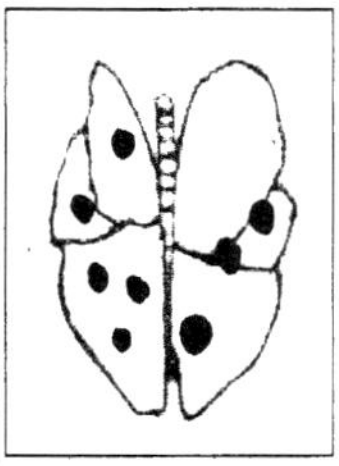

16. Cow-often gritty parenchyma, mostly of dorsal diaphragmatic lobes; uremic pneumonitis, Vit D toxicity, Vit A deficiency, lymphosarcoma

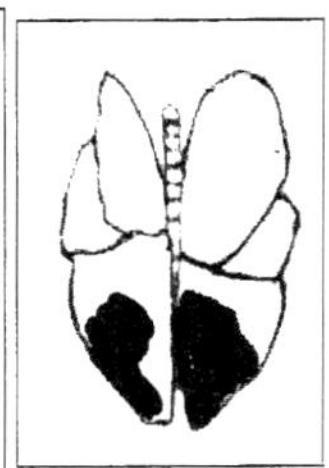

17. Cow-lung worms (D. viviparous) in airways of dorsal diaphragmatic lobes, most may move forward after death

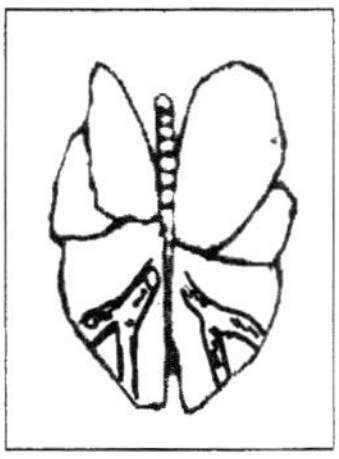

18. Calf-unilateral, diffuse, proliferative pneumonia. No known cause

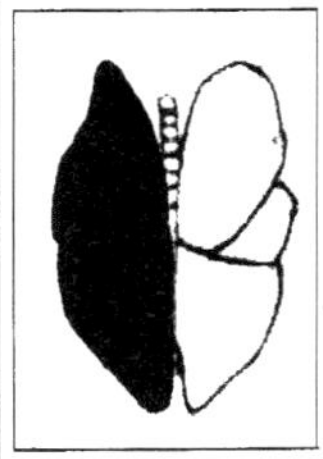

19. Newborn-scattered areas of dark, uninflated lobes, soft and collapsed, 1) fetal atelectasis, 2) similar areas that are firm-pneumonia with airways obstructed with mucus, fetal pneumonia

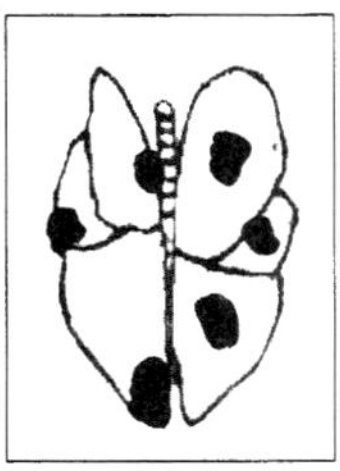

20. Focally extensive, firm areas, hard to tell from Shipping fever or Contagious pleuropneumonia or tuberculosis. TB often has liquid pus in swollen nodes.

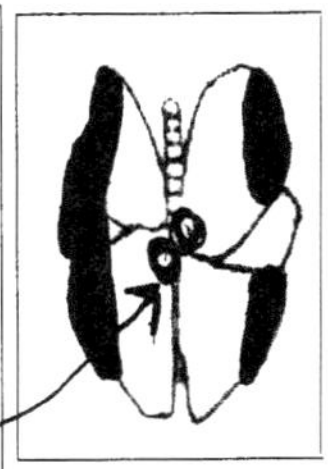

21. Sheep-inhalation pneumonia because sheep wormed after placing it on its' rear end and drenched

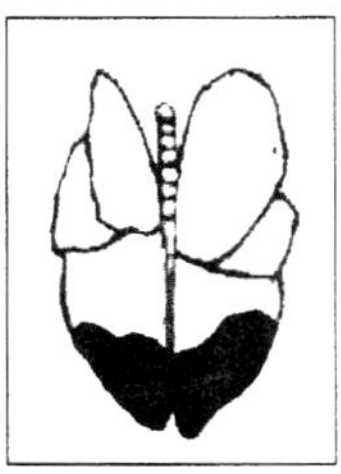

22. Horse-multifocal emphysematous bulla at edges, common and even normal

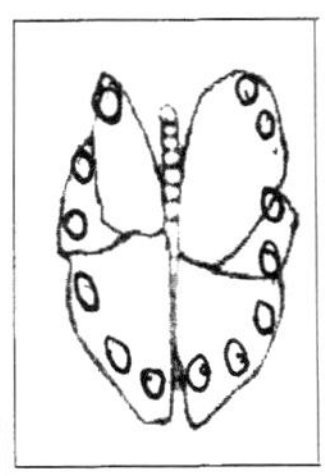

23. Horse-diffuse emphysematous lungs, enlarged- chronic heaves with and without evidence of perilobular bronchitis

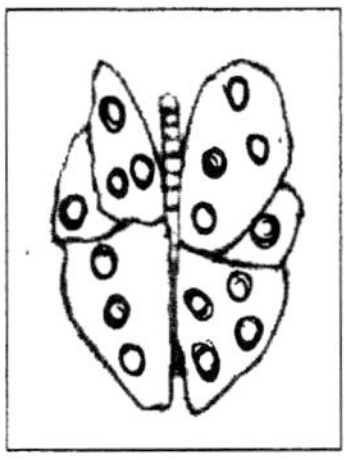

24. Horse-often no emphysema but disseminated, pale, firm nodules with mucus in bronchi and bronchioles; mucoid bronchiolitis-acute heaves

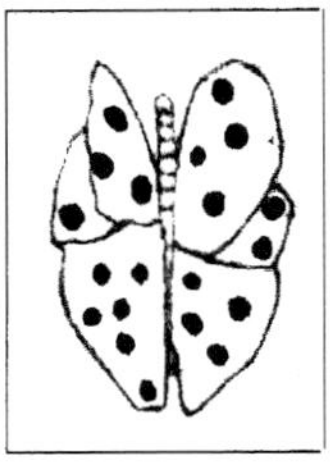

25. Horse and others-usually well-delineated line of sepsis in both pleural cavities and on lung but may be unilateral; may find causative abscess by careful palpation; purulent pleuritis, pyothorax

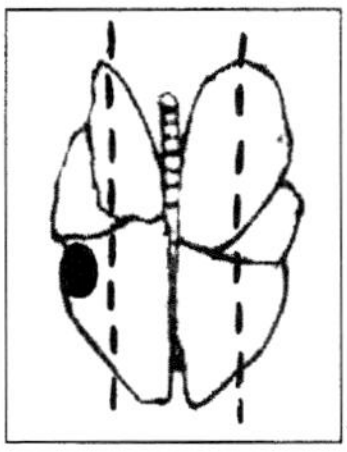

26. Horse-firm, even hard, locally extensive areas in cranioventral lobes of slight, mild septic pneumonia. Shipping fever of horses-secondary inhalation pneumonia from heads tied up during transport. The most common type of pneumonia in horses.

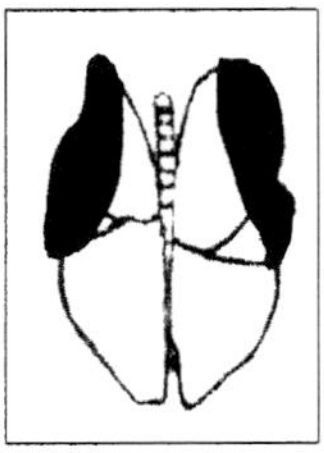

27. Septic centers with dark zone of parenchyma around them that on histopathology are inflammatory areas of *Pneumocystis carinii*; secondary *Pneumocystis* pneumonitis

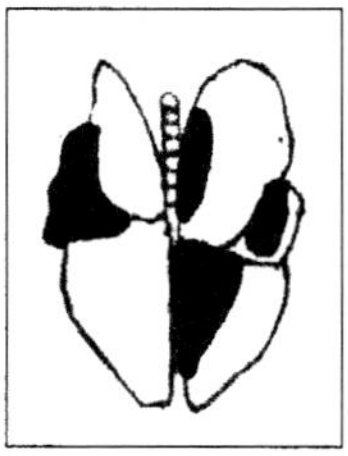

28. Locally extensive pneumonia, very septic, probably due to inhalation of ingesta with CNS problem of swallowing; rabies or even equine herpes infections.

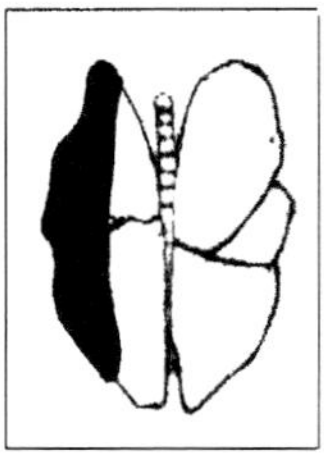

29. Cat-fine red hair, *Aleurostrongylus* scattered in lung parenchyma and under pleural surface of mostly diaphragmatic lobes

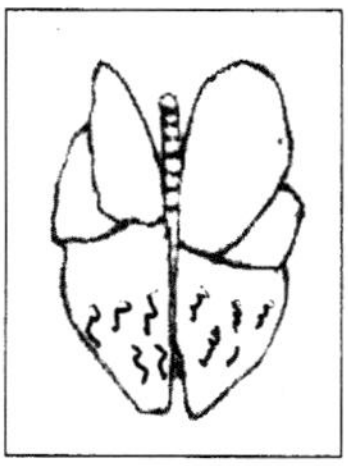

30. Cat and horse-Large areas of pale lung parenchyma suggesting emphysema but oil (mineral oil treatment) inhalation may be noticed on cut sections or floating oil drops in formalin; mineral oil inhalation, also in horses for same reason

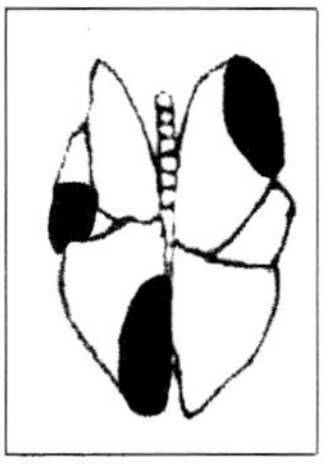

Odds and Ends

Tribute at Cornell Campus

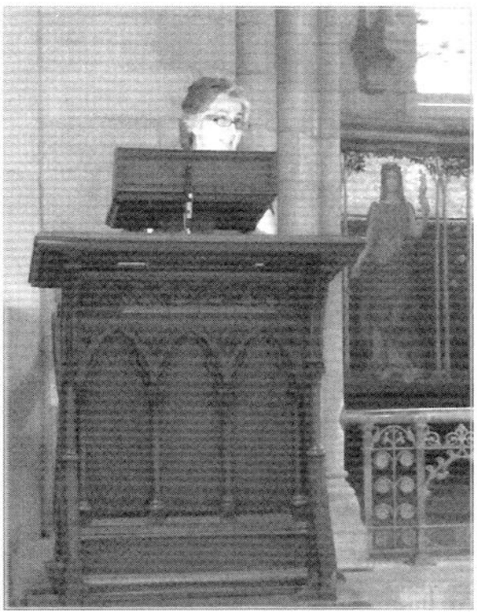 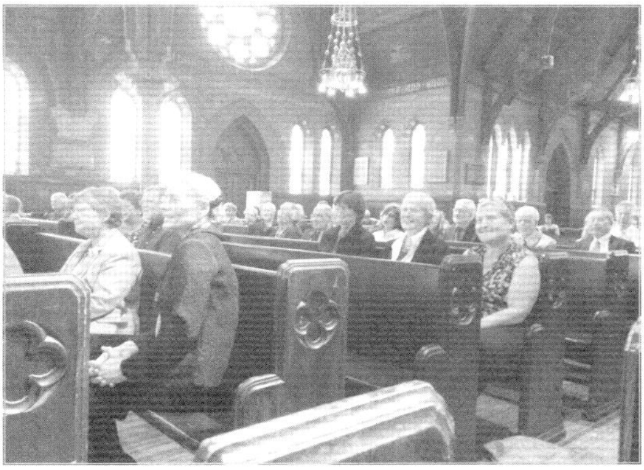

On Thursday, May 12th, Dr. John King was remembered in a memorial service at Sage Chapel on the Cornell campus by members of the veterinary pathology community as well as friends and colleagues from around the country.

In a 1996 interview, John King said he wanted to be remembered for the teaching. At the service, 12 of his former students and colleagues (Ana Alcaraz, Cory Brayton, Helen Han Hsu, Ron Minor, Don Schlafer, Mark Butt, Claus Buergelt, Don Meuten, Page Bouchard, Wanda Haschek, Judy St. Leger, and Bruce Williams honored the man, telling stories of how he had changed each of our lives. The almost 2-hour tribute was a mixture of laughter and and a few tears, and began with members of the Ithaca Veterans of Foreign Wars providing a reverent salute, taps and presenting a flag to John's widow Marie, in honor of John's WWII service in Germany.

It was a tribute but not a farewell to the man, who will live on in so many of the students he trained, and the colleagues he inspired.

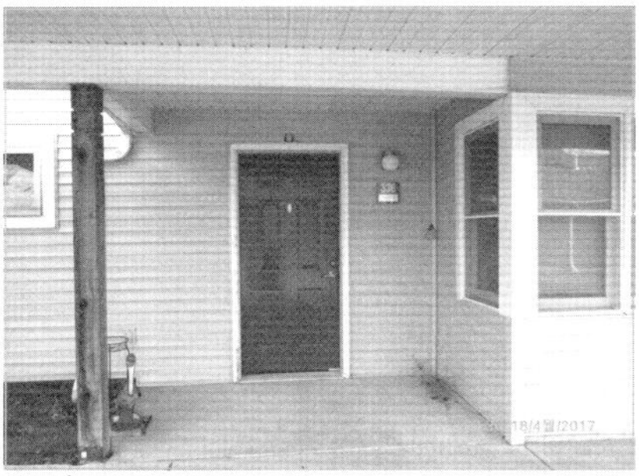

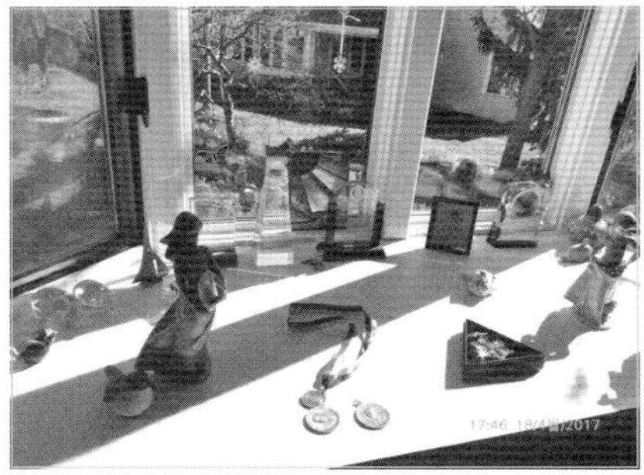
17:46 18/4월/2017

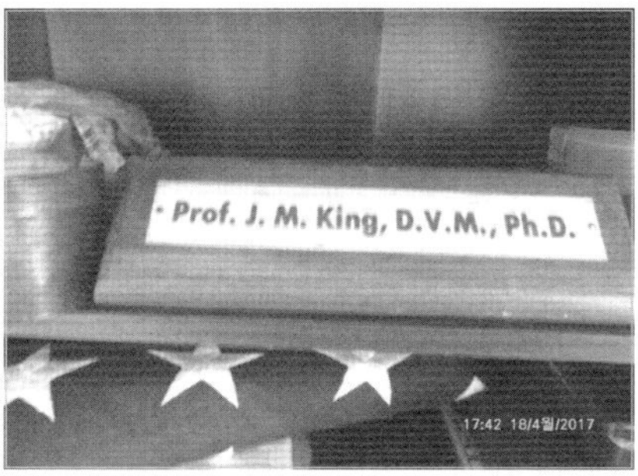
Prof. J. M. King, D.V.M., Ph.D.
17:42 18/4월/2017

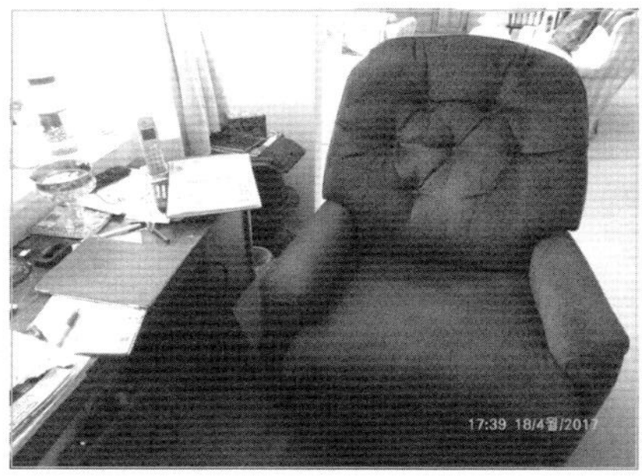
17:39 18/4월/2017

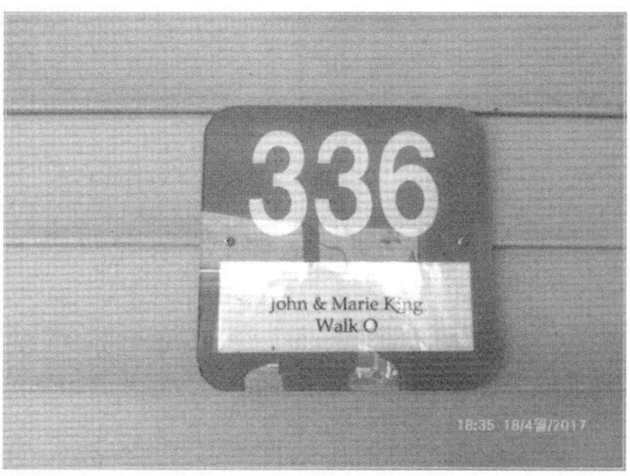
336
John & Marie King
Walk O
18:35 18/4월/2017

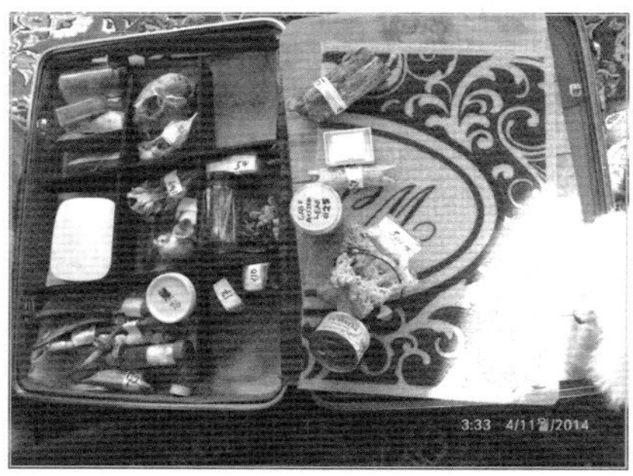
3:33 4/11월/2014

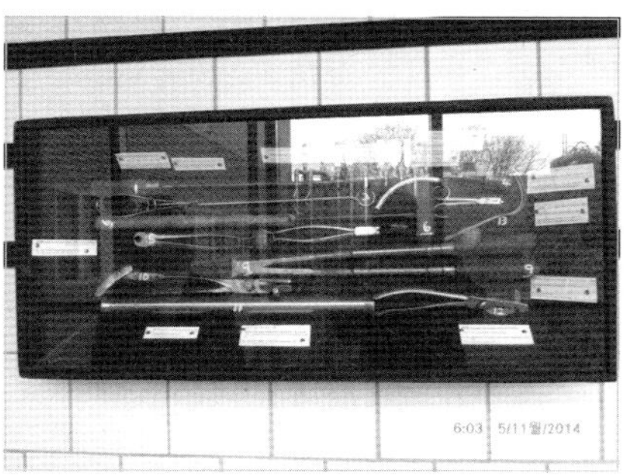
6:03 5/11월/2014

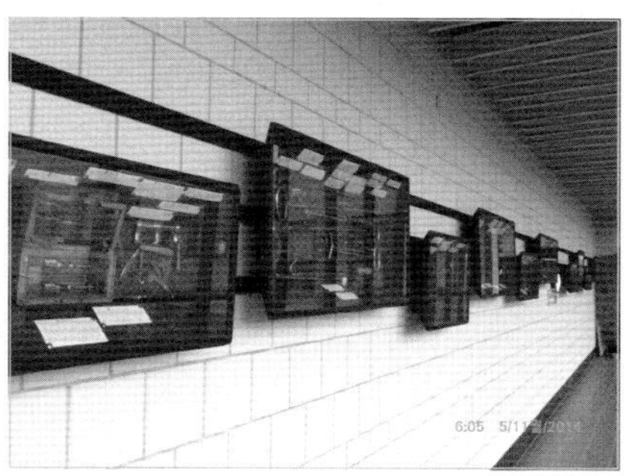

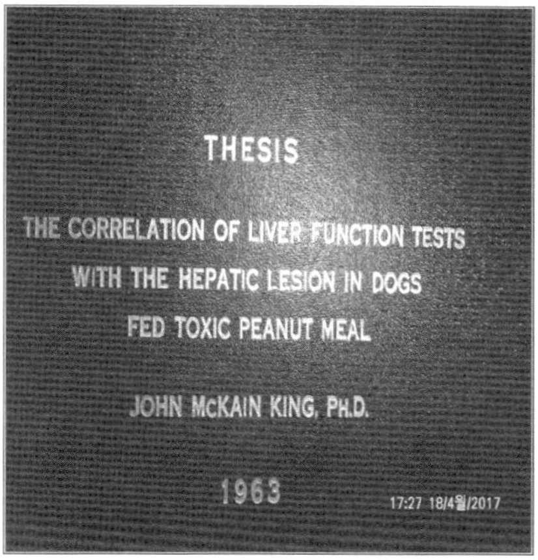

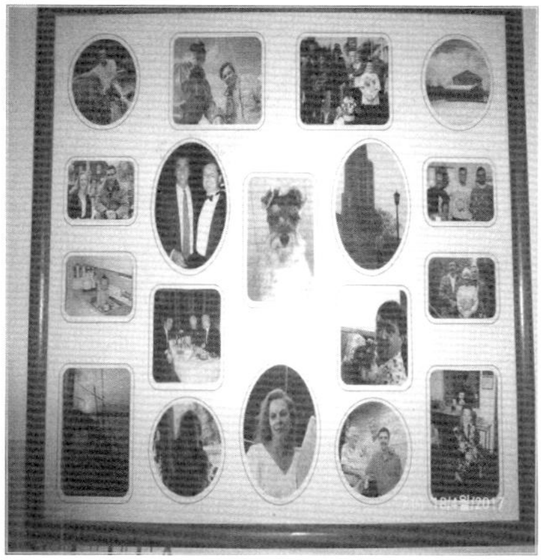

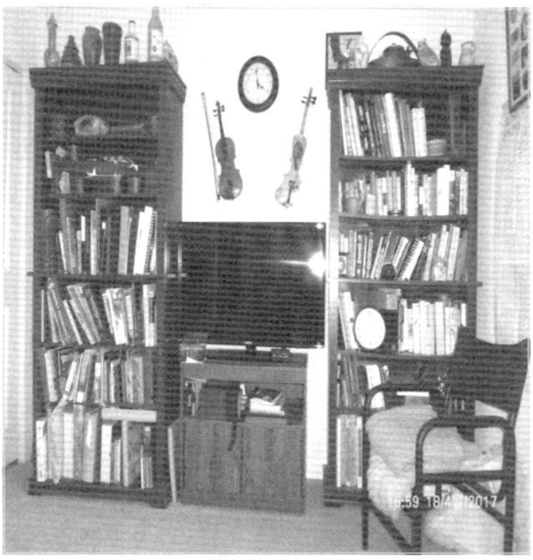

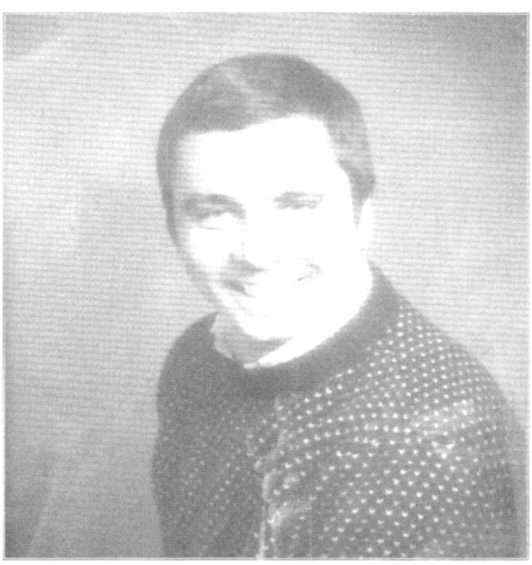

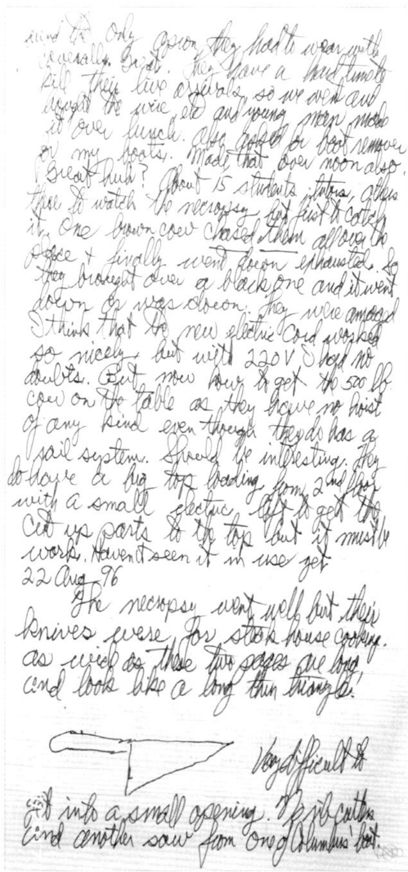
and the only gown they had to wear with overalls. Great. They have a hard time to kill their live animals, so we went and bought the wire etc and young man made it over lunch. Also asked for boot remover for my boots. Made that over noon also. Great huh? About 15 students, tutors, others there to watch the necropsy but first to catch it. One brown cow chased them all over the place + finally went down exhausted. So they brought over a black one and it went down & was down. They were amazed I think that the new electric cord worked so nicely, but with 220V I had no doubts. But now how to get the 500 lb. cow on the table as they have no hoist of any kind even though they do has a rail system. Should be interesting. They do have a big top loading from 2nd floor with a small electric lift to get the cut up parts to the top but it must be work. Haven't seen it in use yet

22 Aug 96

The necropsy went well but their knives were for steak house cooking. as well as these two saws are long and look like a long thin triangle!

Very difficult to get into a small opening. Rib cutters and another saw from one of Columbus' boat.

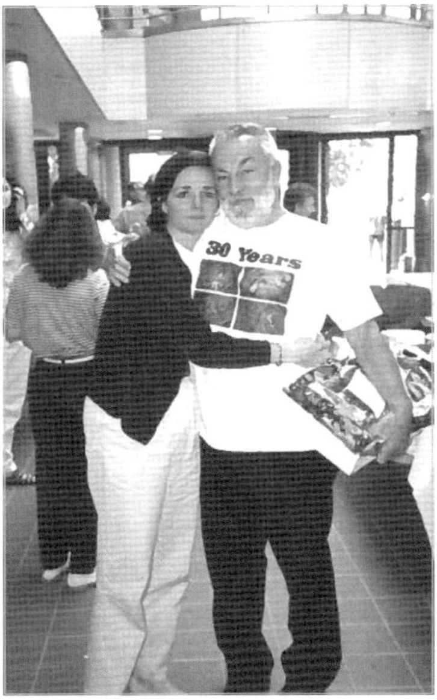
30 Years

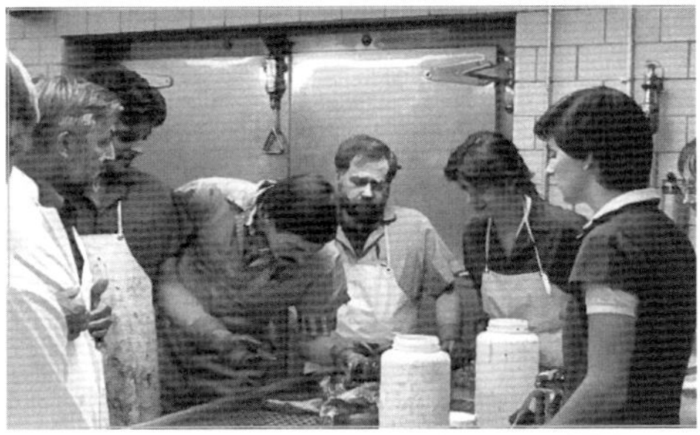

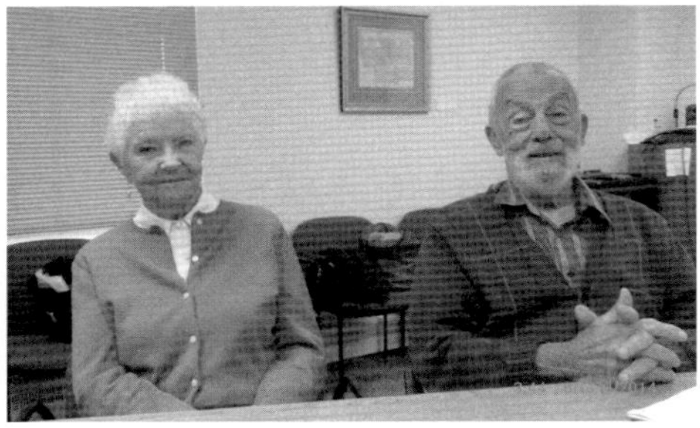

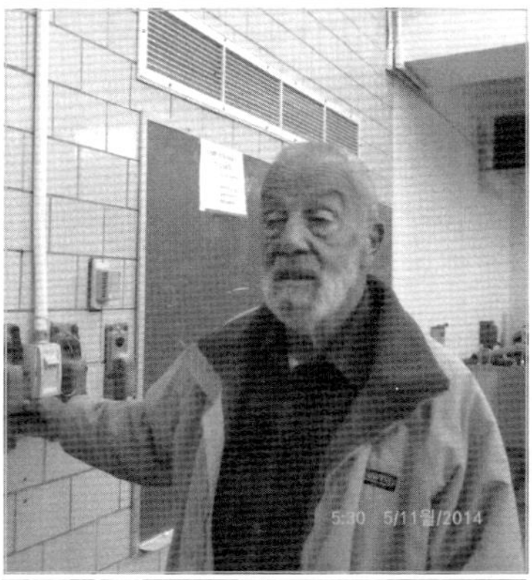

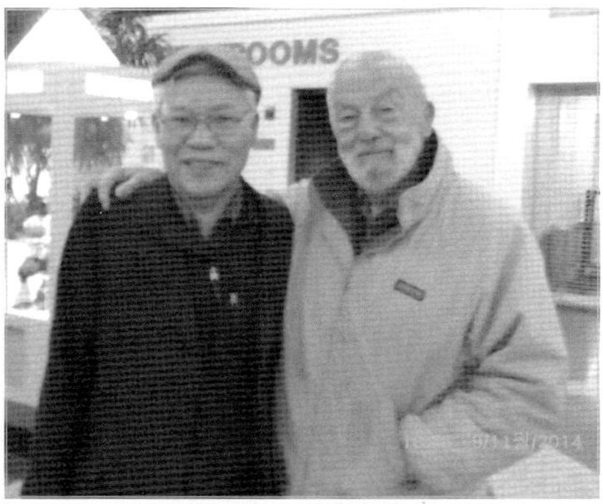

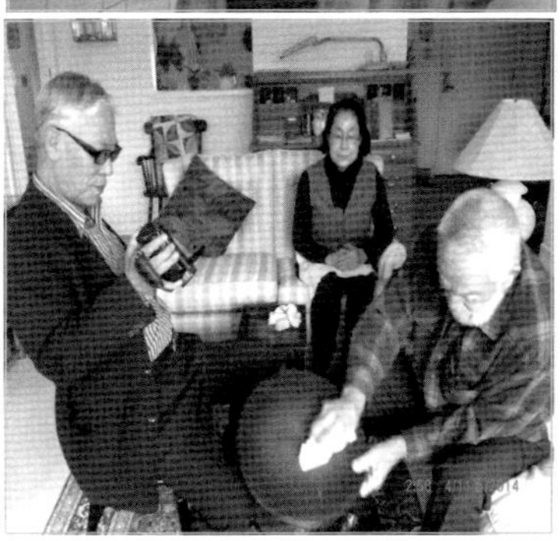

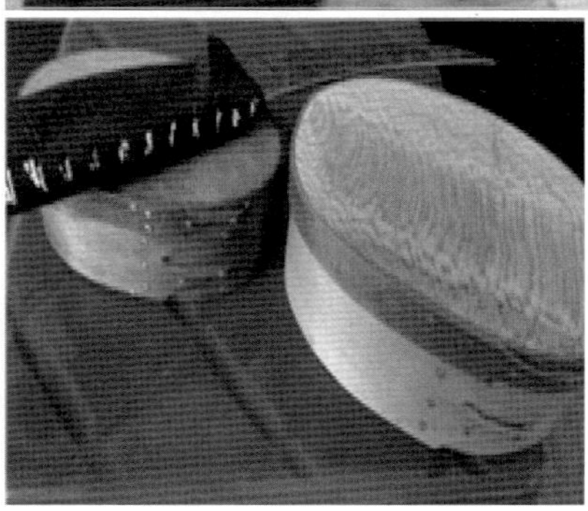

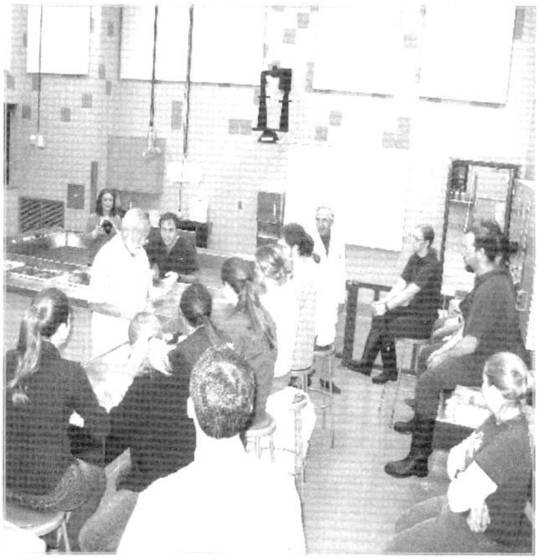

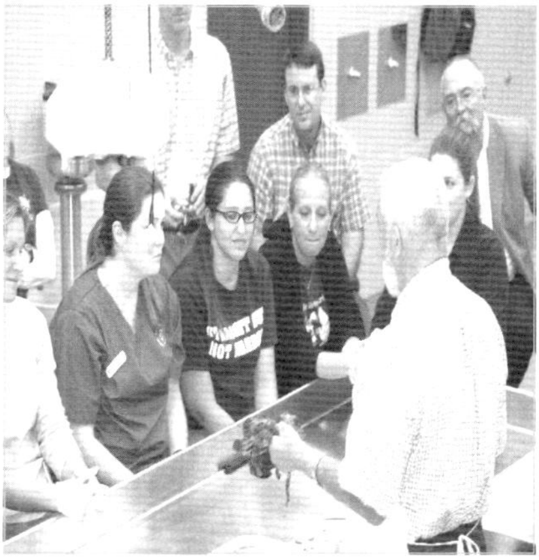

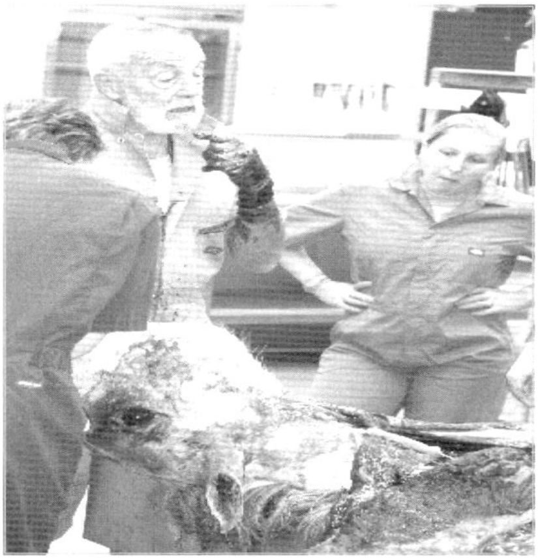

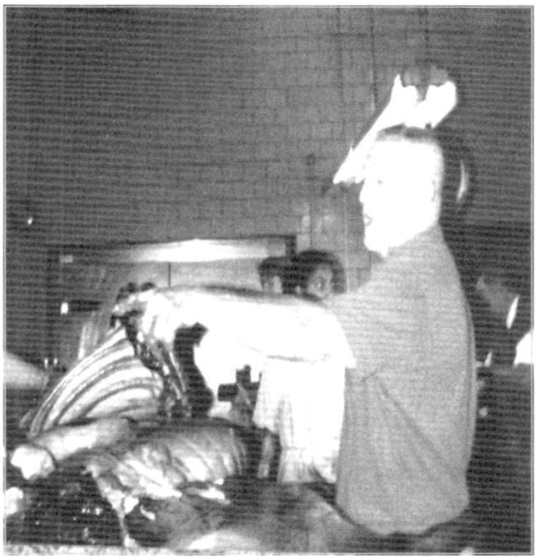

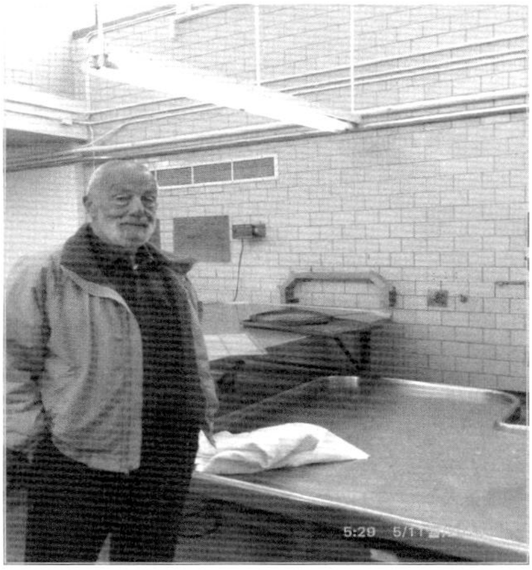

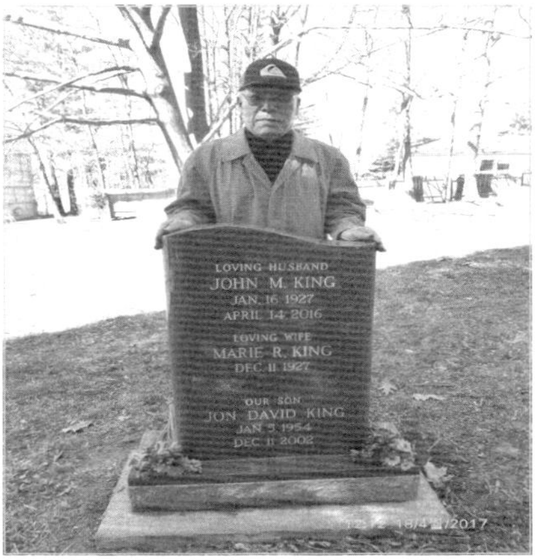
LOVING HUSBAND
JOHN M. KING
JAN. 16 1927
APRIL 14 2016
LOVING WIFE
MARIE R. KING
DEC. 11 1927
OUR SON
JON DAVID KING
JAN 3 1954
DEC 11 2002

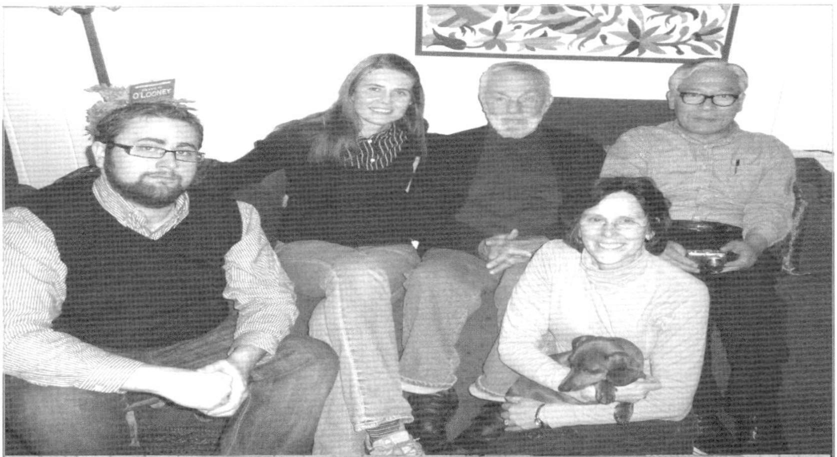

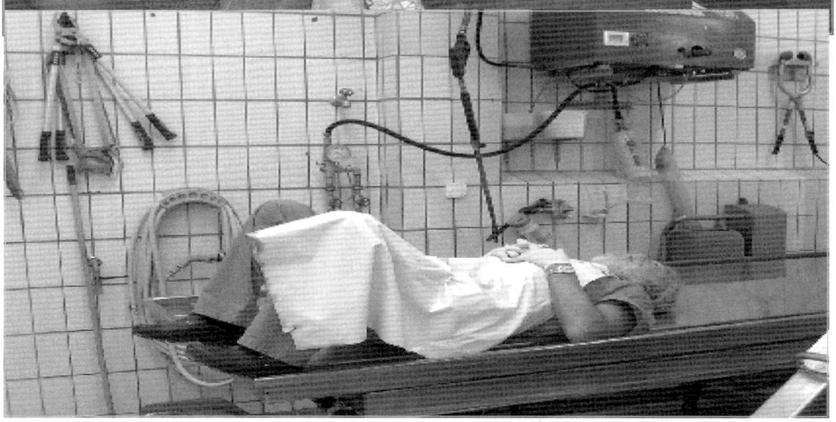

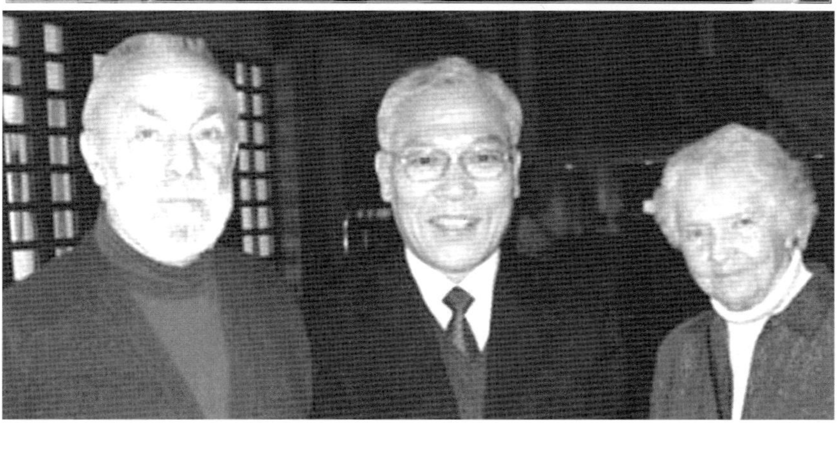

To John:

Calm winds gently rocks the boat,
Seldom an exciting moment,
Small the tales of adventure,
Few the shores to explore!

Come the harsh winds of Hurrican John,
Waves clash tossing the boat as but a toy,
Adventures abound,
Drawing mates from distant shores,
All struggling, yearning to earn the right
To utter those sacred few words,

PROVE ME WRONG!

Talmage T. Brown

CHARLES LOUIS DAVIS D.V.M. FOUNDATION

THE ADVANCEMENT OF VETERINARY AND COMPARATIVE PATHOLOGY

Senoir Editor: S.W. Thompson, D.V.M.
Associate Editor: P.F. Wadrworth, B.V.M.S., Ph.D
Associate Editor: R. Mueller, D.V.M., Ph.D.

Managing Editor: A.P. Gendron, D.V.M., Ph.D.
Copy Editor: P.C. Mann, D.V.M.
Production Editor: K. O'Donnell

Volume 26 Issue 1 **JANUARY/FEBRUARY 1998**

The Foundation

Wishes Its Members And Supporters

A Happy And Healthy

New Year

THE FOUNDATION RECEIVED THE FOLLOWING LETTER IT WISHES TO SHARE WITH YOU ALL:

To: Dr. Samuel Thompson and the C.L. Davis Foundation

This is to thank you all for the kind, fantastic award you have recently given to me in the form of the Harold W. Casey Teaching Award. I had an idea that maybe some consideration was afoot but I was dumbfounded by the honor and consider it a major highlight of my career.

Marie, my wife cried for me at the table and everyone stood up to honor me and I am so proud.

Thank you from the bottom of my heart.

Again sincere thanks for this award and honor.

I get a phone call once or twice a day to congratulate me.

Thanks so much,
John M. King
(Recipient of the 1997 Harold W. Casey Teaching Award)

In This Issue:

PETER OLAFSON, DVM

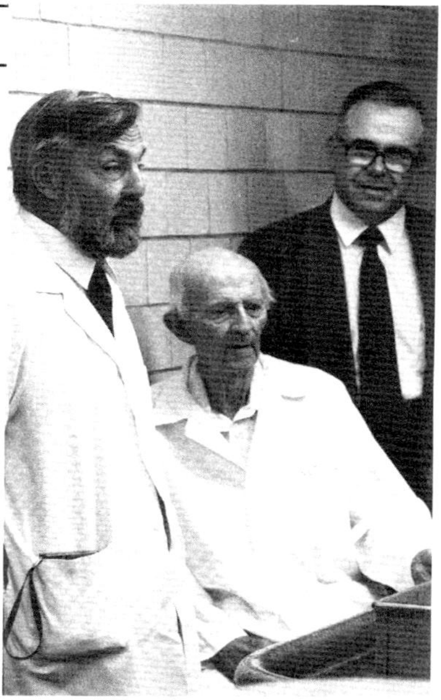

Photo: K. Redmond

Dr. John King, Dr. Olafson (seated), and Dr. Francis Fox during the 1984 Pathology Short Course.

PETER OLAFSON, Doctor of Veterinary Medicine and Professor Emeritus, died on September 3, 1985, after a long illnes. He was 88 years old.

Dr. Olafson was one of the leading veterinary pathologists in the United States, contributing to the definition and development of the field. His research included work on pyelonephritis in dogs, pseudoleukemia in calves, brain tumors in small animals, muscular dystrophy of lambs, equine wobbler disease, bovine listeriosis, toxoplasmosis, cardiac anomalies, and sterility in bulls. During the 1940's he was one of the first to recognize and describe bovine virus diarrhea and hyperkeratosis of cattle.

Born on a large farm in the Red River Valley, near Gardar, North Dakota, he was a rural school teacher before serving as an assistant in the Veterinary Department of the North Dakota Agricultural College where he went on to earn his undergraduate degree in 1924. That same year he began his studies at the New York State Veterinary College, graduating in 1926 with a DVM degree. He was appointed an instructor in Veterinary Pathology at Cornell, teaching in the department of pathology while he earned his masters degree, also from Cornell. In 1927, Dr. Olafson was appointed an Assistant Professor and in 1936 he earned the title of full Professor in the Department of Pathology. He continued to teach and conduct research until his retirement in 1965.

Dr. Olafson was a member of the American Veterinary Medical Association, the American Association of Pathologists and Bacteriologists, the International Association of Medical Museums, the New York State Veterinary Medical Society, and the Southern Tier Veterinary Medical Association. He was also a member of Sigma Xi, Phi Kappa Phi, and Phi Zeta. An annual Short Course in Pathology at the New York State College of Veterinary Medicine is named in his honor, and the James Law Distinguished Lecturer Series is dedicated to him as an "eminent veterinary teacher and pathologist, whose endeavors continue in the tradition of James Law." Dr. Olafson is survived by four daughters and several grandchildren.

Veterinary Viewpoint Vol. 4, No. 4, 1985

Classic Doonesbury (1978)

by Garry Trudeau

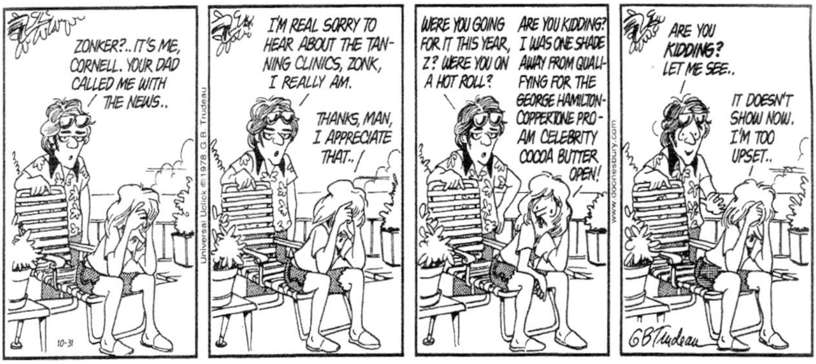

ZONKER?.. IT'S ME, CORNELL.. YOUR DAD CALLED ME WITH THE NEWS..
I'M REAL SORRY TO HEAR ABOUT THE TANNING CLINICS, ZONK, I REALLY AM.
THANKS, MAN, I APPRECIATE THAT..
WERE YOU GOING FOR IT THIS YEAR, Z? WERE YOU ON A HOT ROLL?
ARE YOU KIDDING? I WAS ONE SHADE AWAY FROM QUALIFYING FOR THE GEORGE HAMILTON-COPPERTONE PRO-AM CELEBRITY COCOA BUTTER OPEN!
ARE YOU KIDDING? LET ME SEE..
IT DOESN'T SHOW NOW. I'M TOO UPSET..

Mr. Gnu

by Travis Dandro

Johnny Woodruff

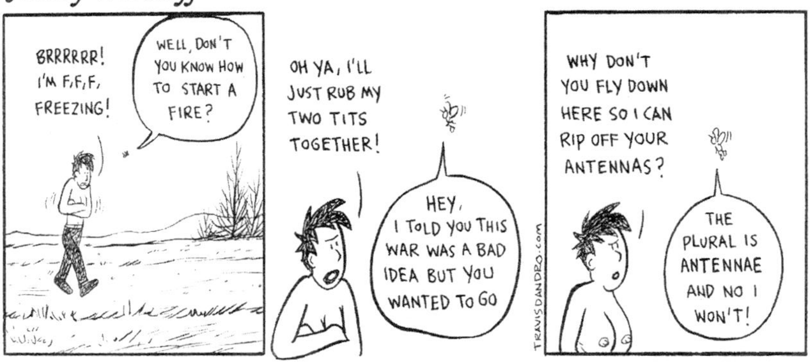

BRRRRRR! I'M F,F,F, FREEZING!
WELL, DON'T YOU KNOW HOW TO START A FIRE?
OH YA, I'LL JUST RUB MY TWO TITS TOGETHER!
HEY, I TOLD YOU THIS WAR WAS A BAD IDEA BUT YOU WANTED TO GO
WHY DON'T YOU FLY DOWN HERE SO I CAN RIP OFF YOUR ANTENNAS?
THE PLURAL IS ANTENNAE AND NO I WON'T!
TRAVISDANDRO.com

Mr. Gnu *Mr. Gnu and Barry enjoy nature's seasonal rhythms*

by Travis Dandro

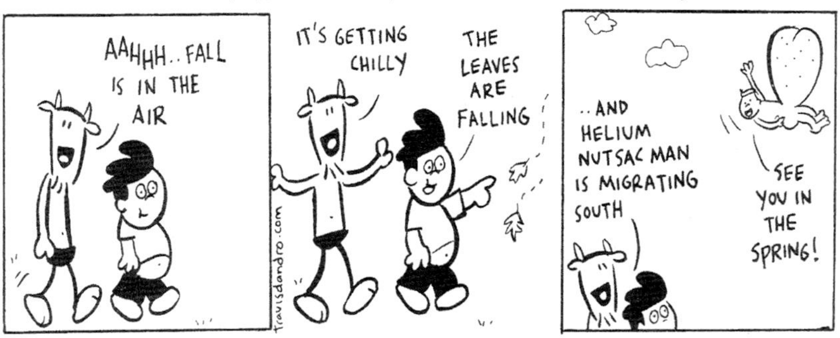

AAHHH.. FALL IS IN THE AIR
IT'S GETTING CHILLY
THE LEAVES ARE FALLING
..AND HELIUM NUTSAC MAN IS MIGRATING SOUTH
SEE YOU IN THE SPRING!
travisdandro.com

THE CORNELL DAILY SUN Friday Octobar 31, 2014

Interesting Anecdotes from Talking with John King : Nam-Yong Park

■ Episode 1

On July 29, 2000, I had the pleasure of meeting John King, a renowned Professor at Cornell University whom I had always wanted to meet and get to know better. Neither I was his disciple nor had I ever attended Cornell University as a student. As soon as I saw him, I was struck by a kind of oriental affection. Compared to Professor Koehler, who was head of the Pathology Institute at Vienna Veterinary University in Austria, where I first studied in 1980, Professor John King was so much more relaxed and approachable.

On April 22, 2008, Professor John King, Dr. Bruce Williams and Dr. Claus Buergelt arrived at Seoul National University Hoam Hotel, while Dr. Professor Corrie Brown arrived later. An 81-year-old professor must have been so tired after a long-distance trip, around 14-hour flight, so I tried to help him unload his luggage from the trunk of the taxi. My hand was tapped immediately by him and he said "Don't touch, Why you would you want to kill me!" I realized that they were very different from Asians elders. The next day, we went to a Korean folk village for sightseeing. There was a wide walking area. I bought a cane which he refused to use first, but he finally broke his stubbornness.

■ Episode 2

After giving a lecture at KVMA in Seoul, he traveled to Gwangju and attended a lovely dinner party with a group of 10 people, including four Indonesian professors at the hotel restaurant. During the party, John King suddenly loosened his belt, opened the zipper and pulled out 200$, showing it off as a secret safe. Every time

I went to the bathroom, I was worried about him losing this emergency fund. I didn't want to miss this opportunity, so I took photographs, which I later used to create a comparison table for the elderly in the East and West, which I presented to the audience before the next day's lesson.

In December 2009, Professor John King was waiting for me at Atlanta Airport, watching football TV putting his airport cart next to him. It was his favorite sport. He used a portable navigation to find our way to Athens/UGA, however it kept slipping over his hand in front of the knees, so I was anxious. "Is this navigator commonly used in Korea as well?", he asked. "In South Korea, you can use any Samsung cellular phone and directly speak a destination through its microphone to find a way instead of bringing portable navigator", I replied. I continued, "Hyundai and Kia vehicles usually have navigation systems with large screens." "All stations for public transportation basically have GPS system with very fast Wi-Fi Internet connections that are faster than those in the United States." Although his TV, refrigerator, washing machine, and cellular phone were product from LG, he would not know that LG is a Korean company like Samsung.

▪ Episode 3

"Attention!", he suddenly shouted, while eating pizza for lunch with a group of people in the UGA Seminar room. He asked us to shout out loudly on his phone so that her wife could hear it, since it was her birthday. "Happy birthday to you!!" He would gladly be a henpecked husband to his wife who had spent 60 years living together. He was at the wheel, picking up Dr. Corrie Brown and Dr. Keits Harris at their places and heading to Gainesville to meet Claus Buergelt··· What an impeccable driving skill for his age of 81 years old! I greatly admired him. We stopped by UGA/Tifton campus where 7-8 people were running a seminar. He opened the door, went in and asked, "Someone who knows who I am?" Most of the young people were dazed and unanswered. Among them, the chief pathologist answered, "John King!" he was a voracious reader every night. He would love to read thriller novels like Dale Brown's Plan of Attack on the bed without his glasses in dim lights. In the morning, he would bring to my place a loaf of bread displayed at the hotel, saying "Dr. park, my Korean son!", which were supposedly illegal.

In December 2012, he was going to be a guest lecturer at the ACVP meeting in Seattle and he wanted to meet me there. When I asked to share a hotel room with me, he liked the idea. He had a hearing problem and carried a German hearing aid worth about three-thousand-dollar which he would brag. To speak a funny story, he never failed to take it, but he left his toothbrush at the toilet instead. He sometimes forget things, but it was not dementia.

■ Episode 4

After traveling with John King for six days in the southeastern United States, he arrived at his winter home near Jacksonville, Florida. During the cold season, many people leave Ithaca to live in the warm southern part of the country.

"You know? In life, I've cried out loud twice. One for the first night I arrive at the farm home for boys, a kind of orphanage because my parents split up when I was at 7. And the other for when in December 2002 I got a phone call from someone that my son Jon David died suddenly of a cardiomyopathy at the age of 48."

■ Episode 5

In November 2014, he was interviewed by me in a seminar room at Kendal at Ithalia. I had spent a week at Econo Lodge near to his home and he paid out for whole accommodation.

He showed us where he would like to be buried. He asked me if I would like to plant a tree in front of his tomb later. I answered "Of course I can. It wouldn't cost much, but it seems more meaningful to plant it with some of your disciples with the assistance of the cemetery complex office."

He said, "In my wife's will, she wishes that her ashes is blown away into Mother Nature after death. When she was young, she suffered from slight poliomyelitis and could not get around on her own... But I am not sure about who would die first and what should be supposed to happen..."

He also showed a self-dedicated warehouse-type workshop in a nearby hill. It was a studio where numerous objects were collected. A place where you can learn about Professor John King's hobbies and character... I did not ask if the old instruments frame displayed on the wall of the Cornell University library was also made here.

9 November 2014, 4 AM at Ithaca Airport. Professor John King woke up early in the morning and picked me up. This is going to be the last... In his hands, a booklet of Food Animal Practice/ Necropsy techniques which was signed and dated.

"Please stop the laborious necropsy in the heaven. Without the pacemaker and stent in your heart and away from COVID-19 Pandemic, you might be living well ever with 68 years of your love, Mrs. Marie and your son Jon, singing Karoaoke which I have given you for a gift."

Index